Cancer
Home Exercise Guide & Workbook

Plus

Exercise Benefits & Precautions

Lost Temple Fitness & Rehab

Karen Cutler: LPTA, ACE Certified Personal Trainer

Medical, Cancer, Arthritis & Lymphedema Specialist

It is advised that you always check with your medical doctor or physical therapist before starting an exercise program or change in diet.

Websites

LostTempleFitness.com

LostTempleFitnessCancer.com

LostTemplePets.com

LostTempleArt.com

INTRODUCTION

It has been proven that exercise is one of the main factors that you can control for a healthy lifestyle. Many people do not know how to start or progress an exercise program. There are hundreds of pictures for beginner, intermediate and advanced exercise programs, as well as a list of equipment that you can use in the home. This section also includes worksheets and exercise precautions for those at risk for peripheral neuropathy or lymphedema.

This edition also includes 16 different types of cancer with possible exercise precautions after surgery, treatments, such as chemotherapy and radiation and side effects.

This book is for:

- Those that currently have or are cancer survivors that:
    - o Are currently or may have had treatments, such as chemotherapy or radiation
    - o Are planning or have had surgeries and/or at risk for lymphedema or peripheral neuropathy
- The beginner who has never exercised before or the individual that has mastered the basics but wants to know how to advance to the next level.
- The personal trainer, physical therapist, or other coaches who would like to know more about precautions with cancer patients or clients.

This book is not for or may need modification:

- Chronic or acute disorders/injuries that is not being followed by a health care professional. This book can be used in conjunction with a rehab program.
- If you are over 40 and have never exercised before, it is advised that a physician clears you first.
- Undiagnosed pain.
- The person that does not feel they can safely modify their individual program, although can be used in conjunction with rehab or coaches/personal trainers.
- People going through current treatments, lymphedema or other medical issues that have not been cleared by an MD for an exercise program. Other issues that may be addressed in future volumes: Cardiac, Respiratory , Arthritis and Diabetes.

What is covered in this book?

- **Cancer**
    - o Cancer and Exercise, Exercise Contraindications / Precautions after Surgery
    - o Lymph Nodes and Lymphedema
    - o 16 types of cancers plus a section on breast cancer, including description, treatment, side effects and possible recommendations/exercise precautions
    - o Sentinel and Axillary node dissection.
    - o Treatments: *Chemotherapy, Radiation, Hormone therapy, Targeted therapy, Immunotherapy, Stem Cell*
    - o Side effects of treatments and how to manage
    - o Eating Hints Before, During and After Cancer Treatments (National Cancer Institute)
- **Home Exercise Programs** – pictures and explanations with lymphedema and peripheral neuropathy precautions.
    - o Myofascial release
    - o Flexibility – Stretching
    - o Core Stability
    - o Strengthening - Lower extremity (Lying and Seated) and Upper extremity
    - o Balance with progression to Standing Strengthening exercises
    - o Agility and Endurance
- Benefits and Factors to consider before starting an exercise program
- Vital signs and how to monitor exercise intensity
- Temperature – Heat and Cold; Dehydration
- Equipment needed for home exercise
- Warm up/cool down
- Duration, Frequency, Intensity and Primary Movement Patterns

Lost Temple Fitness

LOST TEMPLE FITNESS & REHAB

INTRODUCTION

CANCER

See Sections for Specific TOC

Cancer TOC 1

Cancer 2

Cancer and Exercise 3
    Guidelines including Benefits, Risks, When to Avoid or Modify Exercise
    Routine Starting an Exercise Program
    Guidelines for Type of Exercise, Including Balance, Aerobic/Endurance, Strengthening, Flexibility/ROM

Lymph Nodes and Lymphedema / Exercises 10

Breast Cancer 25
    Breast Cancer Types, Surgeries (and Comparisons), Reconstruction, Implants, Tissue Flap Surgery
    Risks after Surgery – Axillary Web Syndrome, Scar Tissue /Adhesions, Seroma

Sentinel and Axillary Lymph Nodes / Dissection 64

Breast Cancer Exercises and Risk/Precautions 71

15 Cancer Types 94
    Bladder (Kegel), Bone, Brain, Colo-Rectal, Endometrial, Kidney, Leukemia, Liver, Lung,
    Lymphoma, Melanoma, Pancreatic, Prostate, Stomach, Thyroid

Cancer Treatments/ Therapies 199
    Including Surgery, Chemotherapy, Radiation, Hormone therapy, Stem Cell Transplant, Targeted therapy,
    Immunotherapy

Side Effect and Late Effects 230
    Possible cause and Ways to Manage

Eating Hints Before, During and After Cancer Treatments (National Cancer Institute)...................... 257

REFERENCES

HOME EXERCISE PROGRAM
See Section for Specific TOC

HOME EXERCISE PROGRAMS TOC 262

SAFETY FIRST 263

Benefits / Before Starting a Routine

Averages – Body Temperature, Respiration, Blood Pressure, Heart Rate

How to Monitor Intensity of Heart Rate

Temperature – Heat and Cold

Dehydration

Altitude

COMPONENTS OF A CONDITIONING PROGRAM 268

Warm up/cool down

Duration, Frequency, Intensity & Movement Patterns

Breathing –Diaphragmatic, Purse lipped and with Resistance training

Anatomy - Positions, Directions, Muscle - joint action, Skeletal ROM

Equipment that may be needed

Self-Tests – Prior to starting program

Worksheets – Exercise Section/Numbers, Reps, Sets, x-day and Holds

EXERCISES and WORKSHEETS 287

Exercise Section/Numbers and Notes

Myofascial Release 310

    Lymphedema Risks

Flexibility/Stretches / ROM 318

Core/Abdominal 344

Strengthening 367

Lower Extremity – Range of Motion > Isometric > Strengthening (Lying/Seated) 369

Upper Extremity - Range of Motion > Isometric > Strengthening 394

Balance > Lower Extremity Standing Exercises 431

Agility 461

Endurance/Aerobic Capacity. 464

    Calorie

REFERENCES

Quick Summary

Cancer:

- Cancer is a disease in which some of the body's cells grow uncontrollably and spread to other parts of the body.

Cancer and Exercise:

- Exercise in Healthy Adults versus Cancer Patients
- Guidelines
- Risks for Cancer Patients
- Starting an Exercise Program

Lymph Nodes & Lymphedema & Exercises/ROM:

- Lymph nodes are part of the lymphatic and immune system, which protects your body against infection and disease.

Breast Cancer:

- Breast cancer is a disease in which cells in the breast grow out of control.
- There are different kinds of breast cancer

Sentinel & Axillary Lymph Nodes/Dissection:

- A sentinel lymph node is defined as the first lymph node to which cancer cells are most likely to spread from a primary tumor.

Cancer Types:

- Fifteen types of cancer and their description, treatment, side effects
- Possible recommendations post-surgery / exercise precautions

Therapies for Cancer:

- Therapy includes, but not limited to, chemotherapy, radiation, hormone, targeted, immunotherapy, stem cell

Side Effects and Late Side Effects:

- Side Effects and Late Side Effects of therapies and surgeries

Eating Hints: Before, during, and after Cancer Treatment:

- Clear Liquids, Full Liquid Diet, Foods and Drinks that are Easy on the Stomach, Low Fiber, High Fiber, High Protein, Foods and Drinks that are Easy to Chew and Swallow

References

HOME EXERCISE GUIDE

CANCER
Information and pictures from *National Cancer Institute* unless otherwise specified

Definition	Cancer is a disease in which some of the body's cells grow uncontrollably and spread to other parts of the body.
	• Cancer can start almost anywhere in the human body, which is made up of trillions of cells. Normally, human cells grow and multiply (through a process called cell division) to form new cells as the body needs them. When cells grow old or become damaged, they die, and new cells take their place.
	• Sometimes this orderly process breaks down, and abnormal or damaged cells grow and multiply when they shouldn't. These cells may form tumors, which are lumps of tissue. Tumors can be cancerous or not cancerous (benign).
	• Cancerous tumors spread into, or invade, nearby tissues and can travel to distant places in the body to form new tumors (a process called metastasis). Cancerous tumors may also be called malignant tumors. Many cancers form solid tumors, but cancers of the blood, such as leukemias, generally do not.
	• Benign tumors do not spread into, or invade, nearby tissues. When removed, benign tumors usually don't grow back, whereas cancerous tumors sometimes do. Benign tumors can sometimes be quite large, however. Some can cause serious symptoms or be life threatening, such as benign tumors in the brain.
How Does Cancer Develop?	Cancer is a genetic disease—that is, it is caused by changes to genes that control the way our cells function, especially how they grow and divide.
	• Genetic changes that cause cancer can happen because:
	○ of errors that occur as cells divide.
	○ of damage to DNA caused by harmful substances in the environment, such as the chemicals in tobacco smoke and ultraviolet rays from the sun. (Our Cancer Causes and Prevention section has more information.)
	○ they were inherited from our parents.
	• The body normally eliminates cells with damaged DNA before they turn cancerous. But the body's ability to do so goes down as we age. This is part of the reason why there is a higher risk of cancer later in life.
	• Each person's cancer has a unique combination of genetic changes. As the cancer continues to grow, additional changes will occur. Even within the same tumor, different cells may have different genetic changes.

How Cancer Spreads	**There are three ways that cancer spreads in the body** **Tissue.** The cancer spreads from where it began by growing into nearby areas **Blood.** The cancer spreads from where it began by getting into the blood. The cancer travels through the blood vessels to other parts of the body **Lymph system.** The cancer spreads from where it began by getting into the lymph system. The cancer travels through the lymph vessels to other parts of the body
When Cancer Spreads	A cancer that has spread from the place where it first formed to another place in the body is called metastatic cancer. The process by which cancer cells spread to other parts of the body is called metastasis. Metastatic cancer has the same name and the same type of cancer cells as the original, or primary, cancer. For example, breast cancer that forms a metastatic tumor in the lung is metastatic breast cancer, not lung cancer. Under a microscope, metastatic cancer cells generally look the same as cells of the original cancer. Moreover, metastatic cancer cells and cells of the original cancer usually have some molecular features in common, such as the presence of specific chromosome changes. In some cases, treatment may help prolong the lives of people with metastatic cancer. In other cases, the primary goal of treatment for metastatic cancer is to control the growth of the cancer or to relieve symptoms it is causing. Metastatic tumors can cause severe damage to how the body functions, and most people who die of cancer die of metastatic disease.
References	National Cancer Institute (NCI) - What is Cancer? *https://www.cancer.gov/about- cancer/understanding/what-is-cancer*

Cancer and Exercise

It is beneficial for people who are currently undergoing treatment for cancer or survivors to engage in an exercise program. As shown in the first part of this book, exercise can help with endurance, muscle strengthening and flexibility. It is advised that you glance through the following sections: *Safety First* and *Components of a Conditioning Program*, before starting an exercise program. The Home Exercise Guide has general information regarding myofascial release, flexibility/stretches/ROM, core stability, strengthening, balance, agility, and endurance.

Things you should know before starting a program:
* If you had any number lymph nodes removed or radiation, this puts you at risk for lymphedema.
* What type of surgery, if any, was performed.
* If you are currently or have had radiation or chemotherapy, you may want to know the side effects and precautions, i.e. chemo can cause peripheral neuropathy (increases risk of falling) and radiation can put you at risk for lymphedema (swelling in the neck, arm, legs or trunk depending on the area treated).
* Any other risk factors, such as, but not limited to, diabetes, cardiac or pulmonary issues, neurological issues, poor bone density/osteopenia/arthritis or autoimmune disorders.

Most of the research is from the **National Cancer Institute** – Please see *References*.

This book is not meant to substitute an exercise program prescribed by a health care professional but is designed to accompany their recommendations.

Please consult with your oncologist or team before starting any exercise program.

Who is this section recommended for?

- Patients currently undergoing treatment for cancer to be used in conjunction with the oncologist or other health care provider and/or physical therapist recommendations.
- Cancer survivors that are trying to get back into a healthy exercise program.
- Physical therapists and other health care providers, such as a cancer exercise specialist, to be used to prescribe a home exercise program.

Who is this section not for?

- Those who are not able to follow or modify a program without supervision.
- Those who have other medical issues, such as respiratory, cardiac, fracture risks or other acute/chronic issues that have not been cleared by an MD.
- *Also see Introduction*

Exercise in Healthy Adults versus Cancer Patients

Fitness and exercise is the same for cancer patients as it is for the average adult. You can follow the exercise routines suggested in the first section of this book prior to, during and after treatments. In fact, it is recommended that you start reading or at least scanning this section, as suggestions for muscle strengthening, endurance, flexibility, and balance will be the same.

What makes the program different are the various side effects from chemotherapy, surgery, radiation, and other cancer treatments. For example, after a mastectomy you will need to get range back in the arm and have precautions, as well as possible complications, such as lymphedema. Chemotherapy can cause excessive fatigue where you may have to push yourself to get off the couch and make a meal. Radiation can also cause fatigue, and puts you at risk for lymphedema, as well as having localized pain or burning. Everybody's treatment and reaction will be different. This will all depend on the treatment itself, your physical condition prior to treatment and any other issues, such as diabetes or heart disease that may cause other complications.

Although this book is about Home Exercise Programs, it is extremely important to follow your oncology team's prescription, especially after surgery. All cancer treatments are different, and each doctor will have their particular protocol to follow. It may be necessary to participate in physical therapy first and use this book as a guide along with their program. It is also very important to be cleared from a specialist for other complications, such as, but not limited to, heart disease, pulmonary disease, diabetes, bone disease, immune disorders, obesity or neurological conditions.

If you had lymph nodes removed or radiation this puts you at risk for lymphedema, no matter how long ago. Please consult with a certified lymphedema specialist, esp. before adding resistance to your exercise routine.

About me, and the importance of keeping a chart of your daily symptoms.

In 2017 I was diagnosed with breast cancer with a right mastectomy followed by chemotherapy for 16 weeks, and then radiation, and finally reconstruction over a year later. I was exercising 6 days a week and was on fairly healthy diet prior to getting the cancer diagnosis. With that said, chemotherapy wiped me out where I had to push myself to walk in the driveway and eat, as I had no appetite. One of the best things I did was make myself a daily chart to see my ups and downs between chemotherapy treatments, which were every two weeks. Below is an example of a chart I did to show my mental and physical symptoms and how much I did each day. This does not show what I did around the house, but you can certainly make a chart that shows this as well. Again, this example is only my first two weeks of chemo treatments. As the treatments went on and they changed my medication, my symptoms also changed, some for the better, some for the worse.

First 2 weeks of Chemotherapy:

Day	Walk/Time of Day	Other	Eat	Info
Thursday		First Session	Grilled cheese and crackers	Chemo 1
Friday	Chemo Center	Neulasta Injection	Most crackers, grilled cheese, Jello	Nausea – extreme
Saturday	Driveway 10 & 1		Most crackers, grilled cheese, Jello	Nausea
Sunday	Driveway 11& 1		Most crackers, grilled cheese, Jello	Nausea
Monday		Went to oncology chemo center due to nausea / dehydration	Added soup	Added Zofran for nausea and took off Compazine (caused nausea / tremors) Went to oncology due to nausea / dehydration – put on Saline IV
Tuesday	Driveway 1:00		Crackers & soup, cereal grilled cheese	Nausea
Wednesday			Crackers & soup, cereal, grilled cheese, egg whites	Nausea, increased fatigue
Thursday	½ mile 3:00		Prior & peanut butter on toast	Nausea
Friday	1 mile 1:00	Bicep 5 lbs./Triceps 3 lbs.	Prior	Nausea
Saturday	1 mile 3:00		Prior	Decreased nausea
Sunday	2 miles 5:00		Spinach quiche ½ chicken breast	No nausea
Monday	2 ½ mile 5:00		Normal eating – non spicy, eggs	No nausea
Tuesday	2 ½ mile 1:00 1 mile 5:00	Biceps 5 lbs. Triceps 3 lbs. & 5 lbs.	Chicken, rice, broccoli, eggs	Started noticing hair falling out
Wednesday	3 miles 4:30		Turkey Burger Sweet potato pancakes	Hair falling out – depressed Food starting to taste burnt.

Exercise Guidelines

The following information includes research from:

American Cancer Society - *Physical Activity and the Cancer Patient*

Cancer Research UK - *Exercise guidelines for Cancer Patients*

Benefits for Cancer Patients

- May help to decrease nausea during chemotherapy
- May relieve constipation by stimulating digestion and elimination systems
- Increases endurance due to fatigue
- Help to keep or improve your physical abilities (how well you can use your body to do things)
- Improve balance, which may lower risk of falls and broken bones
- Keep muscles from wasting due to inactivity
- Decrease the risk of heart disease
- Decrease the risk of osteoporosis – helps to strength bones
- Improving blood flow to the legs, reducing the risk of blood clots
- Make you less dependent on others for help with normal activities of daily living
- Lower the risk of being anxious and depressed
- Help you control your weight

What Is your Current Activity Level or Was your Activity Level before Treatment?

This makes a big difference in deciding how you will proceed with your exercise program. If you lead a sedentary lifestyle before the cancer, this is not the time to start a moderate aerobic exercise program. This does not mean you should not start an exercise program at all; you will just need to start at a basic level. On the other hand, if you were an athlete before your diagnosis, this will mean you need to cut back during treatment and eventually move forward to regain your strength.

Pain, fatigue and possibly nausea are the most limiting factors during your treatment. Other factors could be peripheral neuropathy, which may alter your balance, dehydration, or lymphedema, etc. Some people also have a pre- existing, or cancer caused comorbidities, (*the presence of one or more additional diseases or disorders co-occurring with a primary disease or disorder*), which could include heart disease, pulmonary disease, obesity, diabetes, neurological conditions, or bone disease, among others. In this instance, you will have to speak to the team of doctors to discuss which exercises will be best suited for not only the cancer, but any other comorbidity.

What is your current performance level? (Chart adapted from *Clinical Exercise Physiology*, pg. 440)

Activity level	Exercise Duration	Exercise Frequency
Active, no limitations	15-20 min	Daily
Able to walk. Decreased leisure activity. Can perform self-care	15-20 min	Daily
Able to walk more than 50% of the time. Moderate fatigue. Limited assistance with ADL's (activity of daily living)	5-10 min	Two sessions daily
Able to walk less than 50% of the time. Fatigue with mild exertion. Requires assistance with ADL	5-10 min	Daily
Confined to bed **Italic not from Clinical Exercise Physiology chart*	*May be able to do ROM in bed with or without assistance.*	**ROM (Range of Motion) Daily*

Guideline for Type of Exercise. Remember to always warm up before exercising and cool down if needed. This is especially true with flexibility training.

Type	Purpose / Benefit	Intensity / Frequency / Duration	Suggestions
Endurance / Aerobic *How to Monitor Heart Rate (HR) Intensity*	*Improves blood flow *Increases stamina *Reduces fatigue *Boosts mood *Controls body weight	*Low - Based on symptoms – can do walking everyday *Moderate 40-60% of HR * 3-5 days a week * 20-60 min. sessions	*Start with walking if possible, outside or on treadmill *Stationary bike if available, especially with neuropathy or balance issues *See balance for standing endurance exercises. *See strengthening exercises without resistance for general movements and Range of Motion (ROM)
Strength Lower *(Resistance information)*	*Improves muscle and contractile strength *Improves bone, tendon & ligament strength *Improves nervous system function	*Limited by Symptoms and Precautions *40-60% of 1 RM *2-3 days per week – Alternate days for UE/LE. *1-3 sets / 3-5 reps. Progress to 8-12 reps as tolerated	**It is important to follow a regiment designed by the oncology team during treatment due to risk of injury, especially after surgery.** *Start by not using any weight and complete Range of Motion if you have never used resistance before. * Increase to light hand weights or resistance bands as tolerated. *During treatment it is better to do high reps with light weights instead of trying to 'bulk up' with heavy weights. Your body needs to heal and should not be focused on repairing a torn muscle.
Strength – Upper *(Resistance information)*	*Improves function for ADLs (Activity Daily Living)	*Limited by Symptoms and Precautions *40-60% of 1 RM *2-3 days per week – Alternate days for UE/LE. *1-3 sets / 3-5 reps. Progress to 8-12 reps as tolerated	
Strength – Core	*Strengthens trunk, which is your foundation *Maintaining a stable core will assist with balance	*Limited by Symptoms and Precautions *2-3 days per week *1-3 sets / 3-5 reps. Progress to 8-10 reps as tolerated	**It is important to follow a regiment designed by the oncology team during treatment due to risk of injury, especially after surgery.** *It is important to follow progression and understand any precautions you may have. *Breathing correctly during abdominal or core exercises are very important.
Flexibility / ROM	*Helps to maintain ROM *Increases flexibility / ROM after certain surgeries *Decreases stiffness & tension *Increases blood supply to joints *Increases neuromuscular coordination	*20-30 second hold *5-7 days a week *2-4 reps per stretch	*Always warm up before stretching a muscle *Dynamic stretching can be a part of your warmup or even be used in conjunction with your endurance exercises. *Try doing arm stretches while walking to increase intensity.
Balance *(Also see Core, Lower Extremity Strengthening, Agility, Endurance)*	*Decreases risk for falls *Helps improve gait pattern *See Purpose for Endurance and Strength above)	*Limited by symptoms and standing tolerance *5-7 days a week *1 set / 2-4 reps 5-10 second hold *Can also be used in place of some Endurance & Strengthening Exercises	*Follow progression program for Balance *Can be used in place of some endurance and strengthening exercises if able to tolerate standing. *Must be able to stand to perform balance. *Sitting balance can strengthen the core. *Make sure you have a chair or sturdy object to hold or nearby in case of loss of balance. *Requires leg strength for progression.

Risks for Cancer Patients

Avoid Exercise:

- Low red blood cell count (anemia).
- Low white blood cell counts or if you take medicines that make you less able to fight infection and impair your immune system. Stay away from public gyms and other public places until your counts are at a safe level.
- Abnormal levels of minerals in your blood, such as sodium and potassium. This can happen if you have had a lot of vomiting or diarrhea.
- Unrelieved pain, nausea/vomiting, or any other symptom that causes you concern. Call your doctor.
- Do not exercise above a moderate level of exertion without talking with your doctor first. Remember, moderate exertion is about as much effort as a brisk walk.
- If you have a catheter or feeding tube, do not do resistance training that uses muscles in the area of the catheter to keep from dislodging it. Talk with your cancer team about what's safe for you. Avoid pools, lakes, or ocean water and other exposures that may cause infections

Modification or Recommendations:

- Skin irritation - people getting radiation should not expose skin in the treatment area to chlorine in swimming pools. Avoid direct sunlight, even after radiation treatments are over due to burning. For radiation to the upper part of the body, suggest wearing a rash guard (shirt that has UV sun protection).
- Stay away from uneven surfaces or any weight-bearing exercises that could cause you to fall and hurt yourself.
- If you have cancer affecting your bones, you might be more at risk of a break or fracture. You must avoid putting too much strain on the affected bones. You could try swimming or exercising in water, as the water supports your body weight, so the skeleton isn't stressed.
- Watch for swollen ankles, unexplained weight gain, or shortness of breath while at rest or with a small amount of activity. Let your doctor know if you have any of these problems.
- Watch out for lymphedema *(see Lymphedema)*.
- Watch for bleeding, especially if you are taking blood thinners. Avoid any activity that puts you at risk of falling or injury. If you notice swelling, pain, dizziness, or blurred vision, call your doctor right away.
- Peripheral neuropathy - Loss of sensation or feelings of pins and needles in your hands and feet due to cancer treatments. Because this puts you at a higher risk of falling, it might be better to use a stationary bike than to do other types of weight bearing exercise. *(Also, see Balance section)*

CETI Contraindications or Recommendations for Exercise

PICC line
- Avoid resistance exercises around the PICC site
- Do not swim or play contact sports
- Avoid repetitive movements in the affected arm

Chemotherapy or Immunotherapy
- IV Chemotherapy – No exercise for 24 hours
- Hematocrit less than 25% - No Exercise
- Hemoglobin less than 24% 8g/dl due to anemia – No Exercise
- White blood cell counts less than 300 mm3 – No Exercise
- White blood cell counts – Avoid public gyms unless blood cell count is above 500 mm3
- Platelet count less than 5000 mm3 – No resistance training – risk of internal bleeding/hemorrhage
- Platelet count less than 30,000 mm3 – Gentle Active Range of Motion *(CETI)*

Starting an Exercise Program

Although this book is about Home Exercise Programs, it is extremely important to follow your oncology team's prescription, especially after surgery. All cancer treatments are different, and each doctor will have their particular protocol to follow.

It may be necessary to participate in physical therapy first and use this book as a guide along with their program. It is also very important to be cleared from a specialist for other complications, such as, but not limited to, heart disease, pulmonary disease, diabetes, bone disease, immune disorders, obesity or neurological conditions.

Exercise Guidelines for Cancer patients currently receiving treatment

The following information includes research from:
> National Comprehensive Cancer Network (NCCN) – Exercising During Cancer
> Treatments American Cancer Society - *Physical Activity and the Cancer Patient*

- American Cancer Society: *"To make your exercise effort most effective (give you the best results), it's important that you work your heart.*
    - *Notice your heart rate, your breathing, and how tired your muscles get. If you get short of breath or very tired, rest for a few seconds, and start exercising again as you are able.*
    - *When you first start, the goal is to exercise for at least 10 minutes at a time. Go slow at first, and over the next few weeks, increase the length of time you exercise.*
    - *Be careful if you're taking blood pressure medicine that controls your heart rate. Your heart rate will not go up, but your blood pressure can get high. Ask your doctor, nurse, or pharmacist about this if you're not sure about your medicines.*
    - *We don't know the best level of exercise for someone with cancer. The goal is to have your exercise program help you keep up your muscle strength and keep you able to do the things you want and need to do. The more you exercise, the better you'll be able to exercise and function. But even if planned exercise stops, it's good to keep being active by doing your normal activities as much as you can".* (See How to Monitor Exercise Intensity)
- Goal: At least 30 minutes of aerobic exercise five days a week or more.
- Start slowly and work your way up. For example, if you are taking a walk, try short periods and rest frequently. Start at a slow 5–10-minute walk, rest, and try a brisk 5 minutes. You can also split up your sessions into 10 minutes throughout the day to equal 30. You don't have to start out at 30 minutes but work up to it.
- Keep track of when your energy levels are at their highest. Pain and fatigue can change daily but take advantage of the times when you are feeling the best. Try to keep on a daily routine.
- When you are feeling moderately fatigued, try getting up and doing something around the house to help with your endurance. It can be something as simple as walking up and down the hallway.
- Try getting up and walking hourly for circulation when you are not sleeping/napping.
- Balance activity with rest that does not interfere with nighttime sleep.
- Be flexible and listen to your body. Although you should keep some type of a schedule, don't feel like you need to
  follow it strictly. If you are feeling ill, extremely fatigued or running a fever let your body rest.
- If you don't feel like doing a regimented routine, try gardening, housework or any other physical hobby you may enjoy. Ask someone to walk with you or use headphones while exercising or walking.
- Drink about 8 to 10 glasses of water a day unless your doctor tells you not to. Unless you are told otherwise, eat a balanced diet that includes protein (meat, milk, eggs, and legumes such as peas or beans).
- Dress comfortably, especially in either cold or humid weather. *(See Temperature).*

Lymph Nodes & Lymphedema TOC / Quick Summary
Information and pictures from *National Cancer Institute* unless otherwise specified

Lymph nodes:

- Lymph nodes are part of the lymphatic and immune system, which protects your body against infection and disease.

Lymphatic System:

- The lymph system is a network of lymph vessels, tissues, and organs that carry lymph throughout the body.

Anatomy of Lymphatic System:

- When the lymph system is working as it should, lymph flows through the body and is returned to the bloodstream.

Lymphedema and Cancer:

- Lymphedema can occur after any cancer or treatment that affects the flow of lymph through the lymph nodes, such as removal of lymph nodes or radiation.

Stages of Lymphedema:

- *Stage 0:* A subclinical state where swelling is not evident despite impaired lymph transport..
- *Stage I or Reversible*: The limb (arm or leg) is swollen and feels heavy. Pressing on the swollen area leaves a pit (dent).
- *Stage II or Spontaneous Irreversible:* The limb is swollen and feels spongy. Pressing on the swollen area does not leave a pit.
- *Stage III or Lymphostatic Elephantiasis:* This is the most advanced stage. The swollen limb may be very large.

Possible Signs of Lymphedema:

- Other conditions may cause the same symptoms and when a doctor should be consulted.

Preventative Measures:

- Skin care
- Avoid blocking fluids/pooling.

Treatment:

- Complete Decongestive Therapy (CDT) or Combined therapy
- Manual Lymph Drainage
- Bandaging
- Pressure Garments / Compression Devices
- Exercise
- Axillary Reverse Mapping

Upper and Lower Extremity Lymphedema Exercises

References

Lymph nodes	Lymph nodes are part of the lymphatic and immune system, which protects your body against infection and disease. • Lymph nodes are small, round organs that are clustered in many areas of the body, such as the underarm. • It consists of a network of vessels and organs that contain lymph, a clear fluid that carries infection-fighting white blood cells as well as fluid and waste products from the body's cells and tissues. • Cancer cells can spread to lymph nodes and other parts of the body through lymph vessels. In a person with cancer, lymph can also carry cancer cells that have broken off from the main tumor. • Once lymph nodes are removed, they will be checked for cancer. Knowing whether cancer is in the underarm lymph nodes can help the doctor decide if you need any treatment in addition to surgery. *NIH NCI (11)* and *NIH NCI (13)*
Sentinel and Axillary Lymph Node / Dissection	**Please see Sentinel and Axillary Lymph Node / Dissection at the end of the Breast Cancer Section**

Lymphatic System – *National Cancer Institute*

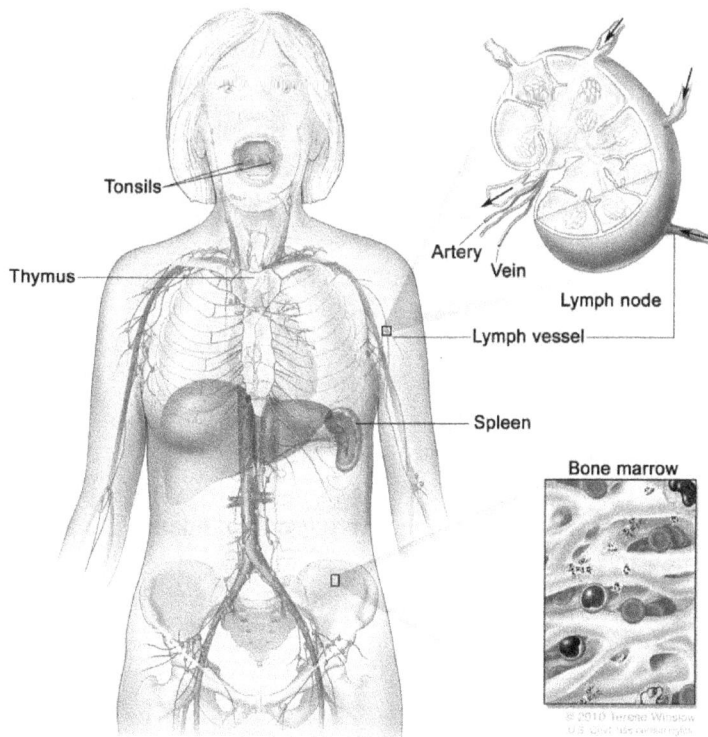

NIH NCI (12) https://www.cancer.gov/about-cancer/treatment/side-effects/lymphedema/lymphedema-pdq)

Lymphatic System	The lymph system is a network of lymph vessels, tissues, and organs that carry lymph throughout the body.
	• The parts of the lymph system that play a direct part in lymphedema include the following:
	   ◦ Lymph: Colorless, watery fluid that travels through the lymph vessels and carries T and B lymphocytes.
	      ▪ Lymphocytes are a type of white blood cell.
	   ◦ Lymph vessels: A network of thin tubes that collect lymph from different parts of the body and return it to the bloodstream.
	   ◦ Lymph nodes: Small, bean-shaped structures that filter lymph and store white blood cells that help fight infection and disease.
	      ▪ Lymph nodes are found along a network of lymph vessels throughout the body.
	      ▪ Groups of lymph nodes are found in the neck, underarm, mediastinum, abdomen, pelvis, and groin.
	• Lymph (clear fluid) and lymphocytes travel through the lymph vessels and into the lymph nodes where the lymphocytes destroy harmful substances. The lymph enters the blood through a large vein near the heart.
	• The spleen, thymus, tonsils, and bone marrow are also part of the lymph system but do not play a direct part in lymphedema.
	NIH NCI (12)

Anatomy of Lymphatic System	When the lymph system is working as it should, lymph flows through the body and is returned to the bloodstream.
	• Fluid and plasma leak out of the capillaries (smallest blood vessels) and flow around body tissues so the cells can take up nutrients and oxygen.
	• Some of this fluid goes back into the bloodstream. The rest of the fluid enters the lymph system through tiny lymph vessels.
	   ◦ These lymph vessels pick up the lymph and move it toward the heart.
	   ◦ The lymph is slowly moved through larger and larger lymph vessels and passes through lymph nodes where waste is filtered from the lymph.
	• The lymph keeps moving through the lymph system and collects near the neck, then flows into one of two large ducts:
	   ◦ The right lymph duct collects lymph from the right arm and the right side of the head and chest.
	   ◦ The left lymph duct collects lymph from both legs, the left arm, and the left side of the head and chest.
	• These large ducts empty into veins under the collarbones, which carry the lymph to the heart, where it is returned to the bloodstream.
	
	➢ **When part of the lymph system is damaged or blocked, fluid cannot drain from nearby body tissues.**
	➢ **Fluid builds up in the tissues and causes swelling/edema.**
	NIH NCI (12)

Cervical lymph nodes

Lymphatics of the mammary gland

Cisterna chyli

Lumbar lymph nodes

Pelvic lymph nodes

Lymphatics of the lower limb

Thoracic duct

Thymus

Axillary lymph nodes

Spleen

Lymphatics of the upper limb

Inguinal lymph nodes

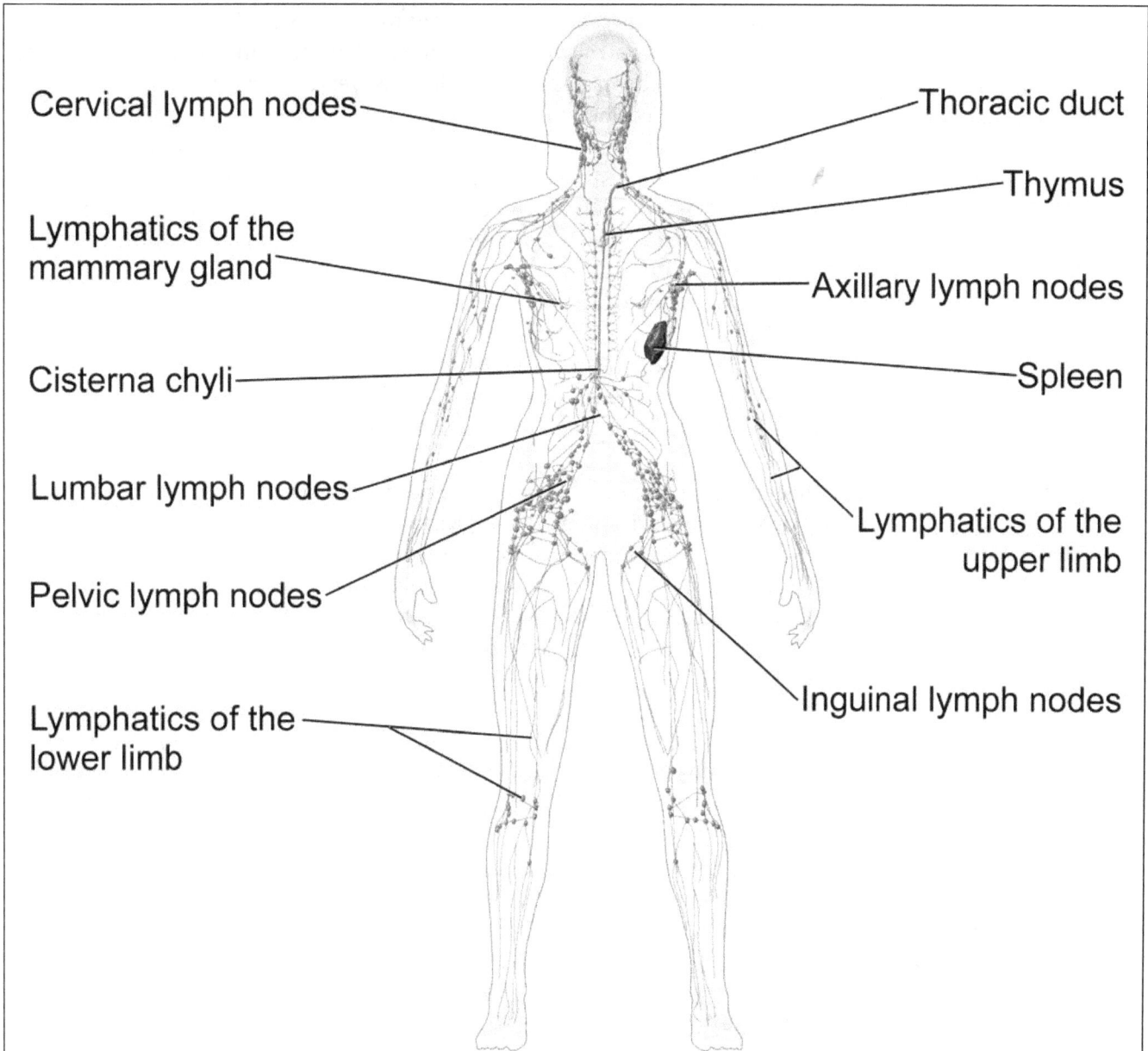

Medical gallery of Blausen Medical 2014". WikiJournal of Medicine

Lymphedema	**Lymphedema** is swelling caused by excess protein-rich lymph trapped within the interstitium and subcutaneous tissues. This is caused by dysfunction of the lymphatic system or pathology. Lymphedema occurs when the lymph system is damaged or blocked. Fluid builds up in soft body tissues and causes swelling. It is a common problem that may be caused by cancer and cancer treatment. Lymphedema usually affects an arm or leg, but it can also affect other parts of the body. Lymphedema can cause long-term physical, psychological, and social problems for patients. *NIH NCI (12)*

Lymphedema and Cancer	Lymphedema can occur after any cancer or treatment that affects the flow of lymph through the lymph nodes, such as removal of lymph nodes. It may develop within days or many years after treatment. Most lymphedema develops within three years of surgery.
	Risk factors for lymphedema include the following:
	• Removal and/or radiation of lymph nodes in the underarm, groin, pelvis, or neck.
	   o The risk of lymphedema increases with the number of lymph nodes affected.
	   o There is less risk with the removal of only the sentinel lymph node (the first lymph node in a group of lymph nodes to receive lymphatic drainage from the primary tumor).
	• Being overweight or obese.
	• Slow healing of the skin after surgery.
	• A tumor that affects or blocks the left lymph duct or lymph nodes or vessels in the neck, chest, underarm, pelvis, or abdomen.
	• Scar tissue in the lymph ducts under the collarbones, caused by surgery or radiation therapy.
	• Lymphedema often occurs in breast cancer patients who had all or part of their breast removed and axillary (underarm) lymph nodes removed. *(See below)*
	• Lymphedema in the legs may occur after surgery for uterine cancer, prostate cancer, lymphoma, or melanoma. It may also occur with vulvar cancer or ovarian cancer. Lymphedema occurs frequently in patients with cancers of the head and neck due to high-dose radiation therapy and combined surgery.
	NIH NCI (12)

Lymphedema and Breast Cancer	Lymphedema is swelling caused by a build-up of lymph. You may have this type of swelling in the hand, arm, chest, or back on the side of your body where lymph nodes were removed by breast cancer surgery or damaged by radiation therapy. Some important facts to know about lymphedema are: • Lymphedema can show up soon after surgery. • Sometimes, lymphedema can last for years. • Lymphedema can show up months or years after cancer treatment is over. • Lymphedema might develop after an insect bite, minor injury, or burn on the arm where lymph nodes were removed or damaged. • Lymphedema can cause pain and other problems. *NIH NCI (11)*

Stages of Lymphedema	• **Stage 0:** A subclinical state where swelling is not evident despite impaired lymph transport. This stage may exist for months or years before edema becomes evident.
	• **Stage I or Reversible:** The limb (arm or leg) is swollen and feels heavy. Pressing on the swollen area leaves a pit (dent).
	   o This stage of lymphedema may diminish with elevation.
	   o Subjective complaints are common.
	• **Stage II or Spontaneous irreversible**: The limb is swollen and feels spongy. Pressing on the swollen area does not leave a pit.
	   o A condition called tissue fibrosis may develop and cause the limb to feel hard.
	• **Stage III or Lymphostatic elephantiasis**: This is the most advanced stage. The swollen limb may be very large.
	   o Stage III lymphedema rarely occurs in breast cancer patients.
	     NIH NCI (12) and other

Possible Signs of Lymphedema	Other conditions may cause the same symptoms. A doctor should be consulted if any of the following problems occur: • Swelling of an arm or leg, which may include fingers and toes. • A full or heavy feeling in an arm or leg. • A tight feeling in the skin. • Trouble moving a joint in the arm or leg. • Thickening of the skin, with or without skin changes such as blisters or warts. • A feeling of tightness when wearing clothing, shoes, bracelets, watches, or rings. • Itching of the legs or toes. • A burning feeling in the legs. • Trouble sleeping. • Loss of hair. *NIH NCI (12)*
PREVENTATIVE MEASURES	Tell your doctor right away if you have any of the above symptoms. • The chance of improving the condition is better if treatment begins early. • Untreated lymphedema can lead to problems that cannot be reversed. *NIH NCI (12)*
Skin Care	Suggestions for Skin Care: • Keep skin and nails clean and cared for, to prevent infection. • Bacteria can enter the body through a cut, scratch, insect bite, or other skin injury. • Fluid that is trapped in body tissues by lymphedema makes it easy for bacteria to grow and cause infection. • Look for signs of infection, such as redness, pain, swelling, heat, fever, or red streaks below the surface of the skin. • Call your doctor right away if any of these signs appear. Careful skin and nail care helps to prevent infection: • Use cream or lotion to keep the skin moist. • Treat small cuts or breaks in the skin with an antibacterial ointment. • Avoid needle sticks of any type into the limb (arm or leg) with lymphedema. This includes shots or blood tests. • Use a thimble for sewing. • Avoid testing bath or cooking water using the limb with lymphedema. There may be less feeling (touch, temperature, pain) in the affected arm or leg, and skin might burn in water that is too hot. • Wear gloves when gardening and cooking. • Wear sunscreen and shoes outdoors. • Cut toenails straight across. See a podiatrist (foot doctor) as needed to prevent ingrown nails and infections. • Keep feet clean and dry and wear cotton socks. *NIH NCI (12)*

Avoid blocking fluids and pooling in Affected Limb	Avoid blocking the flow of fluids through the body. It is important to keep body fluids moving, especially through an affected limb or in areas where lymphedema may develop. • Do not cross your legs while sitting. • Change sitting position at least every 30 minutes. • Wear only loose jewelry and clothes without tight bands or elastic. • Do not carry handbags on the arm with lymphedema. • Do not use a blood pressure cuff on the arm with lymphedema. • Do not use elastic bandages or stockings with tight bands. Keep blood from pooling in the affected limb. • Keep the limb with lymphedema raised higher than the heart when possible. • Do not swing the limb quickly in circles or let the limb hang down. This makes blood and fluid collect in the lower part of the arm or leg. • Do not apply heat to the limb. *NIH NCI (12)*
Treatment	Possible Treatments: • Damage to the lymph system cannot be repaired. • Treatment is given to control the swelling caused by lymphedema and keep other problems from developing or getting worse. • Physical (non-drug) therapies are the standard treatment. • Treatment may be a combination of several physical methods. • The goal of these treatments is to help patients continue with activities of daily living, to decrease pain, and to improve the ability to move and use the limb (arm or leg) with lymphedema. • Drugs are not usually used for long-term treatment of lymphedema. *NIH NCI (12)*

Complete Decongestive Therapy or Combined Therapy	Combined physical therapy or complete decongestive therapy is a program managed by a certified lymphedema therapist to include:
	• Manual lymphatic drainage
	• Compression bandaging
	• Exercise
	• Skin care – *see skin care above*
	• Patient education
	• At the beginning of the program, the therapist gives many treatments over a short time to decrease most of the swelling in the limb with lymphedema.
	   • The patient then continues the program at home to keep the swelling down.
	    NIH NCI (12)

Manual Lymphatic Drainage **MLD**	**Manual Lymphatic Drainage (MLD)** • MLD (manual therapy) for lymphedema should begin with someone specially trained in treating lymphedema. • In this type of massage, the soft tissues of the body are lightly rubbed, tapped, and stroked. It is a very light touch, almost like dry brushing. • MLD may help move lymph out of the swollen area into an area with working lymph vessels. • Patients can be taught to do this type of massage therapy themselves by a certified lymphatic therapist. *NIH NCI (12)* **EFFECTS:** • Increases reabsorption of protein rich fluid • Increases lymphatic activity • Promotes relaxation • Creates and analgesic effect *(Klose Education)* When done correctly, massage therapy does not cause medical problems. **Massage should NOT be done on any of the following:** • Open wounds, bruises, or areas of broken skin. • Tumors that can be seen on the skin surface. • Areas with deep vein thrombosis (blood clot in a vein). • Sensitive soft tissue where the skin was treated with radiation therapy. *NIH NCI (12)* **CONTRAINDICATIONS:** • Acute infections, such as cellulitis • Untreated congestive heart failure (CHF) • Malignant disease – cancer • Renal dysfunction • Acute undiagnosed DVT *(Klose education)*

Bandages	**Bandages**
	• Once the lymph fluid is moved out of a swollen limb, bandaging (wrapping) can help prevent the area from refilling with fluid.
	• Bandages also increase the ability of the lymph vessels to move lymph along.
	• Lymphedema that has not improved with other treatments is sometimes helped with bandaging.
	NIH NCI (12)
	
	INDICATIONS:
	• Lymphedema
	• Chronic venous insufficiency (CVI)
	• Combination venous and lymphatic edema
	• Lipedema
	• Post-traumatic edema
	• Post-surgical edema
	• Acute DVT (*with* physician dx)
	
	CONTRAINDICATION:
	• Acute infections (MD must clear patient)
	• Arterial wounds
	• Arterial disease (ABI 0.8 or below)
	• Acute DVT (*without physician dx)*
	• Cardiac edema (untreated CHF)
	• Acute trauma without diagnosis
	
	PRECAUTIONS
	• Sensory deficits
	• Malignancy
	• Diabetes
	    – Small vessel (arteriole) and sensory deficits
	    – Toe bandaging may be contraindicated
	• Paralysis
	• Poor cognition or altered mental status
	• Sensitivity to the products used for bandaging
	(Klose Education)

Pressure Garments	**Pressure Garments** • Pressure garments are made of fabric that puts a controlled amount of pressure on different parts of the arm or leg to help move fluid and keep it from building up. • Some patients may need to have these garments custom-made for a correct fit. • Wearing a pressure garment during exercise may help prevent more swelling in an affected limb. • It is important to use pressure garments during air travel, because lymphedema can become worse at high altitudes. • Pressure garments are also called compression sleeves and lymphedema sleeves or stockings. *NIH NCI (12)*

Compression Device	**Compression Device** • Compression devices are pumps connected to a sleeve that wraps around the arm or leg and applies pressure on and off. The sleeve is inflated and deflated on a timed cycle. • This pumping action may help move fluid through lymph vessels and veins and keep fluid from building up in the arm or leg. • Compression devices may be helpful when added to complete decongestive therapy. • The use of these devices should be supervised by a trained professional because too much pressure can damage lymph vessels near the surface of the skin. *NIH NCI (12)*

Exercise
 	
(Also see Exercise and Breast Cancer)
	Exercise
	Both light exercise and aerobic exercise (physical activity that causes the heart and lungs to work harder) help the lymph vessels move lymph out of the affected limb and decrease swelling.
	• Talk with a certified lymphedema therapist before beginning exercise.
	    o Patients who have lymphedema or who are at risk for lymphedema should talk with a certified lymphedema therapist before beginning an exercise routine.
	    o (*See the Lymphology Association of North America* (https://www.clt-lana.org/) *web site for a list of certified lymphedema therapists in the US*)
	• Wear a pressure garment if lymphedema has developed.
	    o **Patients who have lymphedema should always wear a well-fitting pressure garment during all exercise that uses the affected limb or body part.**
	    o When it is not known for sure if a woman has lymphedema, upper-body exercise without a garment may be more helpful than no exercise at all.
	    o Patients who do not have lymphedema do not need to wear a pressure garment during exercise.
	• Breast cancer survivors should begin with light upper-body exercise and increase it slowly.
	    o Some studies with breast cancer survivors show that upper-body exercise is safe in women who have lymphedema or who are at risk for lymphedema.
	    o Weight-lifting that is slowly increased may keep lymphedema from getting worse.
	    o Exercise should start at a very low level, increase slowly over time, and be overseen by the lymphedema therapist.
	    o If exercise is stopped for a week or longer, it should be started again at a low level and increased slowly.
	    o If symptoms (such as swelling or heaviness in the limb) change or increase for a week or longer, talk with the lymphedema therapist.
	    o It is likely that exercising at a low level and slowly increasing it again over time is better for the affected limb than stopping the exercise completely.
	• More studies are needed to find out if weightlifting is safe for cancer survivors with lymphedema in the legs.
	NIH NCI (12)

Other Treatments	**Weight loss** • In patients who are overweight, lymphedema related to breast cancer may improve with weight loss. **Laser therapy** • Laser therapy may help decrease lymphedema swelling and skin hardness after a mastectomy. A hand-held, battery-powered device is used to aim low-level laser beams at the area with lymphedema. **Drug therapy** • Lymphedema is not usually treated with drugs. Antibiotics may be used to treat and prevent infections. Other types of drugs, such as diuretics or anticoagulants (blood thinners), are usually not helpful and may make the lymphedema worse. **Surgery** • Lymphedema caused by cancer is rarely treated with surgery. *NIH NCI (12)*

Axillary Reverse Mapping (ARM)

The axillary reverse mapping (ARM) technique has been developed to map and preserve arm lymphatic drainage during ALND and/or SLNB, thereby minimizing arm lymphedema. However, the success of ARM in reducing lymphedema has not been exactly determined.

- If ARM can be confirmed to be both effective and oncologically safe in preventing lymphedema, this technique should be recommended in the management of breast cancer treatment.
  NIH – National Library of Medicine. Axillary Reverse Mapping (ARM): Where to Go

- Lymphedema is a major chronic morbidity that occurs in patients undergoing treatment for breast cancer (BC). Surgery for BC includes axillary surgery with either sentinel lymph node biopsy (SLNB) or axillary lymph node dissection (ALND).
- Lymphedema occurs due to removal or disruption of lymphatic drainage of the arm that overlaps with drainage of the breast. The risk of lymphedema increases significantly with adjuvant radiation.
- Axillary reverse mapping (ARM) is a technique where blue dye is injected into the upper arm at surgery, allowing direct visualization of arm lymphatics and nodes during either SLNB or ALND.
  - This allows preservation of arm lymphatics unless there is suspicion of metastatic disease in ARM lymphatics or if the ARM node is/are also the sentinel lymph node.
- Studies to date have largely been observational cohort studies, and mainly with low-risk patients undergoing SLNB only. There is only one published randomized controlled trial, and this included only patients undergoing modified radical mastectomy.
  NIH – National Library of Medicine. Axillary Reverse Mapping (ARM) Technique (ARM)

- Traditionally, the rates of arm swelling after sentinel node biopsy range from 3-8%[1] and from 13-40%[2] after axillary dissection surgery. The studies that looked at ARM show a lymphedema rate that is lower, around 1-3% for the sentinel node surgery and 4-9%[3] for the axillary dissection surgery.
- Sometimes, it is not always possible to do ARM, and the surgeon needs to inject the blue dye in the breast to help identify the correct lymph nodes. This may be the case if you have had previous chemotherapy in the breast, or if the lymph nodes are not accurately found with other methods.
- Additionally, it is possible that the blue lymph nodes and the channels that are identified to drain the arm need to be removed to treat your cancer safely. If this is the case, you may be placed in a special group to watch your arm swelling closely or even have the option of having these channels reconnected. This is usually done by surgeons who are well experienced in lymphatic surgery and may include plastic surgeons also.
  Summit Education: Oncology Rehab Dec 12, 2019

UPPER EXTREMITY LYMPHEDEMA EXERCISES

This routine of 10-12 repetitions should always be done prior to exercises for those with lymphedema or at risk, including those that have had *any* amount of lymph nodes remove in the upper extremity and/or radiation.

Description	Pictures
Other information at beginning of book. UE = Upper Extremity Section Flex = Flexibility Section	See UE or Flex section of book for other pictures
FIST CLENCH *Lymphedema control and circulation* Hands on thighs, open and close hand	
FIST CLENCH *Lymphedema control and circulation* Open and close your hand 15-20x with arm elevated above heart to prevent edema	
FIST CLENCH *Lymphedema control and circulation* Open and close your hand 15-20x with arm elevated above heart to prevent edema **NOT OVERHEAD first 1-2 weeks and/or until drains are out**	
SHRUGS UE #87 Raise your shoulders upward towards your ears as shown. Shrug both shoulders at the same time. Inhale up/exhale down	

Description	Pictures
Description Other information at beginning of book. UE = Upper Extremity Section Flex = Flexibility Section	**Pictures** See UE or Flex section of book for other pictures
SHOULDER ROLLS - Backwards UE #89 Move your shoulders in a circular pattern so that you are moving in an up, back and down direction. Perform small circles if needed for comfort.	
NECK ROTATION and SIDE BENDS Flex #47 SIDE BENDS: (*Top*) Tilt your head as if you are trying to touch your ear to your shoulder. ROTATION: (*Bottom*) Turn you head to the side as if looking over your shoulder.	
NECK FLEXION AND EXTENSION Flex #48 EXTENSION: Look up as if you are looking at the sky moving your neck only. FLEXION: Look down as if you are looking at the floor. For an extra stretch gently put both hands behind your head to move chin towards the chest and hold.	
SHOULDER RAISE / ELBOW CIRCLES Place your fingertips onto your shoulders. Slowly raise the elbow up to the side, then move it forwards, gently circling your arm. You are aiming to get your elbow level with your shoulder. Try to increase the height each time you do the exercises until you get level with your shoulder.	
ISOMETRIC CHEST PRESS Place the palms of your hands together with your elbows bent and arms at shoulder level or below. Exhale while pushing hands together and inhale and relax. 5-10x.	

LOWER EXTREMITY LYMPHEDEMA EXERCISES

This routine of 10-12 repetitions should always be done prior to exercises for those with lymphedema or at risk, including those that have had *any* amount of lymph nodes remove in the upper extremity and/or radiation.

Description	Pictures
Other information at beginning of book. LE = Lower Extremity Section Flex = Flexibility Section	See LE or Flex section of book for other pictures
BICYCLES *Lymphedema control and circulation* Lying on your back, bend the knees at an angle. In a circular motion, complete ~10 repetitions in each direction, as if on a bike	
LEG CIRCLE *Lymphedema control and circulation* Lying on your back, bend one leg and point the opposite leg towards the ceiling. Move the leg in a small circumduction ~10x each way. *Think of drawing a small circle on the ceiling with your foot.* Repeat on the opposite leg.	
LEG FLEXION / EXTENSION *Lymphedema control and circulation* Lying on your back, bend and extend leg ~10x repetitions. You can either alternate or repeat on the same leg and repeat with opposite leg.	
FOOT PLANTAR/ DORSI FLEXION and CIRCLES *Lymphedema control and circulation* Lying on your back, extend the legs towards the ceiling. • Dorsi/plantar flex foot (ankle pump) ~10x. • Foot circles ~10x each direction	

Diaphragmatic Breathing

Lie either on your back with your knees bent or sit up

Inhale through your nose; as you do so, allow your stomach to rise. Limit movement in your chest. Attempt to push your bottom ribs out to the side as you breathe in.

Exhale through your mouth; as you do so, allow your stomach to fall. Limit movement in your chest.

Diaphragmatic breathing 6x a day for 5-10 repetitions

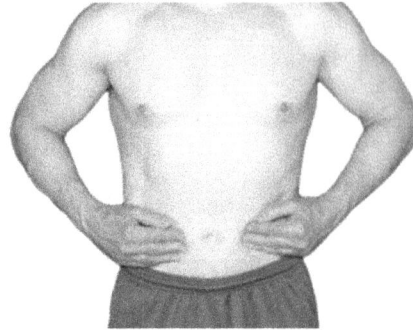

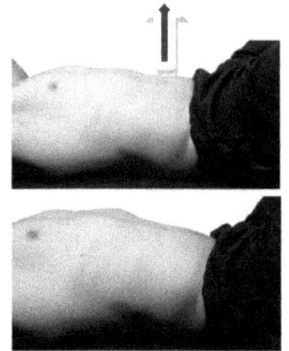

REFERENCES

American Cancer Society - Lymph Node Surgery for Breast Cancer *https://www.cancer.org/cancer/breast-cancer/treatment/surgery-for-breast-cancer/lymph-node-surgery-for-breast-cancer.html*

Medical gallery of Blausen Medical 2014". WikiJournal of Medicine

NIH NCI (11) https://www.cancer.gov/types/breast/surgery-choices/lymphedema

NIH NCI (12) https://www.cancer.gov/about-cancer/treatment/side-effects/lymphedema/lymphedema-pdq NIH

NCI (13) https://www.cancer.gov/about-cancer/diagnosis-staging/staging/sentinel-node-biopsy-fact-sheet

NIH – National Library of Medicine. Axillary Reverse Mapping (ARM): Where to Go *https://pubmed.ncbi.nlm.nih.gov/29961238/*

NIH – National Library of Medicine. Axillary Reverse Mapping (ARM) Technique (ARM) *https://clinicaltrials.gov/ct2/show/NCT03109522*

Pink Ribbon Program©

Summit Education: Oncology Rehab Dec 12, 2019

UPMC Axillary Lymph Node Dissection *https://www.upmc.com/locations/hospitals/magee/services/magee-womens-cancers/breast-cancer-program/treatment/breast-cancer-surgery/axillary-lymph-node*

Wikipedia – Axillary Lymph Nodes - *https://en.wikipedia.org/wiki/Axillary_lymph_nodes*

Wiki McMaster: *Breast Cancer https://wiki.mcmaster.ca/LIFESCI_4M03/_detail/screen_shot_2017-10-02_at_5.51.59_pm.png?id=group_1_presentation_1_-_breast_cancer*

BREAST CANCER

Information and pictures from *National Cancer Institute* unless otherwise specified

Quick Summary this Section

Breast Cancer:
- What is Breast Cancer, Stage Groups, Risk Factors, Protective Factors,

Types:
- DCIS, LCIS, IDC, ILC, Rare, Inflammatory, Paget Disease

Surgeries:
- Mastectomy, Lumpectomy, Nipple Sparing Mastectomy, Total or Simple Mastectomy, Considerations, Comparisons

Reconstruction:
- Factors - Timing and Choice
- Reconstruction: Implants or Autologous Tissue

Breast Implants:
- Implants
- Tissue Expanders

Tissue Flap Surgeries:
- Autologous Tissue & Reconstruction
- TRAM, DIEP, SIEA, LAT, Gluteal, TUG, IGAP
- Nipple Reconstruction

Risks after Breast Surgery:
- Axillary Web Syndrome - AWS (Cording), Scar Tissue / Adhesions, Seroma / Compression

Sentinel and Axillary Lymph Nodes:
- Sentinel Lymph Node Biopsy (SLNB)
- Axillary Lymph Node Dissection (ALND) *- see Lymphedema*

Things to Avoid, Post Op Healing & Mastectomy:
- Avoid 2 - weeks Post op, Post op healing concerns, Recommendations post mastectomy

Exercise Examples - Post Mastectomy:
- Examples of Exercises, Stretches or Edema Control after Mastectomy

Home Exercise Guide Breast and / or Lymphedema:
- Home Exercise Guide For Post Surgery and / or Lymphedema

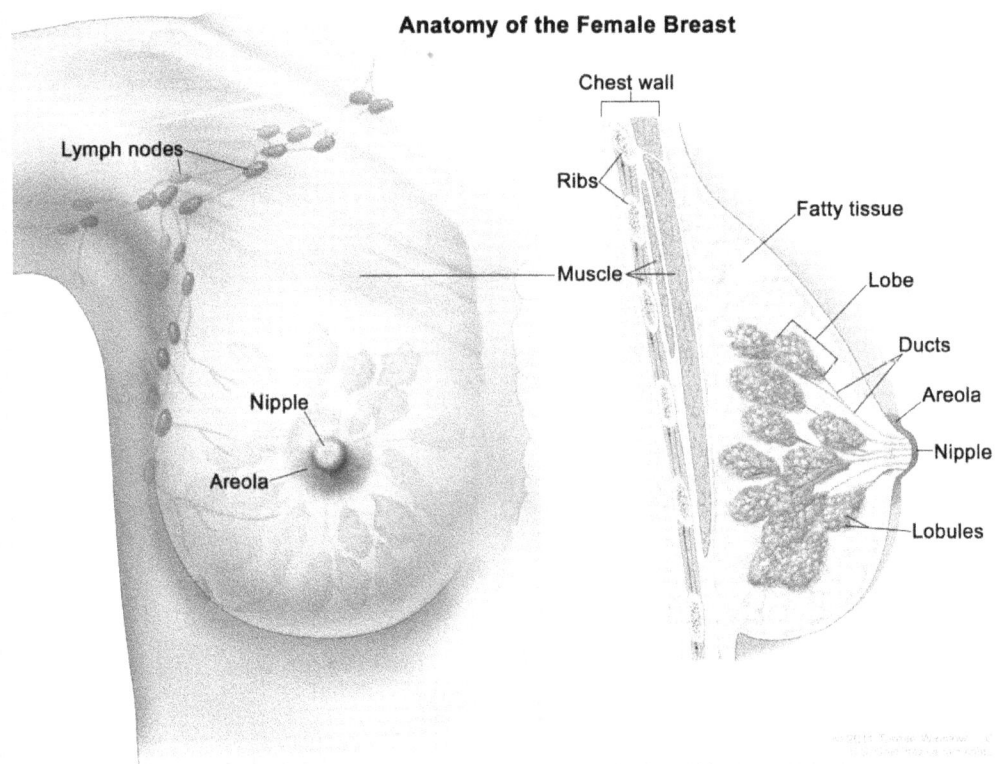

What is Breast Cancer?	Breast cancer is a disease in which cells in the breast grow out of control. There are different kinds of breast cancer. The kind of breast cancer depends on which cells in the breast turn into cancer. • Breast cancer can begin in different parts of the breast. A breast is made up of three main parts: lobules, ducts, and connective tissue. • The lobules are the glands that produce milk. The ducts are tubes that carry milk to the nipple. • The connective tissue (which consists of fibrous and fatty tissue) surrounds and holds everything together. • Most breast cancers begin in the ducts or lobules. • Breast cancer can spread outside the breast through blood vessels and lymph vessels. ○ When breast cancer spreads to other parts of the body, it is said to have metastasized. *CDC (1)* **Anatomy of the Female Breast** *NIH - NCI (National Cancer Institute) https://www.cancer.gov/types/breast/patient/breast- treatment-pdq#_148*

Staging and Stage Groups	Stage refers to the extent of your cancer, such as how large the tumor is, and if it has spread.
	 • A cancer is always referred to by the stage it was given at diagnosis, even if it gets worse or spreads.
	 • New information about how a cancer has changed over time gets added on to the original stage. So, the stage doesn't change, even though the cancer might.
	
	 Systems that Describe Stage
	 There are many staging systems. Some, such as the TNM staging system, are used for many types of cancer. Others are specific to a particular type of cancer.
	
	 Most staging systems include information about:
	 • Where the tumor is located in the body
	 • The cell type (such as, adenocarcinoma or squamous cell carcinoma)
	 • The size of the tumor
	 • Whether the cancer has spread to nearby lymph nodes
	 • Whether the cancer has spread to a different part of the body
	 • Tumor grade, which refers to how abnormal the cancer cells look and how likely the tumor is to grow and spread
	 NIH – NCI (6)
	
	 In breast cancer, stage is based on the size and location of the primary tumor, the spread of cancer to nearby lymph nodes or other parts of the body, tumor grade, and whether certain biomarkers are present.
	
	 To plan the best treatment and understand your prognosis, it is important to know the breast cancer stage. *NIH – NCI (2)*
	
	 • **Clinical Prognostic Stage** is used first to assign a stage for all patients based on health history, physical exam, imaging tests (if done), and biopsies
	     o The Clinical Prognostic Stage is described by the TNM system, tumor grade, and biomarker status (ER, PR, HER2).
	     o In clinical staging, mammography or ultrasound is used to check the lymph nodes for signs of cancer.
	
	 • **Pathological Prognostic Stage** is then used for patients who have surgery as their first treatment.
	     o Prognostic Stage is based on all clinical information, biomarker status, and laboratory test results from breast tissue and lymph nodes removed during surgery
	
	 • **Anatomic Stage** is based on the size and the spread of cancer as described by the TNM system.

Risk Factors	**Risk Factors**
	- A personal history of benign (non-cancer) breast disease.
	- A family history of breast cancer in a first- degree relative (mother, daughter, or sister).
	- Inherited changes in the BRCA1 or BRCA2 genes or in other genes (such as PALB2) that increase the risk of breast cancer.
	- Breast tissue that is dense on a mammogram.
	- Exposure of breast tissue to estrogen made by the body. This may be caused by:
	    o Menstruating at an early age.
	    o Older age at first birth or never having given birth.
	    o Starting menopause at a later age.
	- Taking hormones such as estrogen combined with progestin for symptoms of menopause.
	- Treatment with radiation therapy to the breast/chest.
	- Drinking alcohol.
	- Obesity.
	
	BRCA
	Of all women with breast cancer, 5% to 10% may have a germline mutation of the genes BRCA1 and BRCA2. Specific mutations of BRCA1 and BRCA2 are more common in women of Jewish ancestry.
	- The estimated lifetime risk of developing breast cancer for women with BRCA1 and BRCA2 mutations is 40% to 85%.
	- Carriers with a history of breast cancer have an increased risk of contralateral disease that may be as high as 5% per year.
	- Male BRCA2 mutation carriers also have an increased risk of breast cancer.
	- Mutations in either the BRCA1 or the BRCA2 gene also confer an increased risk of ovarian cancer or other primary cancers.
	- Once a BRCA1 or BRCA2 mutation has been identified, other family members can be referred for genetic counseling and testing. *NIH – NCI (1)*

Protective Factors	**Protective Factors** Protective factors and interventions to reduce the risk of female breast cancer include the following: - Estrogen use (after hysterectomy). - Exercise. - Early pregnancy. - Breast feeding. - Selective estrogen receptor modulators (SERMs). - Aromatase inhibitors or inactivators. - Risk-reducing mastectomy. - Risk-reducing oophorectomy or ovarian ablation. *NIH – NCI (1)*

Breast Cancer Types

Information and pictures from *National Cancer Institute* unless otherwise specified

Quick Summary of Section

Ductal carcinoma in situ (DCIS):

- DCIS is considered a precursor lesion for the subsequent development of invasive carcinoma with a high-risk index factor than that expected in women without DCIS

Lobular carcinoma in situ (LCIS):

- Lobular carcinoma in situ (LCIS) is an uncommon condition in which abnormal cells form in the milk glands (lobules) in the breast. LCIS isn't cancer, but being diagnosed with LCIS indicates that you have an increased risk of developing breast cancer.

Invasive ductal carcinoma (IDC):

- The most common type of invasive breast cancer. It begins in the lining of the milk ducts (thin tubes that carry milk from the lobules of the breast to the nipple) and spreads outside the ducts to surrounding normal tissue. Invasive ductal carcinoma can also spread through the blood and lymph systems to other parts of the body.

Invasive lobular carcinoma (ILC):

- A type of invasive breast cancer that begins in the lobules (milk glands) of the breast and spreads to surrounding normal tissue. It can also spread through the blood and lymph systems to other parts of the body.

Rare cancers:

- For example, male breast cancer, medullary breast cancer, lymphoma of the breast

Inflammatory breast

- Inflammatory breast cancer is a rare and very aggressive disease in which cancer cells block lymph vessels in the skin of the breast. This type of breast cancer is called "inflammatory" because the breast often looks swollen and red, or inflamed.

Paget Disease of the Breast:

- Paget disease of the breast (also known as Paget disease of the nipple and mammary Paget disease) is a rare type of cancer involving the skin of the nipple and, usually, the darker circle of skin around it, which is called the areola.

Ductal Carcinoma in situ (DCIS)	DCIS is considered a precursor lesion for the subsequent development of invasive carcinoma with a high-risk index factor than that expected in women without DCIS Death due to DCIS is extremely rare, but death occurring after initial diagnosis of DCIS is either because of undetected invasive component or due to recurrence of invasive lesion after the treatment. *NCBI - Diversity of Breast Carcinoma* • 85% of breast cancer originates in the ducts • These cancers are considered benign, but eventually will become invasive with time **Symptoms:** DCIS doesn't typically have any signs or symptoms. However, DCIS can sometimes cause signs such as: • A breast lump • Bloody nipple discharge *Mayo Clinic: Ductal carcinoma in situ (DCIS)*
Lobular Carcinoma in situ (LCIS)	Lobular carcinoma in situ (LCIS) is an uncommon condition in which abnormal cells form in the milk glands (lobules) in the breast. LCIS isn't cancer, but being diagnosed with LCIS indicates that you have an increased risk of developing breast cancer. Women with LCIS have an increased risk of developing invasive breast cancer in either breast. • 15% of breast cancer originates in the lobules • These cancers are considered benign but eventually will become invasive with time. **Symptoms:** LCIS usually doesn't show up on mammograms. The condition is most often discovered as a result of a breast biopsy done for another reason, such as a suspicious breast lump or an abnormal mammogram. *Mayo Clinic: Lobular carcinoma in situ (LCIS)*
Invasive Ductal Carcinoma (IDC)	The most common type of invasive breast cancer. It begins in the lining of the milk ducts (thin tubes that carry milk from the lobules of the breast to the nipple) and spreads outside the ducts to surrounding normal tissue. Invasive ductal carcinoma can also spread through the blood and lymph systems to other parts of the body. Also called infiltrating ductal carcinoma. *NIH – NCI – IDC definition* • The cancer cells grow outside the ducts into other parts of the breast tissue. • Invasive cancer cells can also spread, or metastasize, to other parts of the body. **Symptoms:** • A lump in your breast. • Thickened breast skin. • Rash or redness on your breast. • Swelling in your breast. • New pain in your breast. • Dimpling on your breast or the skin of your nipple. • Nipple pain. • Inverted nipple.

Invasive Lobular Carcinoma (ILC)	A type of invasive breast cancer that begins in the lobules (milk glands) of the breast and spreads to surrounding normal tissue. It can also spread through the blood and lymph systems to other parts of the body. Also called infiltrating lobular carcinoma. *NIH- NCI – ILC definition* • Begins in the milk-producing glands (lobules) of the breast. • Cancer cells have broken out of the lobule where they began and have the potential to spread to the lymph nodes and other areas of the body. • Invasive lobular carcinoma makes up a small portion of all breast cancers. • Invasive lobular carcinoma is less likely than other forms of breast cancer to cause a firm or distinct breast lump. **Symptoms:** At its earliest stages, invasive lobular carcinoma may cause no signs and symptoms. As it grows larger, invasive lobular carcinoma may cause: • An area of thickening in part of the breast • A new area of fullness or swelling in the breast • A change in the texture or appearance of the skin over the breast, such as dimpling or thickening • A newly inverted nipple *Mayo Clinic: Invasive lobular carcinoma*
Rare Cancers – not limited to:	• Male Breast Cancer - Cancer that forms in tissues of the breast in men. Most male breast cancer begins in cells lining the ducts. It is very rare and usually affects older men. • Medullary breast cancer • Mucinous (mucoid or colloid) breast cancer • Tubular breast cancer • Adenoid cystic carcinoma of the breast • Metaplastic breast cancer • Lymphoma of the breast • Basal type breast cancer • Phyllodes or cystosarcoma phyllodes • Papillary breast cancer

Inflammatory Breast Cancer	Inflammatory breast cancer is a rare and very aggressive disease in which cancer cells block lymph vessels in the skin of the breast. This type of breast cancer is called "inflammatory" because the breast often looks swollen and red, or inflamed. • Inflammatory breast cancer is rare, accounting for 1 to 5 percent of all breast cancers diagnosed in the United States. Most inflammatory breast cancers are invasive ductal carcinomas, which means they developed from cells that line the milk ducts of the breast and then spread beyond the ducts. • Inflammatory breast cancer progresses rapidly, often in a matter of weeks or months. At diagnosis, inflammatory breast cancer is either stage III or IV disease, depending on whether cancer cells have spread only to nearby lymph nodes or to other tissues as well. • Compared with other types of breast cancer, inflammatory breast cancer tends to be diagnosed at younger ages. • More common and diagnosed at younger ages in African American women than in white women. • Inflammatory breast tumors are frequently hormone receptor negative, which means they cannot be treated with hormone therapies, such as tamoxifen, that interfere with the growth of cancer cells fueled by estrogen. • More common in obese women than in women of normal weight. *NIH – NCI – Inflammatory Breast*
Paget Disease of the Breast	• Paget disease of the breast (also known as Paget disease of the nipple and mammary Paget disease) is a rare type of cancer involving the skin of the nipple and, usually, the darker circle of skin around it, which is called the areola. • Most people with Paget disease of the breast also have one or more tumors inside the same breast. These breast tumors are either ductal carcinoma in situ or invasive breast cancer. • Paget disease of the breast occurs in both women and men, but most cases occur in women. Approximately 1 to 4 percent of all cases of breast cancer also involve Paget disease of the breast. • The average age at diagnosis is 57 years, but the disease has been found in adolescents and in people in their late 80s • Studies have shown that breast-conserving surgery that includes removal of the nipple and areola, followed by whole-breast radiation therapy, is a safe option for people with Paget disease of the breast who do not have a palpable lump in their breast and whose mammograms do not reveal a tumor The symptoms of Paget disease of the breast are often mistaken for those of some benign skin conditions, such as dermatitis or eczema. These symptoms may include the following: • Itching, tingling, or redness in the nipple and/or areola • Flaking, crusty, or thickened skin on or around the nipple • A flattened nipple • Discharge from the nipple that may be yellowish or bloody • Because the early symptoms of Paget disease of the breast may suggest a benign skin condition, and because the disease is rare, it may be misdiagnosed at first. • People with Paget disease of the breast have often had symptoms for several months before being correctly diagnosed. *NIH NCI – Paget*

CDC – Center of Disease Control and Prevention

CDC (1) – What is Breast Cancer? *https://www.cdc.gov/cancer/breast/basic_info/what-is-breast-cancer.htm*

Mayo Clinic: *Mayoclinic.org*

Mayo Clinic: Ductal carcinoma in situ (DCIS) *https://www.mayoclinic.org/diseases-conditions/dcis/symptoms-causes/syc-20371889*

Mayo Clinic: Invasive lobular carcinoma *https://www.mayoclinic.org/diseases-conditions/invasive-lobular-carcinoma/symptoms-causes/syc-20373973*

Mayo Clinic: Lobular carcinoma in situ (LCIS) *https://www.mayoclinic.org/diseases-conditions/lobular-carcinoma-in-situ/symptoms-causes/syc-20374529*

NCBI - Diversity of Breast Carcinoma *https://www.ncbi.nlm.nih.gov/pmc/articles/PMC4689326/*

NIH – NCI – National Cancer Institute

NIH – NCI - IDC definition *https://www.cancer.gov/publications/dictionaries/cancer-terms/def/invasive-ductal-carcinoma*

NIH – NCI (1) - Breast Treatment (professional) *https://www.cancer.gov/types/breast/hp/breast-treatment-pdq*

NIH – NCI (2) Treatment (patient) https://www.cancer.gov/types/breast/patient/breast-treatment-pdq#_181

NIH- NCI - ILC definition- *https://www.cancer.gov/publications/dictionaries/cancer-terms/def/invasive-lobular-carcinoma*

NIH NCI - Paget *https://www.cancer.gov/types/breast/paget-breast-fact-sheet*

NIH – NCI – Inflammatory Breast Cancer *https://www.cancer.gov/types/breast/ibc-fact-sheet*

Breast Surgeries

Information and pictures from *National Cancer Institute* unless otherwise specified

Quick Summary of Section

Mastectomy:

- Surgical removal of the breast that has DCIS or cancer.

Breast Conserving Lumpectomy:

- Breast-sparing surgery means the surgeon removes only the DCIS or cancer and some normal tissue around it.

Considerations for Breast - Conserving surgery:

- Most women with DCIS or breast cancer can choose to have breast- sparing surgery, usually followed by radiation therapy: Choices, what will my breasts look and feel like, returning to activities, will I need more surgery, recurrence.

Nipple-Sparing Mastectomy:

- A nipple-sparing mastectomy is similar to the skin-sparing mastectomy. This procedure is more often an option for women who have a small, early-stage cancer near the outer part of the breast, with no signs of cancer in the skin or near the nipple.

Total Mastectomy or Simple Mastectomy:

- The surgeon removes your whole breast.

Modified Radical Mastectomy:

- Surgery for breast cancer in which the breast, most or all of the lymph nodes under the arm and the lining over the chest muscles are removed.

Considerations with Mastectomy:

- Most women with DCIS or breast cancer can choose to have a mastectomy: Choices, what will my breasts look and feel like, returning to activities, will I need more surgery, recurrence.

Considerations with Mastectomy and Reconstruction:

- If you have a mastectomy, you might also want breast reconstruction surgery.

Compare the Types of Breast Surgery:

- Mastectomy, Skin sparing mastectomy, Mastectomy with reconstruction:
    - Is this surgery right for me?
    - How long before I can return to normal activities?
    - What other problems might I have?
    - What will my breast look like?
    - Will my breast have feeling?
    - Will I need more surgery?
    - What are the chances that my breast cancer will return in the same area?

Mastectomy	Surgical removal of the breast that has DCIS or cancer. There are different types of mastectomies: • Total mastectomy (also known as simple mastectomy) • Skin-sparing mastectomy • Modified radical mastectomy. ***A mastectomy is most often recommended when:*** • There are multiple areas of cancer within your breast • The tumor is greater than 5cm (2inches) • Your breast is small or shaped such that removal of the entire cancer will leave little breast tissue or a deformed breast • You do not want or cannot have radiation therapy (sometimes radiation is necessary, even if you have a mastectomy). ***Possible Side Effects of Mastectomy*** • Infection, poor wound healing, a reaction to the drugs used in surgery (anesthesia) • A collection of fluid or blood under the skin may occur after a mastectomy *Department of Health NY: Breast Cancer Treatment*
Breast Conserving - Lumpectomy Also called breast-sparing surgery, partial mastectomy, quadrantectomy, and segmental mastectomy.	Breast-sparing surgery means the surgeon removes only the DCIS or cancer and some normal tissue around it. • If you have cancer, the surgeon will also remove one or more lymph nodes from under your arm. • Breast-sparing surgery usually keeps your breast looking much like it did before surgery. • After breast-sparing surgery, most women also receive radiation therapy. Some women will also need chemotherapy, hormone therapy, and/or targeted therapy. • The main goal of this treatment is to keep cancer from coming back in the same breast. *NIH NCI (8)*

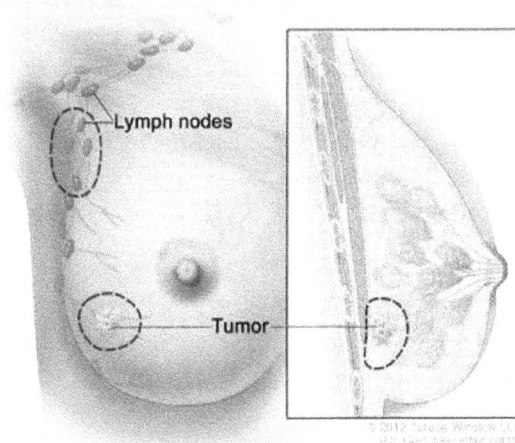

Breast-sparing Surgery

Lymph nodes

Tumor

NHI NCI (8) https://www.cancer.gov/types/breast/surgery-choices

Considerations for Breast-conserving surgery	*Is this surgery right for me?* • Most women with DCIS or breast cancer can choose to have breast-sparing surgery, usually followed by radiation therapy. *How long before I can return to normal activities?* • Most women are ready to return to most of their usual activities within 5 to 10 days. *What other problems might I have?* • You may feel very tired and have skin changes from radiation therapy. *What will my breast look like?* • Your breast should look a lot like it did before surgery. • But if your tumor is large, your breast may look different or smaller after breast-sparing surgery. • You will have a small scar where the surgeon cut to remove the DCIS or cancer. The length of the scar will depend on how large an incision the surgeon needed to make. *Will my breast have feeling?* • Yes. You should still have feeling in your breast, nipple, and areola (the dark area around your nipple). *Will I need more surgery?* • If the surgeon does not remove all the DCIS or cancer the first time, you may need more surgery. *What are the chances that my breast cancer will return in the same area?* • There is a chance that your cancer will come back in the same breast. But if it does, it is not likely to affect how long you live. • About 10% of women (1 out of every 10) who have breast-sparing surgery along with radiation therapy get cancer in the same breast within 12 years. If this happens, you can be effectively treated with a mastectomy. *NIH NCI (8)*
Nipple-sparing mastectomy	A nipple-sparing mastectomy is similar to the skin-sparing mastectomy. This procedure is more often an option for women who have a small, early-stage cancer near the outer part of the breast, with no signs of cancer in the skin or near the nipple. • The surgeon often removes the breast tissue beneath the nipple (and areola) during the procedure, to check for cancer cells. If cancer is found in this tissue, the nipple must be removed. *Department of Health NY: Breast Cancer Treatment*

Total Mastectomy or **Simple Mastectomy**	The surgeon removes your whole breast. • Sometimes, the surgeon also takes out one or more of the lymph nodes under your arm.

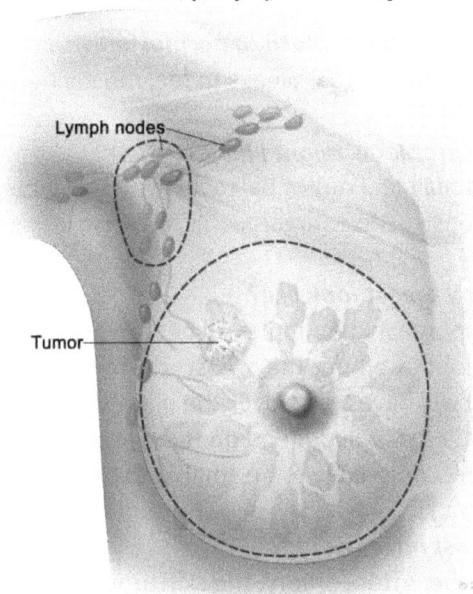

NHI NCI (8) https://www.cancer.gov/types/breast/surgery-choices

Modified Radical Mastectomy	Surgery for breast cancer in which the breast, most or all of the lymph nodes under the arm, and the lining over the chest muscles are removed. • Sometimes the surgeon also removes part of the chest wall muscles.

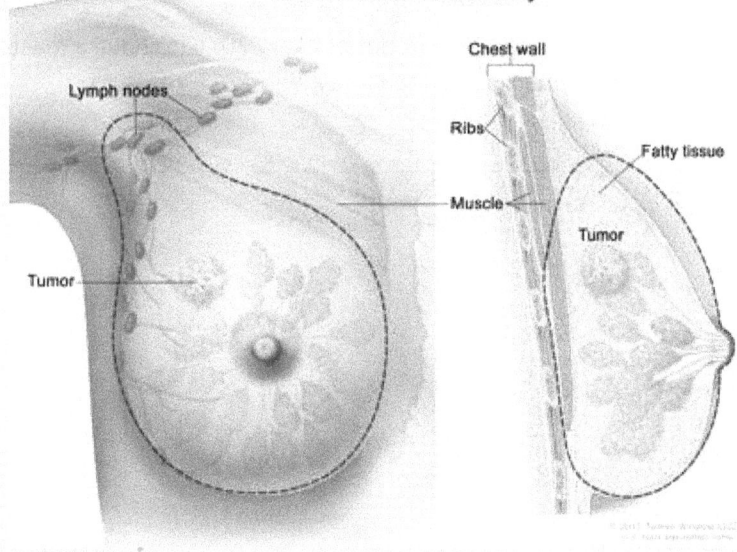

NHI NCI (8) https://www.cancer.gov/types/breast/surgery-choices

Considerations with Mastectomy	*Is this surgery right for me?* Most women with DCIS or breast cancer can choose to have a mastectomy. A mastectomy may be a better choice for you if: • You have small breasts and a large area of DCIS or cancer. • You have DCIS or cancer in more than one part of your breast. • The DCIS or cancer is under the nipple. • You are not able to receive radiation therapy. *How long before I can return to normal activities?* • It may take 3 to 4 weeks to feel mostly normal after a mastectomy. *What other problems might I have?* • You may feel out of balance if you had large breasts and do not have reconstruction surgery. This may also lead to neck and shoulder pain. *What will my breast look like?* • Your breast and nipple will be removed. You will have a flat chest on the side of your body where the breast was removed. • You will have a scar over the place where your breast was removed. The length of the scar will depend on the size of your breast. If you have smaller breasts, your scar is likely to be smaller than if you have larger breasts. *Will my breast have feeling?* • Maybe. After surgery, the skin around where the surgeon cut and maybe the area under your arm will be numb (have no feeling). • This numb feeling may improve over 1 to 2 years, but it will never feel like it once did. Also, the skin where your breast was may feel tight. *Will I need more surgery?* • If you have problems after your mastectomy, you may need more surgery. *What are the chances that my breast cancer will return in the same area?* • There is a smaller chance that your cancer will return in the same area than if you have breast-sparing surgery. • About 5% of women (1 out of every 20) who have a mastectomy will get cancer on the same side of their chest within 12 years. *NHI NCI (8)*

Considerations with Mastectomy and Reconstruction	*Is this surgery right for me?*
	• If you have a mastectomy, you might also want breast reconstruction surgery.
	• You can choose to have reconstruction surgery at the same time as your mastectomy or wait and have it later.
	
	How long before I can return to normal activities?
	• Your recovery will depend on the type of reconstruction you have. It can take 6 to 8 weeks or longer to fully recover from breast reconstruction.
	
	What other problems might I have?
	• You may not like how your breast-like shape looks.
	• If you have an implant:
	   o Your breast may harden and can become painful.
	   o You will likely need more surgery if your implant breaks or leaks.
	• If you have flap surgery, you may lose strength in the part of your body where a muscle was removed.
	
	What will my breast look like?
	• You will have a breast-like shape, but your breast will not look or feel like it did before surgery. And, it will not look or feel like your other breast.
	• You will have scars where the surgeon stitched skin together to make the new breast-like shape.
	• If you have tissue flap reconstruction, you will have scars around the new breast, as well as the area where the surgeon removed the muscle, fat, and skin to make the new breast-like shape.
	
	Will my breast have feeling?
	• No. The area around your breast will not have feeling.
	
	Will I need more surgery?
	• You will need more than one surgery to build a new breast-like shape. The number of surgeries you need will depend on the type of reconstruction you have and if you choose to have a nipple or areola added.
	• Some women may also decide to have surgery on the opposite breast to help it match the new breast-like shape better.
	• If you have an implant, you are likely to need surgery many years later to remove or replace it.
	
	What are the chances that my breast cancer will return in the same area?
	• Your chances are the same as mastectomy, since breast reconstruction surgery does not affect the chances of the cancer returning.
	
	NHI NCI (8)

Compare the Types of Breast Surgery:

National Cancer institute (NHI NCI (8)

Is this surgery right for me?

Breast-Sparing Surgery	Most women with DCIS or breast cancer can choose to have breast-sparing surgery, usually followed by radiation therapy.
Mastectomy	Most women with DCIS or breast cancer can choose to have a mastectomy. A mastectomy may be a better choice for you if: • You have small breasts and a large area of DCIS or cancer. • You have DCIS or cancer in more than one part of your breast. • The DCIS or cancer is under the nipple. • You are not able to receive radiation therapy.
Mastectomy with Reconstruction	If you have a mastectomy, you might also want breast reconstruction surgery. You can choose to have reconstruction surgery at the same time as your mastectomy or wait and have it later.

How long before I can return to normal activities?

Breast-Sparing Surgery	Most women are ready to return to most of their usual activities within 5 to 10 days.
Mastectomy	It may take 3 to 4 weeks to feel mostly normal after a mastectomy.
Mastectomy with Reconstruction	Your recovery will depend on the type of reconstruction you have. It can take 6 to 8 weeks or longer to fully recover from breast reconstruction.

What other problems might I have?

Breast-Sparing Surgery	You may feel very tired and have skin changes from radiation therapy.
Mastectomy	You may feel out of balance if you had large breasts and do not have reconstruction surgery. This may also lead to neck and shoulder pain.
Mastectomy with Reconstruction	You may not like how your breast-like shape looks. If you have an implant: • Your breast may harden and can become painful. • You will likely need more surgery if your implant breaks or leaks. If you have flap surgery, you may lose strength in the part of your body where a muscle was removed.

What will my breast look like?

Breast-Sparing Surgery	Your breast should look a lot like it did before surgery. But if your tumor is large, your breast may look different or smaller after breast-sparing surgery. You will have a small scar where the surgeon cut to remove the DCIS or cancer. The length of the scar will depend on how large an incision the surgeon needed to make.
Mastectomy	Your breast and nipple will be removed. You will have a flat chest on the side of your body where the breast was removed. You will have a scar over the place where your breast was removed. The length of the scar will depend on the size of your breast. If you have smaller breasts, your scar is likely to be smaller than if you have larger breasts.
Mastectomy with Reconstruction	You will have a breast-like shape, but your breast will not look or feel like it did before surgery. And, it will not look or feel like your other breast. You will have scars where the surgeon stitched skin together to make the new breast-like shape. If you have tissue flap reconstruction, you will have scars around the new breast, as well as the area where the surgeon removed the muscle, fat, and skin to make the new breast-like shape.

Will my breast have feeling?

Breast-Sparing Surgery	Yes. You should still have feeling in your breast, nipple, and areola (the dark area around your nipple).
Mastectomy	Maybe. After surgery, the skin around where the surgeon cut and maybe the area under your arm will be numb (have no feeling).
	This numb feeling may improve over 1 to 2 years, but it will never feel like it once did. Also, the skin where your breast was may feel tight.
Mastectomy with Reconstruction	No. The area around your breast will not have feeling.

Will I need more surgery?

Breast-Sparing Surgery	If the surgeon does not remove all the DCIS or cancer the first time, you may need more surgery.
Mastectomy	If you have problems after your mastectomy, you may need more surgery.
Mastectomy with Reconstruction	You will need more than one surgery to build a new breast-like shape. The number of surgeries you need will depend on the type of reconstruction you have and if you choose to have a nipple or areola added.
	Some women may also decide to have surgery on the opposite breast to help it match the new breast-like shape better.
	If you have an implant, you are likely to need surgery many years later to remove or replace it.

What are the chances that my breast cancer will return in the same area?

Breast-Sparing Surgery	There is a chance that your cancer will come back in the same breast. But if it does, it is not likely to affect how long you live. About 10% of women (1 out of every 10) who have breast-sparing surgery along with radiation therapy get cancer in the same breast within 12 years. If this happens, you can be effectively treated with a mastectomy.
Mastectomy	There is a smaller chance that your cancer will return in the same area than if you have breast-sparing surgery. About 5% of women (1 out of every 20) who have a mastectomy will get cancer on the same side of their chest within 12 years.
Mastectomy with Reconstruction	Your chances are the same as mastectomy, since breast reconstruction surgery does not affect the chances of the cancer returning.

NIH NCI (8:) https://www.cancer.gov/types/breast/surgery-choices

Department of Health NY: Breast Cancer Treatment - What You Should Know
https://www.health.ny.gov/publications/0401/#treatment_options

Breast Reconstruction
Information and pictures from *National Cancer Institute* unless otherwise specified

Quick Summary of Section

Breast Reconstruction:
- Women who choose to have their breasts rebuilt have several options for how it can be done.
- Breasts can be rebuilt using implants (saline or silicone).
- They can also be rebuilt using autologous tissue (that is, tissue from elsewhere in the body).

Factors – Timing:
- What factors can affect the timing of breast reconstruction?.

Factors – Choice:
- What factors can affect the choice of breast reconstruction method?.

Reconstruction with Implants:
- Surgery and recovery; Possible complications.

Reconstruction with Autologous Tissue:
- Surgery and recovery; Possible complications.

Breast Reconstruction	Many women who have a mastectomy—surgery to remove an entire breast to treat or prevent breast cancer—have the option of having the shape of the removed breast rebuilt. <ul><li>Women who choose to have their breasts rebuilt have several options for how it can be done. Breasts can be rebuilt using implants (saline or silicone).</li><li>They can also be rebuilt using autologous tissue (that is, tissue from elsewhere in the body).</li><li>Sometimes both implants and autologous tissue are used to rebuild the breast.</li></ul> Surgery to reconstruct the breasts can be done (or started) at the time of the mastectomy (which is called immediate reconstruction) or it can be done after the mastectomy incisions have healed and breast cancer therapy has been completed (which is called delayed reconstruction). <ul><li>Delayed reconstruction can happen months or even years after the mastectomy.</li><li>In a final stage of breast reconstruction, a nipple and areola may be re-created on the reconstructed breast, if these were not preserved during the mastectomy.</li><li>Sometimes breast reconstruction surgery includes surgery on the other, or contralateral, breast so that the two breasts will match in size and shape. *NIH NCI (9)*</li></ul>

What factors can affect the timing of breast reconstruction?	• One factor that can affect the timing of breast reconstruction is whether a woman will need radiation therapy.
	    ○ Radiation therapy can sometimes cause wound healing problems or infections in reconstructed breasts, so some women may prefer to delay reconstruction until after radiation therapy is completed. However, because of improvements in surgical and radiation techniques, immediate reconstruction with an implant is usually still an option for women who will need radiation therapy.
	    ○ Autologous tissue breast reconstruction is usually reserved for after radiation therapy, so that the breast and chest wall tissue damaged by radiation can be replaced with healthy tissue from elsewhere in the body.
	• Another factor is the type of breast cancer. Women with inflammatory breast cancer usually require more extensive skin removal. This can make immediate reconstruction more challenging, so it may be recommended that reconstruction be delayed until after completion of adjuvant therapy.
	• Even if a woman is a candidate for immediate reconstruction, she may choose delayed reconstruction. For instance, some women prefer not to consider what type of reconstruction to have until after they have recovered from their mastectomy and subsequent adjuvant treatment.
	• Women who delay reconstruction (or choose not to undergo the procedure at all) can use external breast prostheses, or breast forms, to give the appearance of breasts.
	NIH NCI (9)

What factors can affect the choice of breast reconstruction method?	Several factors can influence the type of reconstructive surgery a woman chooses. These include the size and shape of the breast that is being rebuilt, the woman's age and health, her history of past surgeries, surgical risk factors (for example, smoking history and obesity), the availability of autologous tissue, and the location of the tumor in the breast. • Women who have had past abdominal surgery may not be candidates for an abdominally based flap reconstruction. Each type of reconstruction has factors that a woman should think about before making a decision. • All women who undergo mastectomy for breast cancer experience varying degrees of breast numbness and loss of sensation (feeling) because nerves that provide sensation to the breast are cut when breast tissue is removed during surgery. ○ However, a woman may regain some sensation as the severed nerves grow and regenerate, and breast surgeons continue to make technical advances that can spare or repair damage to nerves. • Any type of breast reconstruction can fail if healing does not occur properly. In these cases, the implant or flap will have to be removed. If an implant reconstruction fails, a woman can usually have a second reconstruction using an alternative approach. *NIH NCI (9)* *Some of the more common considerations are listed below*

Reconstruction with Implants	**Surgery and recovery** • Enough skin and muscle must remain after mastectomy to cover the implants • Shorter surgical procedure than for reconstruction with autologous tissue; little blood loss • Recovery period may be shorter than with autologous reconstruction • Many follow-up visits may be needed to inflate the expander and insert the implant **Possible complications** • Infection • Accumulation of clear fluid causing a mass or lump (seroma) within the reconstructed breast • Pooling of blood (hematoma) within the reconstructed breast • Blood clots • Extrusion of the implant (the implant breaks through the skin) • Implant rupture (the implant breaks open and saline or silicone leaks into the surrounding tissue) • Formation of hard scar tissue around the implant (known as a contracture) • Obesity, diabetes, and smoking may increase the rate of complications • Possible increased risk of developing a very rare form of immune system cancer called anaplastic large cell lymphoma **Other considerations** • May not be an option for patients who have previously undergone radiation therapy to the chest • May not be adequate for women with very large breasts • Will not last a lifetime; the longer a woman has implants, the more likely she is to have complications and to need to have her implants removed or replaced • Silicone implants may feel more natural than saline implants to the touch • The Food and Drug Administration (FDA) recommends that women with silicone implants undergo periodic MRI screenings to detect possible "silent" rupture of the implants. *NIH NCI (9)* More information about implants can be found on *FDA's Breast Implants page.* *https://www.fda.gov/MedicalDevices/ProductsandMedicalProcedures/ImplantsandProsthetics/BreastImplants/default.html*

Reconstruction with Autologous Tissue	**Reconstruction with Autologous Tissue** • **Surgery and recovery** o Longer surgical procedure than for implants o The initial recovery period may be longer than for implants o Pedicled flap reconstruction is usually a shorter operation than free flap reconstruction and usually requires a shorter hospitalization o Free flap reconstruction is a longer, highly technical operation compared with pedicled flap reconstruction that requires a surgeon who has experience with microsurgery to re-attach blood vessels • **Possible complications** o Necrosis (death) of the transferred tissue o Blood clots may be more frequent with some flap sources o Pain and weakness at the site from which the donor tissue was taken o Obesity, diabetes, and smoking may increase the rate of complications • **Other considerations** o May provide a more natural breast shape than implants o May feel softer and more natural to the touch than implants o Leaves a scar at the site from which the donor tissue was taken o Can be used to replace tissue that has been damaged by radiation therapy *NIH NCI (9)*

Breast Implants
Information and pictures from *National Cancer Institute* unless otherwise specified

Quick Summary of Section

Breast Implant:

- Implants are inserted underneath the skin or chest muscle following the mastectomy.
- Breast reconstruction with an implant is often done in steps with a tissue expander.
- In some cases, the implant can be placed in the breast during the same surgery as the mastectomy. That is, a tissue expander is not used to prepare for the implant.

Tissue Expanders:

- A breast tissue expander is an inflatable breast implant designed to stretch the skin and muscle to make room for a future, more permanent implant.

Breast Implant *(Also see below)*	Implants are inserted underneath the skin or chest muscle following the mastectomy. (Most mastectomies are performed using a technique called skin-sparing mastectomy, in which much of the breast skin is saved for use in reconstructing the breast.) Implants are usually placed in two parts: <ul><li>The first step is called *tissue expansion*. This is when the plastic surgeon places a balloon expander under the chest muscle (*usually over the pectoralis minor and under the pectoralis major*). Over many weeks, saline (salt water) will be added to the expander to stretch the chest muscle and the skin on top of it by the plastic surgeon. This process makes a pocket for the implant.</li><li>After the chest tissue has relaxed and healed enough, the expander is removed and replaced with an implant (filled with saline or silicone gel). The chest tissue is usually ready for the implant 2 to 6 months after mastectomy. This creates a new breast-like shape. Although this shape looks like a breast, you will not have the same feeling in it because nerves were cut during your mastectomy.</li><li>In some cases, the implant can be placed in the breast during the same surgery as the mastectomy—that is, a tissue expander is not used to prepare for the implant.</li><li>Surgeons are increasingly using material called acellular dermal matrix as a kind of scaffold or "sling" to support tissue expanders and implants.<ul><li>Acellular dermal matrix is a kind of mesh that is made from donated human or pig skin that has been sterilized and processed to remove all cells to eliminate the risks of rejection and infection.</li></ul></li><li>Breast implants do not last a lifetime. If you choose to have an implant, chances are you will need more surgery later on to remove or replace it.</li><li>Implants can cause problems such as breast hardness, pain, and infection. The implant may also break, move, or shift. These problems can happen soon after surgery or years later.</li><li>Chemotherapy or radiation may be recommended to you by your surgical oncologist following your mastectomy. If you choose to have these treatments it will delay the tissue expansion process by approximately four to eight weeks. *John Hopkins Medicine - Tissue Expanders* *NIH NCI (9)* & *(10)*</li></ul>

Tissue Expander

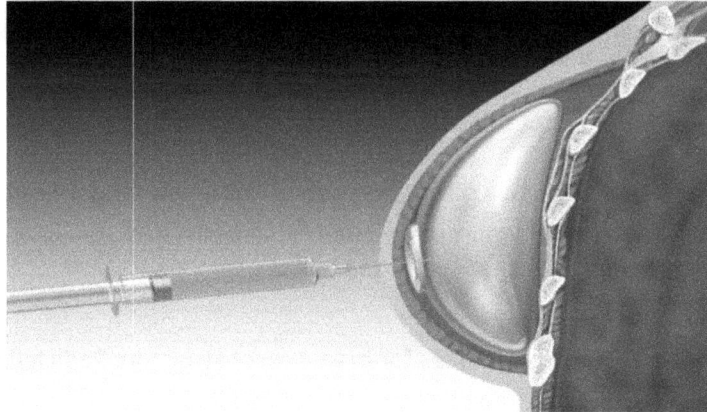

John Hopkins Medicine (YouTube Video)

Tissue Expanders	Tissue expansion involves expansion of the breast skin and muscle using a temporary tissue expander. A few months later, the expander is removed and the patient receives either microvascular flap reconstruction, or the insertion of a permanent breast implant. This type of breast reconstruction requires two separate operations. **What is a breast tissue expander?** • A breast tissue expander is an inflatable breast implant designed to stretch the skin and muscle to make room for a future, more permanent implant. • At the same time your mastectomy is done by our breast surgical oncologist, the breast plastic and reconstructive surgeon will insert a tissue expander beneath your skin and chest muscle. • Through a tiny valve mechanism located inside the expander, the nurse practitioner will periodically inject a salt-water solution to gradually fill the expander over several weeks or months. • You may feel a sensation of stretching and pressure in the breast area during this procedure, but most women find it is not too uncomfortable. • This process will usually begin three to four weeks after your mastectomy, once your drains are removed, and will continue until the size is slightly larger than your other breast. • After the skin over the breast area has stretched enough, the expander will be removed in a second operation and either flap reconstruction or a permanent implant will be inserted. • The nipple and the dark skin surrounding it, called the areola, are reconstructed in a subsequent procedure. *John Hopkins Medicine - Tissue Expanders* ***Expanders could be in for up to a year or more if chemotherapy and radiation are done after surgery. Implants are placed 3-6 weeks after chemotherapy is complete or 6 months after radiation.*** **Common Side Effects:** • Pain and Stiffness • Often numb at fill site • Difficult to lie on side • Postural changes

Tissue Flap Surgery

Information and pictures from *National Cancer Institute* unless otherwise specified

Quick Summary of Section

Tissue Flap Surgery:

- In tissue flap surgery, a reconstructive plastic surgeon builds a new breast-like shape from muscle, fat, and skin taken from other parts of your body (usually your belly, back, or buttock).

Autologous Tissue:

- Different sites in the body can provide flaps for breast reconstruction. Pedicled flap vs free flap.

Reconstruction with Autologous Tissue:

- Surgery and recovery; Possible complications

Abdomen: TRAM flap:

- Tissue comes from the lower abdomen as in a DIEP flap but includes muscle. It can be either pedicled or free.

Abdomen: DIEP flap:

- Tissue comes from the abdomen and contains only skin, blood vessels and fat, without the underlying muscle. This type of flap is a free flap.

Abdomen: SIEA flap:

- Tissue comes from the abdomen as in a DIEP flap but includes a different set of blood vessels. It also does not involve cutting of the abdominal muscle and is a free flap.

Back: Latissimus dorsi flap (LAT flap):

- Tissue comes from the middle and side of the back. This type of flap is pedicled when used for breast reconstruction.

Buttock (gluteal) flap:

- A gluteal flap is a free flap procedure that takes tissue from your buttocks and transplants it to your chest area.

Thigh flaps (TUG) and (IGAP):

- Transverse upper gracilis (TUG) flap, uses muscle and fatty tissue from the bottom of the buttocks to the inner thigh.

Nipple Reconstruction:

- After the chest heals from reconstruction surgery and the position of the breast mound on the chest wall has had time to stabilize, a surgeon can reconstruct the nipple and areola.

References

Tissue Flap Surgery *(Also see below)*	In tissue flap surgery, a reconstructive plastic surgeon builds a new breast-like shape from muscle, fat, and skin taken from other parts of your body (usually your belly, back, or buttock). • This new breast-like shape should last the rest of your life. • Women who are very thin or obese, smoke, or have serious health problems often cannot have tissue flap surgery. • Healing after tissue flap surgery often takes longer than healing after breast implant surgery. • You may have other problems, as well. For example, if you have a muscle removed, you might lose strength in the area from which it was taken. • You may get an infection or have trouble healing. • Tissue flap surgery is best done by a reconstructive plastic surgeon who has special training in this type of surgery and has done it many times before. *NIH NCI (10)*
Autologous Tissue	In autologous tissue reconstruction, a piece of tissue containing skin, fat, blood vessels, and sometimes muscle is taken from elsewhere in a woman's body and used to rebuild the breast. This piece of tissue is called a flap. • Different sites in the body can provide flaps for breast reconstruction. • Flaps used for breast reconstruction most often come from the abdomen or back. However, they can also be taken from the thigh or buttocks. Depending on their source, flaps can be pedicled or free. • With a pedicled flap, the tissue and attached blood vessels are moved together through the body to the breast area. Because the blood supply to the tissue used for reconstruction is left intact, blood vessels do not need to be reconnected once the tissue is moved. • With free flaps, the tissue is cut free from its blood supply. It must be attached to new blood vessels in the breast area, using a technique called microsurgery. This gives the reconstructed breast a blood supply. • Flaps taken from the thigh or buttocks are used for women who have had previous major abdominal surgery or who don't have enough abdominal tissue to reconstruct a breast. These types of flaps are free flaps. With these flaps an implant is often used as well to provide sufficient breast volume. • In some cases, an implant and autologous tissue are used together. For example, autologous tissue may be used to cover an implant when there isn't enough skin and muscle left after mastectomy to allow for expansion and use of an implant. *NIH NCI (10)*

Reconstruction with Autologous Tissue	• **Surgery and recovery**
	    ○ Longer surgical procedure than for implants
	    ○ The initial recovery period may be longer than for implants
	    ○ Pedicled flap reconstruction is usually a shorter operation than free flap reconstruction and usually requires a shorter hospitalization
	    ○ Free flap reconstruction is a longer, highly technical operation compared with pedicled flap reconstruction that requires a surgeon who has experience with microsurgery to re-attach blood vessels
	
	• **Possible complications**
	    ○ Necrosis (death) of the transferred tissue
	    ○ Blood clots may be more frequent with some flap sources
	    ○ Pain and weakness at the site from which the donor tissue was taken
	    ○ Obesity, diabetes, and smoking may increase the rate of complication.
	
	• **Other considerations**
	    ○ May provide a more natural breast shape than implants
	    ○ May feel softer and more natural to the touch than implants
	    ○ Leaves a scar at the site from which the donor tissue was taken
	    ○ Can be used to replace tissue that has been damaged by radiation therapy
	
	• All women who undergo mastectomy for breast cancer experience varying degrees of breast numbness and loss of sensation (feeling) because nerves that provide sensation to the breast are cut when breast tissue is removed during surgery.
	    ○ However, a woman may regain some sensation as the severed nerves grow and regenerate, and breast surgeons continue to make technical advances that can spare or repair damage to nerves.
	
	• Any type of breast reconstruction can fail if healing does not occur properly. In these cases, the implant or flap will have to be removed. If an implant reconstruction fails, a woman can usually have a second reconstruction using an alternative approach.
	NIH NCI (9)

Abdomen: TRAM flap	Tissue comes from the lower abdomen as in a DIEP flap but includes muscle. It can be either pedicled or free. *NIH NCI (9)* • Your surgeon removes tissue — including muscle — from your abdomen in a procedure known as a transverse rectus abdominis muscle (TRAM) flap. • The TRAM flap can be transferred as a free flap or a pedicled flap. • A pedicled TRAM flap uses your whole rectus muscle — one of the four major muscles in your abdomen. • For a muscle-sparing free TRAM flap, your surgeon takes only a portion of your rectus abdominis muscle, which may help you retain abdominal strength after surgery. *Mayo Clinic - Breast reconstruction with flap surgery*

Pedicled Tram Flap (top) and Free TRAM Flap (bottom) – *Pictures from Mayo Clinic*

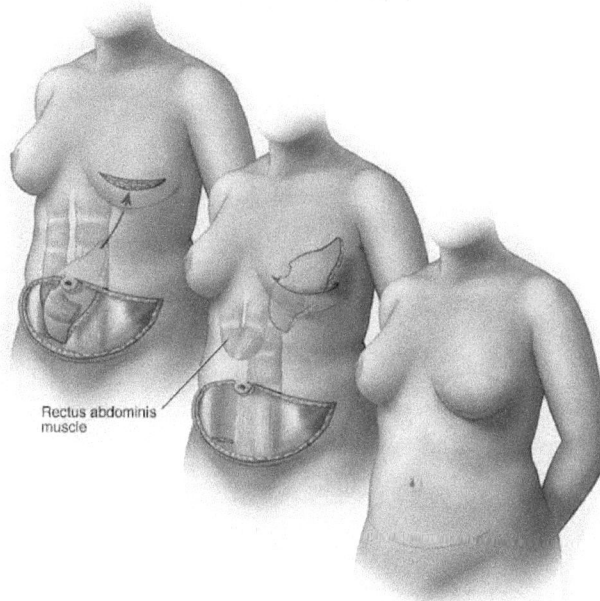

Rectus abdominis muscle

© MAYO FOUNDATION FOR MEDICAL EDUCATION AND RESEARCH. ALL RIGHTS RESERVED.

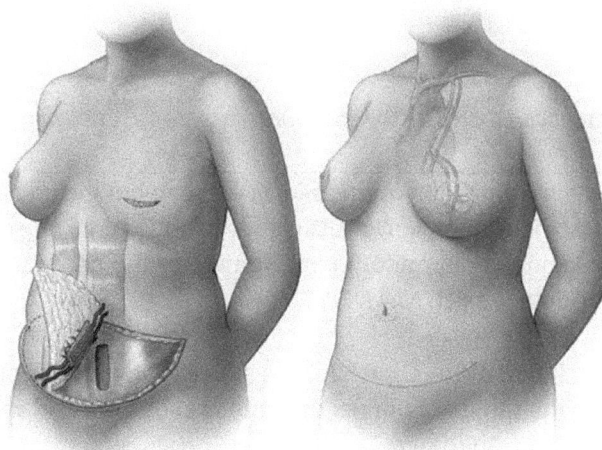

© MAYO FOUNDATION FOR MEDICAL EDUCATION AND RESEARCH. ALL RIGHTS RESERVED.

Mayo Clinic - https://www.mayoclinic.org/tests-procedures/breast-reconstruction-flap/about/pac-20384937

Abdomen: DIEP flap	Tissue comes from the abdomen and contains only skin, blood vessels, and fat, without the underlying muscle. This type of flap is a free flap. *NIH NCI (11)* • A newer procedure, deep inferior epigastric perforator (DIEP) flap, is similar to a TRAM flap, but only skin and fat are removed. • Most of the abdominal muscle is left in place and minimal muscle tissue is taken to form the new breast mound. • Reattaching blood vessels requires expertise in surgery through a microscope (microsurgery). • An advantage to this type of breast reconstruction is that you'll retain more strength in your abdomen. If your surgeon can't perform a DIEP flap procedure for anatomical reasons, he or she might opt for the TRAM procedure instead. *Mayo Clinic - Breast reconstruction with flap surgery*

DIEP flap – *Pictures from Mayo Clinic*

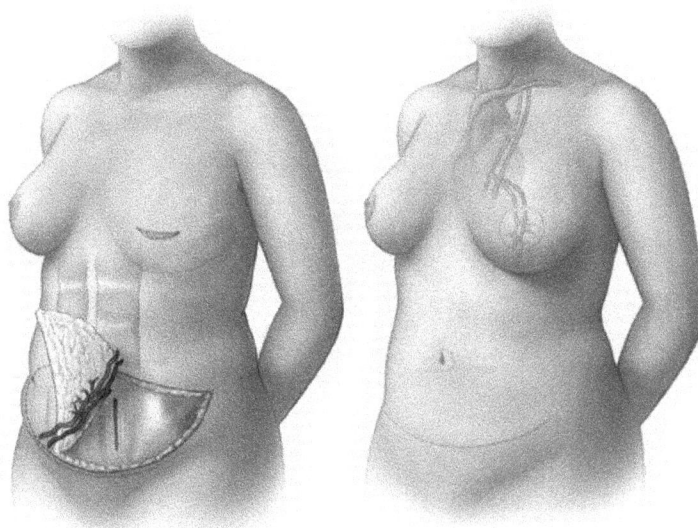

© MAYO FOUNDATION FOR MEDICAL EDUCATION AND RESEARCH. ALL RIGHTS RESERVED.

Mayo Clinic - https://www.mayoclinic.org/tests-procedures/breast-reconstruction-flap/about/pac-20384937

Abdomen: SIEA flap (also called SIEP flap)	Tissue comes from the abdomen as in a DIEP flap but includes a different set of blood vessels. It also does not involve cutting of the abdominal muscle and is a free flap. This type of flap is not an option for many women, as the necessary blood vessels are not adequate or do not exist. *NIH NCI (9)* • A variation of the DIEP flap, the superficial inferior epigastric artery (SIEA) flap uses the same abdominal tissue but relies on blood vessels that aren't as deep within the abdomen. • This provides a less invasive option, but not all women's SIEA blood vessels are adequate for this type of flap surgery. *Mayo Clinic - Breast reconstruction with flap surgery*

Back: Latissimus dorsi flap (LAT flap)	Tissue comes from the middle and side of the back. This type of flap is pedicled when used for breast reconstruction. (LD flaps can be used for other types of reconstruction as well.) *NIH NCI (9)* • This surgical technique takes skin, fat and muscle from your upper back, tunneling it under your skin to your chest. • Because the amount of skin and other tissue is generally less than in a TRAM flap surgery, this approach may be used for small and medium-sized breasts or for creating a pocket for a breast implant. • Although uncommon, some women experience muscle weakness in the back, shoulder or arm after this surgery. *Mayo Clinic - Breast reconstruction with flap surgery*

Latissimus dorsi (LD) flap

Latissimus dorsi muscle

Mayo Clinic - https://www.mayoclinic.org/tests-procedures/breast-reconstruction-flap/about/pac-20384937

Buttock (gluteal) flap	A gluteal flap is a free flap procedure that takes tissue from your buttocks and transplants it to your chest area. A gluteal flap may be an option for women who prefer tissue reconstruction but who don't have enough extra tissue in their backs or abdomens. *Mayo Clinic.org* • PAP flap: Tissue, without muscle, that comes from the upper inner thigh. • SGAP flap: Tissue comes from the buttocks as in an IGAP flap, but includes a different set of blood vessels and contains only skin, blood vessels, and fat. *NIH NCI (9)*
Thigh flaps (TUG) and (IGAP) *NIH NCI (11)*	Inner thigh (TUG). Another newer option, the transverse upper gracilis (TUG) flap, uses muscle and fatty tissue from the bottom of the buttocks to the inner thigh. TUG flap surgery, which isn't available everywhere, may be an option for women whose thighs touch and who have small to medium-sized breasts. *Mayo Clinic.org* • IGAP flap: Tissue comes from the buttocks and contains only skin, blood vessels, and fat. • TUG flap: Tissue, including muscle that comes from the upper inner thigh. *NIH NCI (9)*

Nipple Reconstruction	After the chest heals from reconstruction surgery and the position of the breast mound on the chest wall has had time to stabilize, a surgeon can reconstruct the nipple and areola. • Usually, the new nipple is created by cutting and moving small pieces of skin from the reconstructed breast to the nipple site and shaping them into a new nipple. A few months after nipple reconstruction, the surgeon can re-create the areola, usually using tattoo ink. However, in some cases, skin grafts may be taken from the groin or abdomen and attached to the breast to create an areola at the time of the nipple reconstruction. • Some women who do not have surgical nipple reconstruction may consider getting a realistic picture of a nipple created on the reconstructed breast from a tattoo artist who specializes in 3-D nipple tattooing. • A mastectomy that preserves a woman's own nipple and areola, called nipple-sparing mastectomy, may be an option for some women, depending on the size and location of the breast cancer and the shape and size of the breasts. *NIH NCI (9)*

Nipple Reconstruction

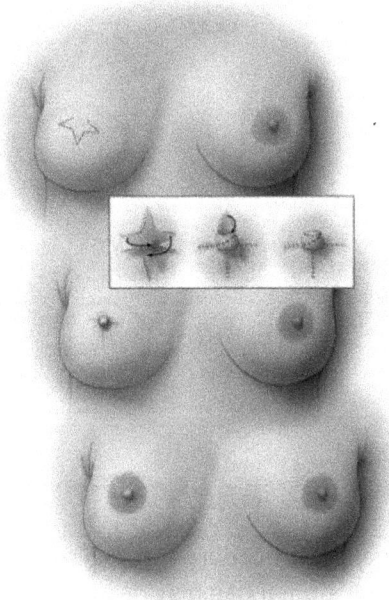

Mayo Clinic - https://www.mayoclinic.org/tests-procedures/breast-reconstruction-flap/about/pac-20384937

John Hopkins Medicine – Tissue Expander *YouTube Video https://www.youtube.com/watch?v=J9B23xnIoTw*

John Hopkins Medicine - Tissue Expanders
https://www.hopkinsmedicine.org/breast_center/treatments_services/reconstructive_breast_surgery/tissue_expanders.html

Mayo Clinic - Breast reconstruction with flap surgery - *https://www.mayoclinic.org/tests-procedures/breast-reconstruction-flap/about/pac-20384937*

NIH NCI (10) https://www.cancer.gov/types/breast/surgery-choices

NIH NCI (11) https://www.cancer.gov/types/breast/reconstruction-fact-sheet

Risks After Breast Surgery

Information and pictures from *National Cancer Institute* unless otherwise specified

Quick Summary of Section

Axillary Web Syndrome (Cording):

- Axillary Web Syndrome (AWS), also known as lymphatic cording, refers to a condition in which a rope-like soft-tissue density develops in the axilla, which may develop as a result of breast cancer treatment.

What causes AWS?

- The etiology of cording is not fully understood. The condition may be related to abnormalities in either the axillary vasculature or the lymphatics.

Who is at Risk for AWS?

- The incidence of cording after axillary lymph node dissection (ALND) has been reported as high as 72%, compared to 20% after sentinel lymph node biopsy (SLNB).

AWS: Pink Ribbon Program®

- Axillary web syndrome is a self-limiting and frequently overlooked cause of significant morbidity in the early post-operative period after breast cancer axillary surgery.

Managing AWS by Breastcancer.org (*Axillary Web Syndrome (Cording*):

- If you have symptoms of AWS, ask your doctor to refer you to a physical therapist or other medical professional (such as a nurse or physician) who specializes in breast cancer rehabilitation.

Scar Tissue / Adhesions / Myofascial Release:

- Breast and axillary surgery, and radiotherapy in breast cancer patients cause scar tissue formation, fibrosis and adhesions at all levels of soft tissues of the upper body.
- Postural restoration through myofascial release (medical massage) is needed by most people, but especially those having significant scarring on the front of the body.

Seroma / Compression:

- A serous fluid collection that develops under the skin flaps during mastectomy or in the axillary dead space.

Resources

	CORDING OR AXILLARY WEB SYNDROME (AWS)
Axillary Web Syndrome (Cording)	Axillary Web Syndrome (AWS), also known as lymphatic cording, refers to a condition in which a rope-like soft-tissue density develops in the axilla, which may develop as a result of breast cancer treatment. It usually appears in the 5 to 8 week period following breast cancer surgery and can lead to shoulder pain and restricted motion. *NCBI: PMC: Atypical presentation of axillary web syndrome* Cords are palpable bands of tissue which can occur in the axilla, across the antecubital fossa into the forearm and wrist, and in the breast or abdominal wall. The incidence of cording following breast cancer treatment ranges from 6 – 72%, and the condition can cause pain and limited range of motion in the upper extremity. *NCBI: PMC: Cording Following Treatment for Breast Cancer* **When does it happen:** • Typically, 3-4 weeks post – op. • Less often 2-4 weeks • Less often over 4 weeks *Klose: Breast Cancer Rehabilitation* ***Mondor disease*** is a rare condition that is characterized by scarring and inflammation of the veins located just beneath the skin of the chest. The affected veins are initially red and tender and subsequently become a painless, tough, fibrous band that is accompanied by tension and retraction of the nearby skin. • In most cases, the condition is benign and resolves on its own; however, Mondor disease can rarely be associated with breast cancer. Although the condition most commonly affects the chest, Mondor disease of other body parts (including the penis, groin, and abdomen) has been described, as well. • Mondor disease is thought to occur when pressure or trauma on the veins causes blood to stagnate. In most cases, the condition arises after recent breast surgery, but it can also be associated with physical strain and/or tight-fitting clothing (i.e. bras). • Treatments are available to help relieve symptoms until the condition resolves. *NIH: NCATS: Mondor Disease*
What causes AWS	The etiology of cording is not fully understood. The condition may be related to abnormalities in either the axillary vasculature or the lymphatics. • Anatomic studies of resected cords reveal that these structures may represent dilated and thrombosed lymphatics and/or thrombosed superficial veins. • The condition is considered to be a variation of (Mondor's disease (*See below*), a rare thrombophlebitis of the subcutaneous veins caused by trauma such as surgery. *NCBI: PMC: Cording Following Treatment for Breast Cancer* • AWS: may be attributed to lymph venous injury during axillary lymph node dissection due to either tissue retraction and/or patient positioning. • Another theory is that because of the interruption in axillary flow, lymphatic vessels are dilating and scalloping to the skin. *Summit Education: Oncology Rehab Dec 12, 2019*

Who is at Risk?	The incidence of cording after axillary lymph node dissection (ALND) has been reported as high as 72%, compared to 20% after sentinel lymph node biopsy (SLNB). • Younger age, lower BMI, and being African-American have also been implicated as potential risk factors. • While cording has been reported to cause limited range of motion, the extent to which this translates into dysfunction performing daily functional reaching activities has yet to be reported. • Little data exists on whether cording is associated with an increased risk of developing upper extremity lymphedema. *NCBI: PMC: Cording Following Treatment for Breast Cancer* **Body habitus:** • Pt's that have AWS were found to be more often of lower weight with a BMI between 23-25. • Pt's that were obese with a BMI between 26-28.9, unlike with lymphedema, tend to have a lower incidence of cording. *Klose: Breast Cancer Rehabilitation.*
Axillary Web Syndrome by *Pink Ribbon Program*®	Axillary web syndrome is a self-limiting and frequently overlooked cause of significant morbidity in the early post-operative period after breast cancer axillary surgery, which is characterized by axillary pain that runs down the medial arm, limited shoulder range of motion affecting mainly shoulder abduction, and cords of subcutaneous tissue extending from axilla into the medial arm, made visible or palpable and painful by shoulder abduction. • In addition, soft tissue may give a cordlike appearance due to increased tension between the skin of the upper arm and adherence of an axillary scar to underlying fascia. • Lymphatic cording is associated with pain and limitation of shoulder movement, and it is common to find shoulder abduction restricted to less than 90°. • Exercise Interventions should typically include supine exercises involving assisted shoulder flexion, active abduction, horizontal abduction, and a trunk rotational stretch with shoulder abduction, stretching exercises for levator scapulae, upper trapezius, pectoralis major, and medial and lateral rotators muscles of the shoulder. *Pink Ribbon Program*®

Managing AWS
 	
by
Breastcancer.org:
Axillary Web
Syndrome
(Cording)
	If you have symptoms of AWS, ask your doctor to refer you to a physical therapist or other medical professional (such as a nurse or physician) *who specializes in breast cancer rehabilitation.* It's not a good idea to wait and see if the condition will resolve on its own. Your natural reaction to the pain of cording will be to avoid moving the arm and shoulder, which can lead to more tightness in the shoulder and chest area. Over time, this may cause more serious problems with function and mobility. Moving and stretching under the guidance of an experienced therapist are the best ways to resolve the condition and stop the pain.
	Together, you and your therapist can develop a treatment plan that's right for you. Your plan may include:
	
	• **Stretching and flexibility exercises:** Your therapist can work with you to help you learn exercises that gently stretch the cords and improve your pain-free range of motion. He or she can teach you exercises to do at home and advise you on how often to do them.
	
	• **Manual therapy:** Your therapist also may gently massage the cord tissue. Using manual therapy, your therapist would gently pull the tissue on your outstretched arm, starting in the upper arm and moving down into the forearm. This sometimes causes the cord to snap or break, and you may even hear a popping sound when that happens. It's usually not painful, and it often brings relief by extending your arm's pain-free range of motion.
	
	• **Moist heat:** Your therapist may apply warm, moist pads directly to the cords as part of therapy. However, it's important that he or she use caution when doing this. Prolonged heat can increase the production of lymph, which can lead to the fluid overload known as lymphedema. If your therapist recommends moist heat, just be sure he or she is experienced in its use for cording.
	
	• **Pain medication:** You may need to take some form of pain medication, such as an NSAID (non-steroidal anti-inflammatory drug, such as Motrin or aspirin), if you experience pain that prevents you from stretching the arm. But remember that the best treatment for the pain is doing the stretching exercises that help the condition get better.
	
	• **Low-level laser therapy:** Some therapists use a small, hand-held device to apply low- level laser beams directly to the skin. Laser therapy can help break down the hardened scar tissue.
	
	• With the exception of pain medication, all of these treatments focus on releasing the tight scar tissue that makes up the cord(s).
	  ○ You may notice that releasing the cord in certain parts of the arm can magnify the tightness in other areas — not because the cording is getting worse, but because the scar tissue is still "stuck" in those other areas. For example, releasing the cord in the upper arm and elbow will reduce pain and improve range of motion, but the wrist and forearm may feel tighter at first.
	  ○ "I describe the cord to my patients as being like a fishing line that is stuck in several places along the fishing rod," says Nicole Stout, MPT, CLT-LANA, physical therapist and lymphedema specialist, the Breast Care Center, National Naval Medical Center. "You can release a few of the stuck spots, but it then magnifies the tightness in the other areas that are still stuck."
	
	Fortunately, cording usually resolves for most people after a few therapy sessions, or at least within a few months.
	
	• It's possible to have limited range of motion for many months or even longer, but that's not typical. For some people, cording may get better and then come back later, but usually cording is a one-time event that doesn't become a persistent problem.
	
	• Experts still aren't exactly sure what happens to the cords after they break down. Some experts believe that they simply get reabsorbed by the body, but other experts say that we simply don't yet know what happens to the cords.
	Breastcancer.org Axillary Web Syndrome (Cording)

SCAR TISSUE / ADHESIONS / MYOFASCIAL RELEASE

Scar Tissue / Adhesions	An adhesion is a band of scar tissue that binds 2 parts of your tissue that are not normally joined together. Adhesions may appear as thin sheets of tissue similar to plastic wrap or as thick fibrous bands. The tissue develops when the body's repair mechanisms respond to any tissue disturbance, such as surgery, infection, trauma, or radiation. *Web MD: Adhesions, General and After Surgery* Breast and axillary surgery, and radiotherapy in breast cancer patients cause scar tissue formation, fibrosis and adhesions at all levels of soft tissues of the upper body. • The occurrence or persistence of upper limb impairments after breast cancer treatment can partially be explained by the presence of myofascial dysfunctions (*fascia surrounding and separating muscle tissue*). • Myofascial dysfunctions are expressed as myofascial trigger points and adhesions or restrictions of the myofascial tissues. • The latter are impairments of gliding of the myofascial tissues relative to each other. • Muscle manipulation during surgery, scar tissue formation, soft tissue adhesions and adaptive postures following surgery or fibrosis from radiotherapy can cause myofascial adhesions. *NCBI: An evaluation tool for Myofascial Adhesions* **According to *Klose (K) and BreastCancer.org (B)*, tissue adhesion can cause:** • Pain *(K)* • Postural changes *(K)* • Impaired shoulder function *(K)* • Movement compensations *(K)* • Nerve pain or numbness if scar tissue forms around nerves. *(B)* • A lump of scar tissue forms in the hole left after breast tissue is removed. If scar tissue forms around a stitch from surgery it's called a suture granuloma and also feels like a lump. *(B)* • Changes in breast appearance. Scar tissue and fluid retention can make breast tissue appear a little firmer or rounder than before surgery and/or radiation. *(B)* *Klose: Breast Cancer Rehabilitation (K)* and *BreastCancer.org: Scar Tissue Formation (B)*
Myofascial Release	Postural restoration through myofascial release (medical massage) is needed by most people, but especially those having significant scarring on the front of the body. • These scars draw the shoulders forward causing the head and neck to also pull forward. This leads to neck and shoulder aches and pains. • The body is meant to be in alignment. When we live and move in non-optimal alignment, serious orthopedic injuries can occur. • Most commonly, I have seen breast cancer survivors develop neck and shoulder impingement. Neck and shoulder impingement can cause shooting pain down the arm and lead to another surgery. Impingement syndromes start with achiness in the neck and shoulders. • Myofascial release is a type of medical massage that is NOT painful. Focus is placed on gently releasing tension along thickenings of fascia and scar tissue. Releasing this tension restores posture and alignment. It also relieves knots and painful areas in all parts of the body. *Breast Cancer Resource Center: Benefits of Myofascial Release Therapy after Mastectomy & Lumpectomy*

	SEROMA / COMPRESSION
Seroma	A serous fluid collection that develops under the skin flaps during mastectomy or in the axillary dead space after axillary dissection. • Incidence of seroma formation after breast surgery varies between 2.5% and 51% . • Although seroma is not life threatening, it can lead to significant morbidity: ○ Flap necrosis ○ Wound dehiscence ○ Predisposes to sepsis ○ Prolonged recovery period ○ Multiple physician visits ○ May delay adjuvant therapy. • Fluid collection is ideally managed by repeated needle aspiration to seal the skin flaps against the chest wall. • Several factors have been investigated as the cause of seroma formation these include ○ Duration of wound drainage ○ Use of pressure garment ○ Postoperative arm activity ○ Preoperative chemotherapy ○ Use of electrocautery *NCBI: Seroma formation after surgery for breast cancer*
Compression	Acute Management with Compression: • Compression with pads and elastic garments • Apply immediate compression after aspiration, when possible Seroma Management Body Shapers: • Avoid shelf bras • Look for wide straps and good trunk coverage • Breast cup vs. flat fabric design (depending on surgery) • Ensure coverage into the axilla • Nighttime use if large breasted: daytime use if supportive enough to be used as a bra • If currently on radiation, consult radiation oncologist *Klose: Breast Cancer Rehabilitation*

Breast Cancer Resource Center: Benefits of Myofascial Release Therapy after Mastectomy & Lumpectomy
https://bcrc.org/benefits-myofascial-release-therapy-mastectomy-lumpectomy/

Breastcancer.org Axillary Web Syndrome (Cording) https://www.breastcancer.org/treatment/side_effects/aws

BreastCancer.org: Scar Tissue Formation *https://www.breastcancer.org/treatment/side_effects/scar_tissue*

Klose: Breast Cancer Rehabilitation

NCBI: Seroma formation after surgery for breast cancer *https://www.ncbi.nlm.nih.gov/pmc/articles/PMC543447/*

NCBI: An evaluation tool for Myofascial Adhesions in Patients after Breast Cancer
*https://www.ncbi.nlm.nih.gov/pmc/articles/PMC5844553/#:~:text=Breast%20and%20axillary%20surgery%20and,
level%20and%20deeper%20myofascial%20structures.*

NCBI: PMC: Atypical presentation of axillary web syndrome (AWS)
https://www.ncbi.nlm.nih.gov/pmc/articles/PMC5178020/

NCBI: PMC: Cording Following Treatment for Breast Cancer
https://www.ncbi.nlm.nih.gov/pmc/articles/PMC3786257/

NIH: NCATS: Mondor Disease: https://rarediseases.info.nih.gov/diseases/7054/mondor-disease

Pink Ribbon Program®

Summit Education: Oncology Rehab Dec 12, 2019

Web MD: Adhesions, General and After *Surgery https://www.webmd.com/a-to-z-guides/adhesion-general-post-surgery#1*

SENTINEL AND AXILLARY LYMPH NODES / DISSECTION

Information and pictures from *National Cancer Institute* unless otherwise specified

Quick Summary of Section

Sentinel Lymph Node:

- A sentinel lymph node is defined as the first lymph node to which cancer cells are most likely to spread from a primary tumor.

Sentinel Lymph Node (SLNB):

- A sentinel lymph node biopsy (SLNB) is a procedure in which the sentinel lymph node is identified, removed, and examined to biopsy determine whether cancer cells are present.

Surgery:

- The surgeon injects a dye, a radioactive tracer, or both into the breast near the tumor. This helps the surgeon see which lymph nodes the lymph from that area of the breast flows to first.

SLNB and Breast Cancer:

- Breast cancer cells are most likely to spread first to lymph nodes located in the axilla, or armpit area, next to the affected breast.

Benefits of SLNB:

- SNLB helps doctors stage cancers and estimate the risk that tumor cells have developed the ability to spread to other parts of the body.

Risks of SLNB:

- All surgery to remove lymph nodes, including SLNB, can have harmful side effects, although removal of fewer lymph nodes is usually associated with fewer side effects, particularly serious ones such as lymphedema.

Axillary Lymph Nodes Dissection (ALND):

- The axillary lymph nodes or armpit lymph nodes are lymph nodes in the human armpit.

Risks of ALND:

- Anywhere from about 10 to 40 (though usually less than 20) lymph nodes are removed from the area under the arm (axilla)and checked for cancer spread.

3 Levels of ALND:

- Least aggressive to most aggressive.

Nerves that may be Damaged during Surgery:

- Several structures, including vessels and muscles with their nerve supply, are related to the breast and should be preserved during mastectomy or axillary node dissection.

Sentinel Lymph Node	A sentinel lymph node is defined as the first lymph node to which cancer cells are most likely to spread from a primary tumor. Sometimes, there can be more than one sentinel lymph node. ● Lymph nodes are small round organs that are part of the body's lymphatic system. The lymphatic system is a part of the immune system. It consists of a network of vessels and organs that contains lymph, a clear fluid that carries infection-fighting white blood cells as well as fluid and waste products from the body's cells and tissues. ● In a person with cancer, lymph can also carry cancer cells that have broken off from the main tumor. *NIH NCI (13)*

Sentinel lymph Node Biopsy (SLNB)

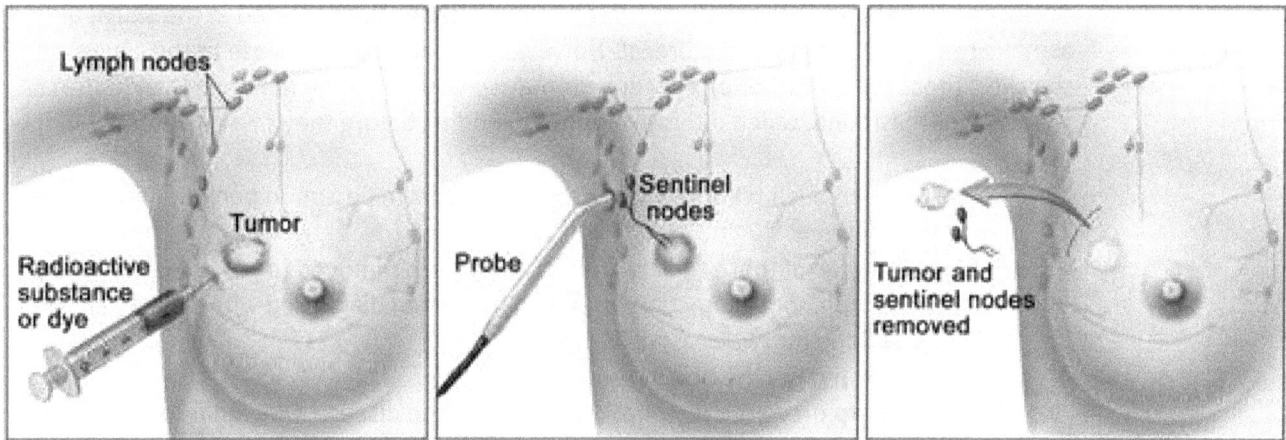

NIH NCI (13) https://www.cancer.gov/about-cancer/diagnosis-staging/staging/sentinel-node-biopsy-fact-sheet

Sentinel Lymph Node Biopsy (SLNB)	A sentinel lymph node biopsy (SLNB) is a procedure in which the sentinel lymph node is identified, removed, and examined to determine whether cancer cells are present. ● It is used in people who have already been diagnosed with cancer. ● A negative SLNB result suggests that cancer has not yet spread to nearby lymph nodes or other organs. ● A positive SLNB result indicates that cancer is present in the sentinel lymph node and that it may have spread to other nearby lymph nodes (called regional lymph nodes) and, possibly, other organs. ○ This information can help a doctor determine the stage of the cancer (extent of the disease within the body) and develop an appropriate treatment plan. *NIH NCI (13)*

Surgery	• First, the surgeon injects a dye, a radioactive tracer, or both into the breast near the tumor. This helps the surgeon see which lymph nodes the lymph from that area of the breast flows to first.
	• Then, he or she removes the node or nodes that contain the dye or radioactive tracer to see if they have cancer.
	   ○ If they do not contain cancer, it is not likely that the other nodes under the arm have cancer. This means that the surgeon usually doesn't have to remove any other lymph nodes.
	   ○ If cancer is found, the surgeon may remove additional lymph nodes, either during the same biopsy procedure or during a follow-up surgical procedure. SLNB may be done on an outpatient basis or may require a short stay in the hospital. *NIH NCI (13)*
	• Fewer lymph nodes are removed with sentinel lymph node biopsy than with standard lymph node surgery.
	• Having fewer lymph nodes removed helps lower the chances that you will develop lymphedema and other problems caused by damage to lymph vessels and lymph nodes.
	NIH NCI (11)

SLNB and Breast Cancer	Breast cancer cells are most likely to spread first to lymph nodes located in the axilla, or armpit area, next to the affected breast. However, in breast cancers close to the center of the chest (near the breastbone), cancer cells may spread first to lymph nodes inside the chest (under the breastbone, called internal mammary nodes) before they can be detected in the axilla.
	• The number of lymph nodes in the axilla varies from person to person; the usual range is between 20 and 40.
	• Historically, all of these axillary lymph nodes were removed (in an operation called axillary lymph node dissection, or ALND) in women diagnosed with breast cancer. This was done for two reasons:
	   ○ Help stage the breast cancer
	   ○ Help prevent a regional recurrence of the disease. (Regional recurrence of breast cancer occurs when breast cancer cells that have migrated to nearby lymph nodes give rise to a new tumor.)
	• However, because removing multiple lymph nodes at the same time increases the risk of harmful side effects, clinical trials were launched to investigate whether just the sentinel lymph nodes could be removed. Two NCI-sponsored randomized phase 3 clinical trials have shown that SLNB without ALND is sufficient for staging breast cancer and for preventing regional recurrence in women who have no clinical signs of axillary lymph node metastasis, such as a lump or swelling in the armpit that may cause discomfort, and who are treated with surgery, adjuvant systemic therapy, and radiation therapy.
	NIH NCI (13)

Benefits of SLNB	SNLB helps doctors stage cancers and estimate the risk that tumor cells have developed the ability to spread to other parts of the body. • If the sentinel node is negative for cancer, a patient may be able to avoid more extensive lymph node surgery, reducing the potential complications associated with having many lymph nodes removed. *NIH NCI (13)*

Risks of SLNB	All surgery to remove lymph nodes, including SLNB, can have harmful side effects, although removal of fewer lymph nodes is usually associated with fewer side effects, particularly serious ones such as lymphedema.
	The potential side effects include:
	
	• Lymphedema *(see lymphedema)*. During lymph node surgery, lymph vessels leading to and from the sentinel node or group of nodes are cut. This disrupts the normal flow of lymph through the affected area, which may lead to an abnormal buildup of lymph fluid that can cause swelling.
	   ○ The risk of lymphedema increases with the number of lymph nodes removed. There is less risk with the removal of only the sentinel lymph node.
	   ○ In the case of extensive lymph node removal in an armpit or groin, the swelling may affect an entire arm or leg.
	   ○ In addition, there is an increased risk of infection in the affected area or limb.
	   ○ Very rarely, chronic lymphedema due to extensive lymph node removal may cause a cancer of the lymphatic vessels called lymphangiosarcoma.
	• Seroma - a mass/ lump caused by the buildup of lymph fluid at the site of the surgery
	• Numbness, tingling, swelling, bruising, or pain at the site of the surgery, and an increased risk of infection
	• Difficulty moving the affected body part
	• Skin or allergic reactions to the blue dye used in SNLB
	• A false-negative biopsy result—that is, cancer cells are not seen in the sentinel lymph node even though they have already spread to regional lymph nodes or other parts of the body. A false-negative biopsy result gives the patient and the doctor a false sense of security about the extent of cancer in the patient's body.
	NIH NCI (13)

Axillary Lymph Nodes	The axillary lymph nodes or armpit lymph nodes are lymph nodes in the human armpit. • Between 20 and 49 in number. • They drain lymph vessels from the lateral quadrants of the breast, the superficial lymph vessels from thin walls of the chest and the abdomen above the level of the navel, and the vessels from the upper limb. • They are divided in several groups according to their location in the armpit. These lymph nodes are clinically significant in breast cancer, and metastases from the breast to the axillary lymph nodes are considered in the staging of the disease. • About 75% of lymph from the breasts drains into the axillary lymph nodes, making them important in the diagnosis and staging of breast cancer. • A doctor will usually refer a patient to a surgeon to have an axillary lymph node dissection to see if the cancer cells have been trapped in the nodes. • For clinical stages I and II breast cancer, axillary lymph node dissection should only be performed after first attempting sentinel node biopsy. *Wikipedia – Axillary Lymph Nodes*

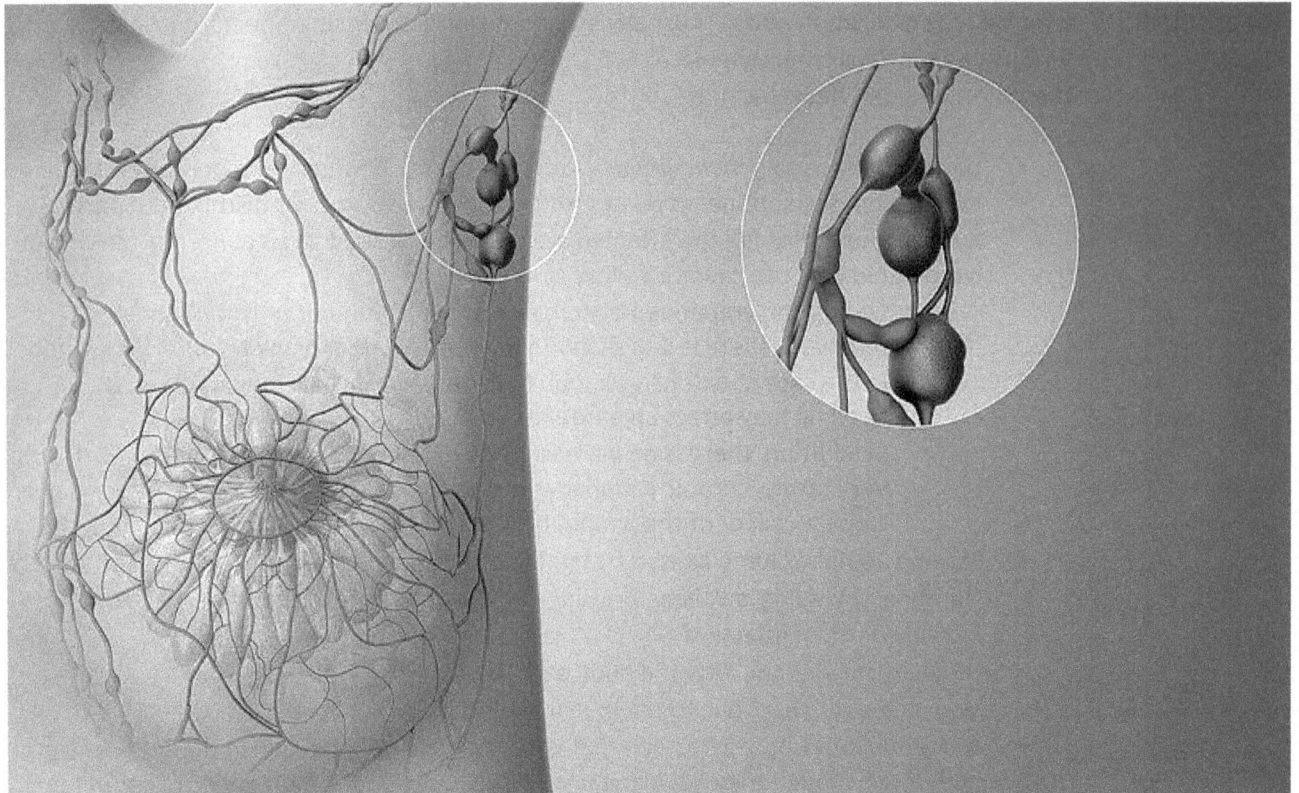

Wikipedia – Axillary Lymph Nodes www.scientificanimations.com

Risks of Axillary Node Dissection	Anywhere from about 10 to 40 (though usually less than 20) lymph nodes are removed from the area under the arm (axilla) and checked for cancer spread.
	
	• ALND is usually done at the same time as a mastectomy or breast-conserving surgery (BCS), but it can be done in a second operation. ALND may be needed:
	   ○ If a previous SLNB has shown 3 or more of the underarm lymph nodes have cancer cells
	   ○ If swollen underarm or collarbone lymph nodes can be felt before surgery or seen on imaging tests and a FNA or core needle biopsy shows cancer
	   ○ If the cancer has grown large enough to extend outside the lymph node(s)
	   ○ If the SLNB is positive for cancer cells after chemotherapy was given to shrink the tumor before surgery. *American Cancer Society*
	
	• Compared with axillary sampling alone, partial or total mastectomy followed by full axillary lymph node dissection significantly increases a patient's chance of developing arm edema.
	
	• In one series of 100 women who underwent partial or total mastectomy and then full axillary lymph node dissection or axillary sampling, arm edema developed in more patients who underwent axillary lymph node dissection compared with sampling alone (30% vs. none). In addition, the extent of axillary lymph node dissection increases the risk for developing arm edema.

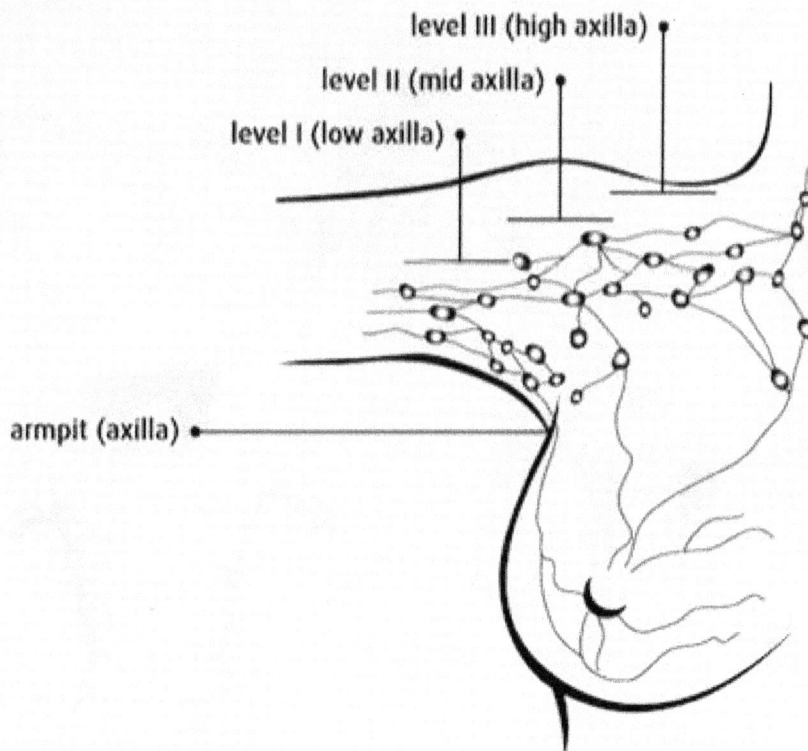

3 Levels of ALND	The three levels of an axillary lymph node dissection, from least aggressive to most aggressive, are: • Level I- The surgical removal of all tissue below the lower edge of the pectoralis minor muscle. • Level II- The surgical removal of the tissue lying underneath the pectoralis minor muscle. • Level III - The most aggressive dissection, and is the surgical removal of tissue lying above the pectoralis minor muscle. A traditional axillary lymph node dissection usually includes removal of the nodes in levels I and II from the "fat pad" under the arm. *UPMC- Axillary Lymph Node Dissection* Surgical Margin for Fat Pad: • Axillary vein – Superior • Thoracodorsal bundle – Lateral • Long thoracic nerve – Medial **Axillary Lymph Nodes** level III (high axilla) level II (mid axilla) level I (low axilla) armpit (axilla) *Wiki McMaster: Breast Cancer*

Nerves that may be Damaged during Surgery *Pink Ribbon Program©*	Several structures, including vessels and muscles with their nerve supply, are related to the breast and should be preserved during mastectomy or axillary node dissection. • The **lateral pectoral nerve** passes medially around the medial pectoralis minor, and the medial pectoral nerve passes laterally around the pectoralis minor. These nerves can be severed during surgery. This results in ***numbness, motor atrophy, decreased sweat production in armpit and arm.*** • The **medial pectoral nerve** innervates pectoralis minor and the lateral portion of the pectoralis major muscles. Preservation of this nerve is particularly important to prevent ***atrophy of the pectoral muscles*** if submuscular implant reconstruction is planned. • The **thoracodorsal nerve** is identifiable medial to the thoracodorsal vein. Injury may result in a ***weakening of the latissimus.*** • The **long thoracic nerve** of Bell is located more medially in the axilla. It runs just beneath the fascia of the serratus anterior, medial to the thoracodorsal complex. Injury to this nerve will result in weakness in the serratus anterior muscle and cause ***winging of the scapula.*** *Pink Ribbon Program©*

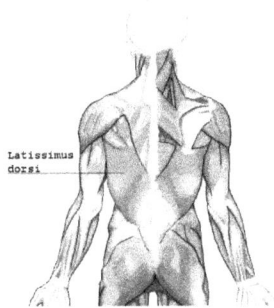

Latissimus dorsi

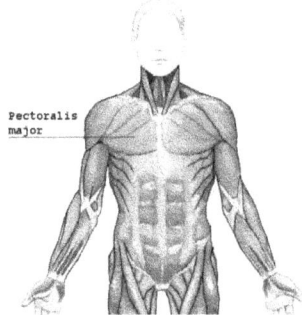

Pec Major

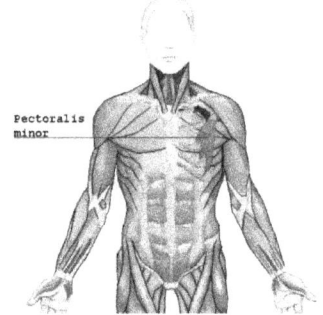

Pec Minor

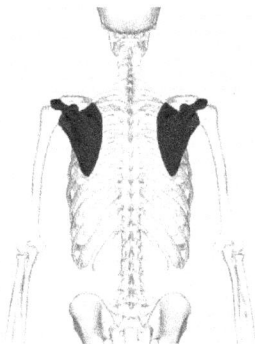

Scapular – normal

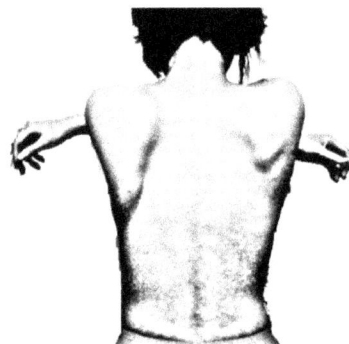

Scapular – winging

Breast Surgery Exercise & Contraindications / Precautions
Information and pictures from *National Cancer Institute* unless otherwise specified

Quick Summary this Section

Exercise Contraindications / Precautions After Breast Surgery
- TRAM Flap Reconstruction
- Latissimus Dorsi Flap Reconstruction
- DIEP Flap Reconstruction
- Tissue Expander
- Lymphedema and Exercise
- Axillary node dissection
- Peripheral Neuropathy
- Nerves that may be Damaged during Surgery

Things to Avoid, Post Op Healing & Mastectomy:
- Avoid 2 - weeks Post op
- Post op healing concerns
- Recommendations post mastectomy

Exercise Examples - Post Mastectomy:
- Examples of Exercises
- Stretches or Edema Control after Mastectomy

Home Exercise Guide Breast and / or Lymphedema:
- Home Exercise Guide For Post Surgery and / or Lymphedema

References

EXERCISE CONTRAINDICATIONS / PRECAUTIONS AFTER BREAST SURGERY

TRAM Flap Reconstruction	TRAM stands for the transverse rectus abdominis muscle, which is located in the lower abdomen, between the waist and the pubic bone. A TRAM flap uses a part of this muscle, its blood vessels, and some belly fat to rebuild the breast. • After TRAM flap surgery, you can start walking the next day, though it will probably hurt because of the incision in your abdomen. • For the first two days, many physical therapists recommend women do calf exercises and deep breathing exercises to help prevent blood clots. • You can start arm rehabilitation exercises 3 or 4 days after surgery. • Once the drains are removed, you can start stretching your chest, shoulders, and arms. It's also a good idea to walk regularly as you recover. • Don't do any abdominal ("abs") exercises until about 6 weeks after surgery or whenever your surgeon says it's OK to start. Start slowly and gently while continuing your stretching exercises and walking or other low-intensity aerobic exercise. • Those with a unilateral TRAM Flap may need minor assistance in lowering themselves back onto the floor. • Bi-lateral Tram Flap, will not be able to roll backwards or subsequently roll back to an upright position without assistance. *BreastCancer.org* and *CETI (Pilates)*
Latissimus Dorsi Flap Reconstruction	The latissimus dorsi is the muscle below the shoulder and behind the armpit. A latissimus dorsi flap uses an oval section of this muscle, skin, and fat to rebuild the breast. • Because this type of reconstruction affects the shoulder muscle, you should wait to start any gentle shoulder stretching until about 2 weeks after surgery. • Wait until about 3 months after surgery to do any resistance/strength exercises. • If you have any shortness of breath, pain, or tightness in your chest, stop exercising immediately. Tell your doctor what happened and work with him or her to develop a plan of movements that are right for you. • LAT Flap - may have noticeable weakness and instability in the affected shoulder(s). • Retract the shoulders prior to initiating the movement. This will help to contract the rhomboids and other scapular stabilizers. • Keep in mind that if you had a LAT Flap that one, or both, of the latissimus muscles are now in their chest wall. Because they are still "attached," they may feel a contraction in their chest when back exercises are performed. *BreastCancer.org* and *CETI (Pilates)*
DIEP Flap Reconstruction	DIEP stands for deep inferior epigastric perforator. In a DIEP flap, fat, skin, and blood vessels, but no muscles, are cut from the wall of the lower belly and moved up to your chest to rebuild your breast. • After DIEP flap surgery, you can start walking the next day, though it will probably hurt because of the incision in your abdomen. • For the first 2 days, many physical therapists recommend women do calf exercises and deep breathing exercises to help prevent blood clots. • You can start arm rehabilitation exercises 3 or 4 days after surgery. • Once the drains are removed, you can start stretching your chest, shoulders, and arms. It's also a good idea to walk regularly as you recover. • Don't do any abdominal ("abs") exercises until about 6 weeks after surgery or whenever your surgeon says it's OK to start. *BreastCancer.org*

Tissue Expander	If you have a tissue expander in (a temporary inflatable implant that stretches the skin to make room for the final implant), you can usually start gentle shoulder stretching exercises about 2 weeks after surgery once your mastectomy scar has started to heal. • Many physical therapists recommend doing these stretches right after a warm shower because the muscles and skin are more flexible. • If you have expanders or breast implants, you will want to begin with limited ROM. It is rare, but possible, that the implants will move out of their "pocket," and need surgical correction. • *No chest exercises when tissue expanders are in place.* *BreastCancer.org* and *CETI (Pilates)*

Lymphedema and Exercise
 	
 If you have lymphedema or are at risk, talk with a certified lymphedema therapist before beginning exercise.
 	
 This includes anyone who has had lymph nodes removed or radiation.
 	
 Increasing resistance too quickly can exacerbate condition.
 	
 (See lymphedema section)
	Both light exercise and aerobic exercise (physical activity that causes the heart and lungs to work harder) help the lymph vessels move lymph out of the affected limb and decrease swelling.
	 • **If you have lymphedema or are at risk, talk with a certified lymphedema therapist before beginning exercise. This includes *anyone* who has had lymph nodes removed or radiation.**
	   o Patients who have lymphedema or who are at risk for lymphedema should talk with a certified lymphedema therapist before beginning an exercise routine. Adding resistance
	     ▪ *(See the Lymphology Association of North America (https://www.clt-lana.org/) web site for a list of certified lymphedema therapists in the US)*
	 • Wear a pressure garment if lymphedema has developed.
	   o Patients who have lymphedema should wear a well-fitting pressure garment during all exercise that uses the affected limb or body part.
	   o When it is not known for sure if a woman has lymphedema, upper-body exercise without a garment may be more helpful than no exercise at all.
	   o Patients who do not have lymphedema do not need to wear a pressure garment during exercise.
	 • Avoid wrapping a band around your hand when using for resistance. This will put you at risk for increased edema by cutting off the circulation. Hold the band or use a band that has handles.
	 • Breast cancer survivors should begin with light upper-body exercise and increase it slowly.
	   o Some studies with breast cancer survivors show that upper-body exercise is safe in women who have lymphedema or who are at risk for lymphedema.
	   o Weight-lifting that is slowly increased may keep lymphedema from getting worse.
	   o Exercise should start at a very low level, increase slowly over time, and *be overseen by the lymphedema therapist*.
	   o If exercise is stopped for a week or longer, it should be started again at a low level and increased slowly.
	   o If symptoms (such as swelling or heaviness in the limb) change or increase for a week or longer, talk with the lymphedema therapist.
	   o It is likely that exercising at a low level and slowly increasing it again over time is better for the affected limb than stopping the exercise completely.
	 • More studies are needed to find out if weight-lifting is safe for cancer survivors with lymphedema in the legs. *NIH NCI (12)*

Axillary Node Dissection	<ul><li>If you have undergone an axillary node dissection, or radiation/dissection to the nodes in the neck, you may struggle with scar tissue/adhesions in that area.</li><li>Gently ease into the stretch and only go as far as you can, with mild discomfort, but NO pain</li><li>Start with a few repetitions and gradually increase as tolerated (no swelling). *CETI (Pilates)*</li></ul>**Also see Lymphedema**
Peripheral Neuropathy	<ul><li>Some cancer treatments cause peripheral neuropathy, a result of damage to the peripheral nerves. These nerves carry information from the brain to other parts of the body.</li><li>Feet or lower extremity – caution with standing on uneven surface, such as a Bosu ball or balance pads due to decreased sensation in feet. Increased risk of falling.</li><li>Hands – caution with holding dumbbells or grasping resistance bands.</li></ul>
Nerves that may be Damaged during Surgery	Several structures, including vessels and muscles with their nerve supply, are related to the breast and should be preserved during mastectomy or axillary node dissection. <ul><li>The **lateral pectoral nerve** passes medially around the medial pectoralis minor, and the medial pectoral nerve passes laterally around the pectoralis minor. These nerves can be severed during surgery. ***This results in numbness, motor atrophy, decreased sweat production in armpit and arm.***</li><li>The **medial pectoral nerve** innervates pectoralis minor and the lateral portion of the pectoralis major muscles. Preservation of this nerve is particularly important to prevent atrophy of the pectoral muscles if submuscular implant reconstruction is planned.</li><li>The **thoracodorsal nerve** is identifiable medial to the thoracodorsal vein. ***Injury may result in a weakening of the latissimus.***</li><li>The **long thoracic nerve** of Bell is located more medially in the axilla. It runs just beneath the fascia of the serratus anterior, medial to the thoracodorsal complex. ***Injury to this nerve will result in weakness in the serratus and cause winging of the scapula.*** *Pink Ribbon Program©*</li></ul>

Neurogenic causes of scapular winging and the physical exam

	Medial winging	Lateral winging	
Injured nerve	Long thoracic	Spinal accessory	Dorsal scapular
Muscle palsy	Serratus anterior	Trapezius	Rhomboids
Physical exam	Arm flexion; push-up motion against a wall	Arm abduction; external rotation against resistance	Arm extension from full flexion
Position of the scapula compared to normal	Entire scapula displaced more medial and superior	Superior angle more laterally displaced	Inferior angle more laterally displaced

NCBI: Scapular winging: anatomical review, diagnosis, and treatments

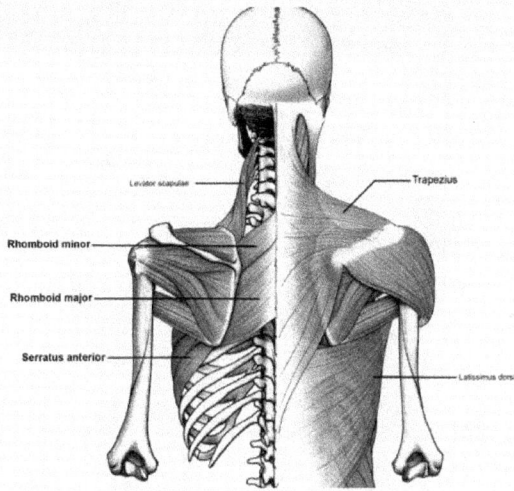

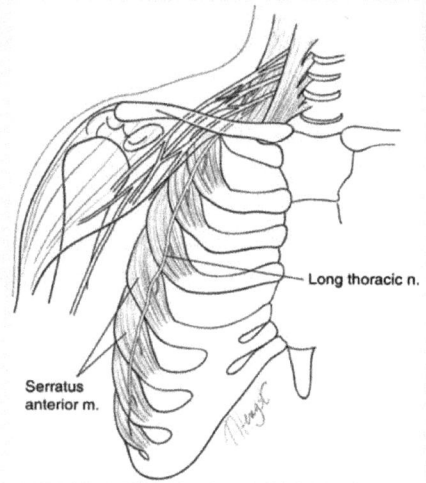

NCBI: Scapular winging: anatomical review, diagnosis, and treatments

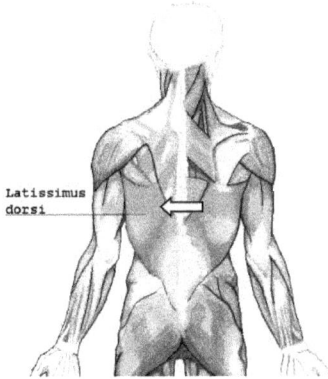

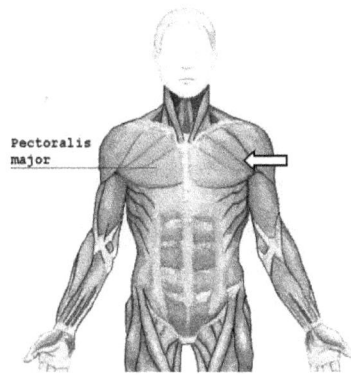

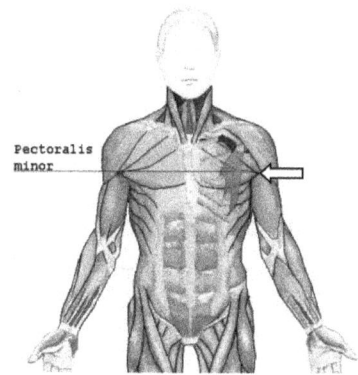

Latissimus dorsl   Pec Major   Pec Minor

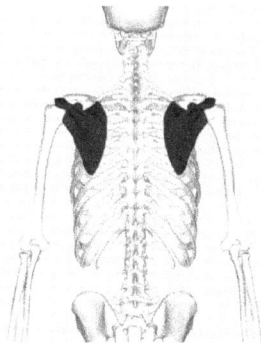

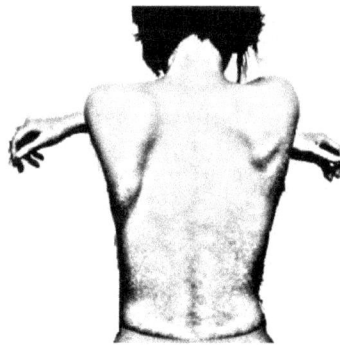

Scapular – normal   Scapular – winging

WikiMedia Commons: *https://commons.wikimedia.org/*

AVOID during the FIRST 2 WEEKS AFTER SURGERY
Cancer Research UK and *Dana Farber*

Your surgeon may suggest slightly different timings, so check if you are unsure.
- Don't lift your arm above the height of your shoulder or stretch behind your back.
- Don't lift anything heavier than a bag of sugar.

You might not realize that some everyday things can strain your muscles. Avoid doing any of the following with your arm on the side of your surgery. Avoiding these things helps your muscles to slowly stretch and heal.

- Pushing yourself up off the bed
- Pushing doors open
- Pulling things towards you, such as pulling washing out of the washing machine

IMPLANT
The implant has been placed under the muscle at the front of your chest. It stretches the chest muscle more than usual. By avoiding the movements listed above, the implant won't move and you won't overstretch the muscle or the wound, so it can all heal and settle down.
- When you are fastening your bra, do it up at the front, swivel it round, and put your arm on the side you had surgery in first. When you put your coat on, make sure you put the side you had surgery in the armhole first.
  Cancer Research UK

If you have a lumpectomy or partial mastectomy with or without a sentinel lymph node biopsy:
- Avoid any activity that bounces or jostles the breast for two weeks after surgery (i.e.: running, jumping, using the elliptical machine).
- Perform shoulder range of motion as tolerated, beginning 1-2 days after surgery.
- If you have an axillary node dissection: You may want to use pillows to elevate your arm at night to decrease swelling during the first week. Putting a pillow between your arm and your side at night will prevent you from rolling on to the surgical site.
- You should avoid repetitive motions with the arm on the surgical side, such as vacuuming, for two weeks after surgery.
- Avoid heavy lifting for 4 weeks.

If you have a mastectomy without reconstruction:
- Perform shoulder range of motion as tolerated, even while the drains are in.
- You may return to low-impact exercises after surgery once your pain is controlled and you feel comfortable.

If you have breast reconstruction:
- You should not lift your arm above shoulder level until cleared by your plastic surgeon.
- You may return to low-impact exercises four weeks after surgery.

Walking is a great exercise to begin immediately to reduce bone loss, counter fatigue and nausea, and prevent muscle atrophy. After surgery, try to walk around for a few minutes 2-3 times per day.

If you've had a mastectomy do not lift your arm past shoulder level while the drains are in.

Dana Farber

POST OP HEALING CONCERNS
©Klose Training: Breast Cancer Rehabilitation

Not Enough Movement	• Tissue adhesions • Shoulder/rib/clavicle stiffness • Decreased lymphangiomotoricity
Not Enough Compression	• Axillary/mastectomy/flap site seroma • Breast edema
Too Much Movement	• Mastectomy skin flaps will not adhere > seroma • ALND > seroma • Lack of lymphatic regeneration > increased risk of lymphedema
Seroma and Lymph Edema Prevention	• To early and/or too aggressive exercise may be increasing the incidence of seroma and lymphedema • ***Avoid wall walks and ROM past shoulder height, at least for the initial 2-3 weeks post-surgery*** • Avoid extreme forward reaching
Post Op Movement Restrictions	• Limit shoulder flexion to 90 degrees for 7-14 days to avoid seroma formation and encourage lymphatic regeneration. • Range of motion in shoulder as far as possible, avoiding pain, after 14 days if no seroma, and per surgeon recommendations. • Encourage using the arm as normally as possible without pain, within surgeons guidelines.

Recommendations Post Mastectomy

3-7 Days
- Avoid lying on side or arm of mastectomy
- Elevate affected side above heart at about a 45 degree angle 2-3x a day to avoid swelling.
- Use your arm to brush hair or trying to reach

First 4 weeks
- Do not use resistance
- Do not do overhead laps in pool
- Do not do body weight exercises or certain yoga poses such as push-ups or downward dog
- Avoid sports, such as skiing, tennis, canoe or any other exercises that extreme stretching of the shoulder.
- Be aware of lymphedema symptoms
- Do stretches in a warm shower or after once cleared to take a shower.
- Do stretches until feeling a slight stretch, not pain.
- Try doing the exercises twice a day 5-7 each.
- You do not have to start with every exercise listed – start with the ones lying down, then move to seated, and then standing.

After 4 – 6 weeks progress as tolerated and/or instructed by MD or physical therapy to include resistance.

Follow MD orders

Examples of Exercises, Stretches or Edema Control after Mastectomy			
1-2 WEEKS POST-OP	**Exercise or Stretch**	**Section**	**Number**
	DIAPHRAGMATIC BREATHING 6x a day for 5-10 repetitions	Duration, Frequency, Intensity	Pg 158
	OPEN AND CLOSE YOUR FIST CLENCH	NA	--
	SHOULDER SHRUGS	Upper Extremity	87
	SHOULDER ROLLS	Upper Extremity	89
	NECK ROTATION and SIDE BENDS	Flexibility	47
	SHOULER RAISE / ELBOW CIRCLES	NA	--
	PENDULUM SHOULDER FORWARD/BACK	Upper Extremity	29
	PENDULUM SHOULDER – SIDE TO SIDE	Upper Extremity	30
	PENDULUM SHOULDER CIRCLES	Upper Extremity	31
	BODY TURNS (rotations)	NA	--
	ELBOW FLEXION EXTENSION – SUPINE Bicep curl without weight on affected side to prevent edema	Upper Extremity	1
	BICEPS CURLS – SEATED Bicep curl without weight on affected side to prevent edema	Upper Extremity	3

3-4 WEEKS POST-OP	Exercise or Stretch	Section	Number
	V RAISE	Upper Extremity	45
	FLEXION – SUPINE - SINGLE OR BILATERAL	Upper Extremity	35
	FLEXION – SUPINE - DOWEL	Upper Extremity	37
	FLEXION - TABLE SLIDE	Flexibility	67
	FLEXION - TABLE SLIDE - BALL	Flexibility	68
	WALL WALK	Flexibility	66
	WALL WALK – Lateral	NA	--
	TRUNK ROTATION – SEATED	Flexibility	61
	CHEST STRETCH – SEATED or STANDING	Flexibility	71
	CHEST STRETCH – SUPINE	NA	--
	SCAPULAR RETRACTIONS - BILATERAL	Upper Extremity	92

4-6 WEEKS POST-OP Or Per MD order	Exercise or Stretch	Section	Number
	SHOULDER EXTENSION - STANDING	Upper Extremity	51
	SHOULDER EXTENSION – BILATERAL Standing dowel without weight	Upper Extremity	53
	LYING DOWN EXTENSION - TABLE or BED	Flexibility	77
	SHOULDER EXTENSION – DOWEL - STANDING	Flexibility	78
	EXTERNAL ROTATION - SUPINE – DOWEL *INTERNAL ROTATION ON OPPOSITE ARM*	Flexibility	69
	EXTERNAL ROTATION - 90-90 – DOWEL	Flexibility	70
	EXTERNAL ROTATION – SEATED – DOWEL *INTERNAL ROTATION ON OPPOSITE ARM*	Flexibility	71
	SCAPULAR PROTRACTION - SUPINE – BILATERAL	Upper Extremity	9
	ABDUCTION - TABLE SLIDE – BALL	Flexibility	75
	ABDUCTION WITH DOWEL	Flexibility	76
	CHEST STRETCH - STEP THROUGH	Flexibility	80

HOME EXERCISE GUIDE FOR POST SURGERY AND/OR LYMPHEDEMA

Breathing Patterns

Diaphragmatic Breathing

Lie either on your back with your knees bent or sit up

Inhale through your nose; as you do so, allow your stomach to rise. Limit movement in your chest. Attempt to push your bottom ribs out to the side as you breathe in.

Exhale through your mouth; as you do so, allow your stomach to fall. Limit movement in your chest.

Diaphragmatic breathing 6x a day for 5-10 repetitions

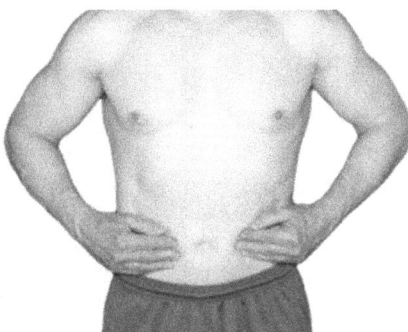

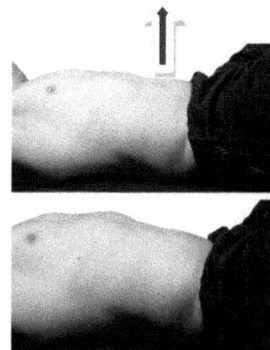

Purse Lip Breathing – Shortness of Breath

(PLB) is a breathing technique that consists of inhaling through the nose with the mouth closed and then exhaling through tightly pressed (pursed) lips. This technique is frequently in those with cardiac or respiratory issues. "*Smell the Roses then Blow Out the Candle*".

Breathing with Exercise

Exhale on the exertion. For example exhale when you are lying on your back and pushing a weight up or when bending your arm doing a bicep curl,. Inhale as you bring the weight slowly to your chest or when you straighten your arm with a bicep curl..

1-2 WEEKS POST OP or PER MD ORDERS

Description	Pictures
Other information at beginning of book. UE = Upper Extremity Section Flex = Flexibility Section	See UE or Flex section of book for other pictures
FIST CLENCH *Lymphedema control and circulation* Hands on thighs, open and close hand	
FIST CLENCH *Lymphedema control and circulation* Open and close your hand 15-20x with arm elevated above heart to prevent edema	
FIST CLENCH *Lymphedema control and circulation* Open and close your hand 15-20x with arm elevated above heart to prevent edema **NOT OVERHEAD first 1-2 weeks and/or until drains are out**	
SHRUGS UE 87 Raise your shoulders upward towards your ears as shown. Shrug both shoulders at the same time. Inhale up/exhale down	

Description	Pictures
Other information at beginning of book. UE = Upper Extremity Section Flex = Flexibility Section	See UE or Flex section of book for other pictures
SHOULDER ROLLS - Backwards UE 89 Move your shoulders in a circular pattern so that you are moving in an up, back and down direction. Perform small circles if needed for comfort.	
NECK ROTATION and SIDE BENDS Flex 47 SIDE BENDS: (*Top*) Tilt your head as if you are trying to touch your ear to your shoulder. ROTATION: *(Bottom)* Turn you head to the side as if looking over your shoulder.	
NECK FLEXION AND EXTENSION Flex 48 EXTENSION: Look up as if you are looking at the sky moving your neck only. FLEXION: Look down as if you are looking at the floor. For an extra stretch gently put both hands behind your head to move chin towards the chest and hold.	
SHOULDER RAISE / ELBOW CIRCLES Place your fingertips onto your shoulders. Slowly raise the elbow up to the side, then move it forwards, gently circling your arm. You are aiming to get your elbow level with your shoulder. Try to increase the height each time you do the exercises until you get level with your shoulder.	
ISOMETRIC CHEST PRESS Place the palms of your hands together with your elbows bent and arms at shoulder level or below. Exhale while pushing hands together and inhale and relax. 5-10x.	

Description	Pictures
Other information at beginning of book. UE = Upper Extremity Section Flex = Flexibility Section	See UE or Flex section of book for other pictures
PENDULUM SHOULDER FORWARD/BACK UE 29 *Start in a standing position and lean forward as allowed by MD – First picture* Shift your body weight forward then back to allow your injured arm to swing forward and back freely. Your affected arm should be fully relaxed.	
PENDULUM SHOULDER – SIDE TO SIDE UE 30 *Start in a standing position and lean forward as allowed by MD as above* Shift your body weight side to side to allow your injured arm to swing side to side freely. Your affected arm should be fully relaxed.	
PENDULUM SHOULDER CIRCLES UE 31 *Start in a standing position and lean forward as allowed by MD as above* Shift your body weight in circles to allow your injured arm to swing in circles freely. Your injured arm should be fully relaxed. REVERSE PENDULUM SHOULDER CIRCLES Shift your body weight in reverse circles to allow your injured arm to swing in circles freely. Your injured arm should be fully relaxed.	

Description	Pictures
Other information at beginning of book. UE = Upper Extremity Section Flex = Flexibility Section	See UE or Flex section of book for other pictures
BODY TURNS / ROTATIONS Cross your arms across your body so that your hands are placed lightly on your elbows. Slowly turn to look to the left and then to the right.	
ELBOW FLEXION EXTENSION – SUPINE UE 1 Lie on your back and rest your elbow on a small rolled up towel. Bend at your elbow and then lower back down.	Extension Flexion
BICEPS CURLS UE 3 Bend your elbow and move your forearm upwards and lower back down. Bicep curl without weight on affected side to prevent edema	

3-4 WEEKS POST OP or PER MD ORDERS

Description	Pictures
Other information at beginning of book. UE = Upper Extremity Section Flex = Flexibility Section	See UE or Flex section of book for other pictures
V RAISE UE 45 Start with your arms down by your side, palms facing inward, thumbs up and your elbows straight. Raise up your arms in the form of a V to shoulder height as shown keeping elbows straight then return to starting position	
FLEXION – SUPINE - SINGLE OR BILATERAL UE 35 Lie on your back with your arm at your side. Slowly raise arm up and forward towards overhead until you feel a stretch – not pain. Can bend your knees for comfort. **NOT OVERHEAD first 2 weeks and/or until drains are out**	
FLEXION – SUPINE - DOWEL UE 37 Can use a broom handle, cane etc. Lie on your back holding dowel with both hands. Slowly raise up and forward towards overhead until you feel a stretch. Your unaffected arm will help lift the wand higher. Hold for 5 seconds, then gently lower arms. Return to starting position. Repeat. **NOT OVERHEAD first 2 weeks and/or until drains are out**	

Description	Pictures
Other information at beginning of book. UE = Upper Extremity Section Flex = Flexibility Section	See UE or Flex section of book for other pictures

Description	Pictures
FLEXION - TABLE SLIDE Shoulder blade stretch Flex 67 Stand rest your affected / target arm on a table either palm down or on side and gently slide it forward and then back. You should feel your shoulder blade move as you do this	
FLEXION - TABLE SLIDE - BALL Flex 68 Stand and rest your target arm on top of a ball on a table. Gently roll the ball forward and then back. You should feel your shoulder blade move as you do this	
WALL WALK - Front Flex 66 Place your target hand on the wall with the palm facing the wall. Walk your fingers up the wall towards overhead. Slide or walk your hand back down the wall to the starting position. You may feel tight, but it shouldn't be painful. If it is very painful, tell your specialist physiotherapist or breast care nurse. **NOT OVERHEAD first 2 weeks and/or until drains are out**	
WALL WALK – Lateral Walk your fingers up the wall sideways – Stand with the side you had the operation next to the wall. Walk your fingers up the wall so that the palm of your hand is facing the wall. **NOT OVERHEAD first 2 weeks and/or until drains are out**	

Description	Pictures
Other information at beginning of book. UE = Upper Extremity Section Flex = Flexibility Section	See UE or Flex section of book for other pictures
TRUNK ROTATION – SEATED Flex 61 Sit up as tall with erect posture. Rotate in one direction, using your hand to press against the opposite thigh to aide in further rotation. Exhale to increase the rotation and stretch. Return to the starting position, maintain an upright posture -repeat in the opposite direction.	
CHEST STRETCH – SEATED or STANDING Flex 71 TOP: Bend arms at a 90-degree angle. Move elbows back until feeling a stretch in front of shoulders/chest. BOTTOM: Clasp hands in back of head. Move elbows back until feeling a stretch in front of shoulders/chest.	
CHEST STRETCH – SUPINE Lie on your back. Put your fingers lightly on your ears or behind your head, with your elbows pointing up towards the ceiling. Slowly let your elbows fall back towards the floor/bed to feel a stretch in the chest and front of the shoulders. Should feel a stretch – not pain.	

Description	Pictures
Other information at beginning of book. UE = Upper Extremity Section Flex = Flexibility Section	See UE or Flex section of book for other pictures

SCAPULAR RETRACTIONS - Bilateral UE 92 Draw your shoulder blades back and down. Squeeze your shoulder blades together, bringing your elbows behind you toward your spine. Elbows will move with you, but don't force the motion with your elbows. Keep your shoulders level as you do this. Do not lift your shoulders up toward your ears. Return to the starting position and repeat 5 to 7 times. CHEST STRETCH Stand up, keeping your arms relaxed and straight by your side. Then slowly take your arms behind you, as if you are trying to touch your hands together at the back. UK **CAREFUL WITH CHEST EXPANDER OR NEW IMPLANTS**	

OTHER EXERCISES PER PHYSICAL THERAPY, CERTFIED CANCER EXERCISE SPECIALIST or OTHER TRAINED SPECIALIST

Description	Pictures
Other information at beginning of book. UE = Upper Extremity Section Flex = Flexibility Section	See UE or Flex section of book for other pictures
SHOULDER EXTENSION - STANDING UE 51 Start with arms by your side. Draw your arm back behind your waist. Keep your elbows straight.	
SHOULDER EXTENSION - STANDING UE 53 Hold a dowel or cane behind your back with both arms. Draw your arms back.	
LYING DOWN EXTENSION - TABLE or BED Flex 77 Lie on your back and gently let target arm drop off table or bed. May want to have someone there to guard or have strap and hold with the other hand.	

Description	Pictures
Other information at beginning of book. UE = Upper Extremity Section Flex = Flexibility Section	See UE or Flex section of book for other pictures
SHOULDER EXTENSION – DOWEL - STANDING Flex 78 Stand and hold a dowel/cane. Use the unaffected arm to help push the target arm back to a stretch, not pain. The elbow should remain straight the entire time. Can cup affected arm in back of dowel if unable to grasp *(see 2nd picture)*	
EXTERNAL ROTATION - SUPINE – DOWEL *INTERNAL ROTATION ON OPPOSITE ARM* Flex 69 Lie on your back holding a dowel/cane with both hands. On the target side, maintain approx. 90-degree bend at the elbow with your arm approximately 30-45 degrees away from your side. Use your other arm to push the dowel/cane to rotate the affected arm back into a stretch, not pain. Hold and then return to the starting position.	
EXTERNAL ROTATION - 90-90 – DOWEL Flex 70 Lie on your back and hold a dowel with your elbows out to the side and rested down. Roll your arms back towards overhead until a stretch is felt, not pain. Keep elbows bent at a 90-degree angle.	

Description	Pictures
Other information at beginning of book. UE = Upper Extremity Section Flex = Flexibility Section	See UE or Flex section of book for other pictures

EXTERNAL ROTATION – SEATED – DOWEL *INTERNAL ROTATION ON OPPOSITE ARM* Flex 71 Using the unaffected arm, push the dowel into the hand of the target arm. Keep the arm at a 90-degree angle and push until a stretch is felt, not pain. Hold and repeat. If needed, use towel under arm for positioning *(see 2nd picture)*	
SCAPULAR PROTRACTION - SUPINE SINGLE OR BILATERAL UE 9 Lie on your back with your arms extended out in front of your body and towards the ceiling. While keeping your elbows straight, protract your shoulders reaching forward towards the ceiling. Keep your elbows straight the entire time.	
ABDUCTION - TABLE SLIDE – BALL Flex 75 Stand and rest your target arm on top of a ball on a table and gently roll it to the side and back.	

Description	Pictures
Other information at beginning of book. UE = Upper Extremity Section Flex = Flexibility Section	See UE or Flex section of book for other pictures
ABDUCTION WITH DOWEL Flex 76 Hold a dowel/cane in front. Slowly push the dowel of the unaffected arm towards the target arm upward and to the side until a stretch is felt, not pain.	
CHEST STRETCH - STEP THROUGH Flex 80 Stand with arms in doorway at a 90-degree angle. Step through until you feel a stretch through the chest and hold. No pain should be felt. Keep shoulders down and back. Take another step to increase stretch. Can modify starting with arms lower and bring up **as tolerated**.	

NCBI: Scapular winging: anatomical review, diagnosis, and treatments:
https://www.ncbi.nlm.nih.gov/pmc/articles/PMC2684151/

CETI: Pilates https*: //www.thecancerspecialist.com/*

Dana Farber - *https://www.dana-farber.org/*

Klose Training ©: Breast Cancer Rehabilitation - *https://klosetraining.com/*

American Cancer Society - Physical Activity and the Cancer Patient - *https://www.cancer.org/treatment/survivorship-during-and-after-treatment/staying-active/physical-activity-and-the-cancer-patient.html*

Cancer Research UK - Exercise guidelines for Cancer Patients
https://www.cancerresearchuk.org/about-cancer/coping/physically/exercise-guidelines Clinical Exercise Physiology, pg. 440

NIH NCI (12) https://www.cancer.gov/about-cancer/treatment/side-effects/lymphedema/lymphedema-pdq

Pink Ribbon Program© - *https://www.pinkribbonprogram.com/*

Cancer Types
Information and pictures from *National Cancer Institute* unless otherwise specified

Quick Summary this Section

Cancer Types:
- Fifteen types of cancer and their description, treatment, side effects
- Possible recommendations post-surgery / exercise precautions
    - Bladder
        - Kegal Exercises – Also for Prostate and Endometrial
    - Bone
    - Brain
    - Colorectal
    - Endometrial
        - See Bladder for Kegal Exercises
    - Kidney
    - Leukemia
    - Liver
    - Lung
    - Lymphoma
    - Melanoma
    - Pancreatic
        - Special Considerations for People with Diabetes
    - Prostate
        - See Bladder for Kegal Exercises
    - Stomach
    - Thyroid
- References following each section

BLADDER (Kegel Exercise)
Information and pictures from *National Cancer Institute* unless otherwise specified

Description	Bladder cancer is a disease in which malignant (cancer) cells form in the tissues of the bladder.

The bladder is a hollow organ in the lower part of the abdomen. It is shaped like a small balloon and has a muscular wall that allows it to get larger or smaller to store urine made by the kidneys.

There are two kidneys, one on each side of the backbone, above the waist. Tiny tubules in the kidneys filter and clean the blood. They take out waste products and make urine. The urine passes from each kidney through a long tube called a ureter into the bladder.

The bladder holds the urine until it passes through the urethra and leaves the body.

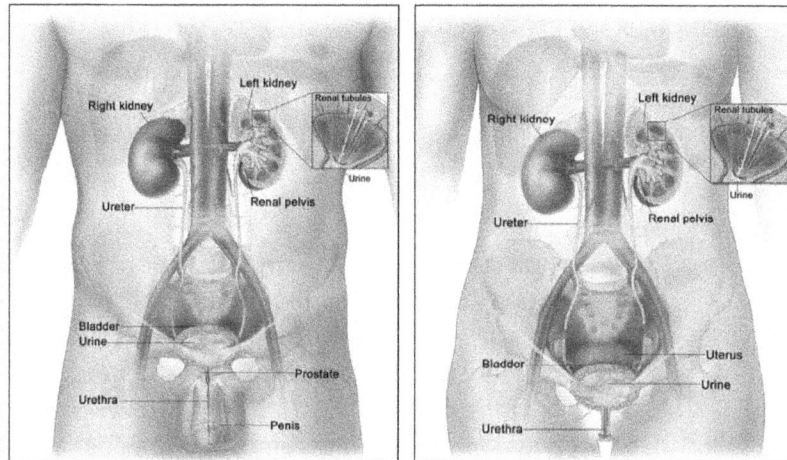

There are three types of bladder cancer that begin in cells in the lining of the bladder. These cancers are named for the type of cells that become malignant (cancerous):

- **Transitional cell carcinoma**: Cancer that begins in cells in the innermost tissue layer of the bladder. These cells are able to stretch when the bladder is full and shrink when it is emptied. Most bladder cancers begin in the transitional cells. Transitional cell carcinoma can be low-grade or high-grade:
  - Low-grade transitional cell carcinoma often recurs (comes back) after treatment but rarely spreads into the muscle layer of the bladder or to other parts of the body.
  - High-grade transitional cell carcinoma often recurs (comes back) after treatment and often spreads into the muscle layer of the bladder, to other parts of the body and to lymph nodes. Almost all deaths from bladder cancer are due to high-grade disease.
- **Squamous cell carcinoma:** Cancer that begins in squamous cells, which are thin, flat cells that may form in the bladder after long-term infection or irritation.
- **Adenocarcinoma:** Cancer that begins in glandular cells that are found in the lining of the bladder. This is a very rare type of bladder cancer.
- **Small cell carcinoma** and **Sarcoma** are rare types of bladder cancer.
- *Superficial bladder cancer:* Cancer that is in the lining of the bladder.
- *Invasive bladder cancer: Cancer* that has spread through the lining of the bladder and invades the muscle wall of the bladder or has spread to nearby organs and lymph nodes

Risk Factors	**Risks Include:** • Using tobacco, especially smoking cigarettes. • Having a family history of bladder cancer. • Having certain changes in the genes that are linked to bladder cancer. • Being exposed to paints, dyes, metals, or petroleum products in the workplace. • Past treatment with radiation therapy to the pelvis or with certain anticancer drugs, such as cyclophosphamide or ifosfamide. • Taking Aristolochia fangchi, a Chinese herb. • Drinking water from a well that has high levels of arsenic. • Drinking water that has been treated with chlorine. • Having a history of bladder infections, including bladder infections caused by Schistosoma haematobium. • Using urinary catheters for a long time.

Treatments	**Chemotherapy**
	Immunotherapy
	Radiation therapy
	
	Surgery
	• **Transurethral resection (TUR) with fulguration**: Surgery in which a cystoscope (a thin lightedtube) is inserted into the bladder through the urethra.
	    o A tool with a small wire loop on the end is then used to remove the cancer or to burn the tumor away with high- energy electricity. This is known as *fulguration*.
	• **Radical cystectomy**: Surgery to remove the bladder and any lymph nodes and nearby organs that contain cancer.
	    o This surgery may be done when the bladder cancer invades the muscle wall, or when superficial cancer involves a large part of the bladder.
	    o In *men*, the nearby organs that are removed are the prostate and the seminal vesicles.
	    o In *women*, the uterus, the ovaries, and part of the vagina are removed.
	    o Sometimes, when the cancer has spread outside the bladder and cannot be completely removed, surgery to remove only the bladder may be done to reduce urinary symptoms caused by the cancer.
	    o When the bladder must be removed, the surgeon creates another way for urine to leave the body.
	• **Partial cystectomy**: Surgery to remove part of the bladder.
	    o This surgery may be done for patients who have a low-grade tumor that has invaded the wall of the bladder but is limited to one area of the bladder.
	    o Because only a part of the bladder is removed, patients are able to urinate normally after recovering from this surgery.
	    o This is also called *segmental cystectomy.*
	• **Urinary diversion**: Surgery to make a new way for the body to store and pass urine.

Possible Side Effects *Cancer Support Community*	**TUR:** • Possible bleeding and pain when you urinate after surgery. **Radical cystectomy** • Women unable to get pregnant and may have early menopause • Men may be impotent **Segmental cystectomy** • Increased urination or unable to hold urine. **Radiation therapy** • Can cause nausea, vomiting, diarrhea, or urinary discomfort. • Can affect sexuality in both men and women. • Women may experience vaginal dryness. • Men may have difficulty with erections. **Chemotherapy** • Certain drugs used in the treatment of bladder cancer may cause kidney damage.
References	Ahlering, Thomas MD – Kegel Exercises for Men - *http://www.urology.uci.edu/prostate/kegel.html* Bladder Cancer Canada - Bladder cancer exercise sample (Kegel)- *https://bladdercancercanada.org/wp- content/uploads/2018/06/Bladder-Cancer-Sample-Exercises.pdf* Cancer Support Community – Bladder Cancer - *https://www.cancersupportcommunity.org/bladder-cancer* CETI- Cancer Exercise Training Institute: *https://www.thecancerspecialist.com/* Medline Plus – Kegel Exercises - *https://medlineplus.gov/ency/patientinstructions/000141.htm* National Cancer Institute (NCI) – Bladder Cancer - *https://www.cancer.gov/types/bladder*

Recovery after Surgery *Information from CETI-* *Cancer Exercise Training Institute* ***Please follow MD/surgeon protocol, as every situation is unique.***	**Transurethral Resection of the Bladder Tumor (TURBT)** ➢ **Hospital Stay:** 1-2 days ➢ **Full Recovery:** 3 weeks ➢ **Restrictions:** No heavy lifting over 10 lbs. or strenuous exercise for at least 6 weeks. ○ No activities such as riding a bike, weightlifting, aerobic exercise or jogging for the first 3-4 weeks ➢ **Exercise:** Walking and Kegel exercises *(see Kegal)* ➢ **Possible Side Effects:** Bleeding or Pain with Urination after Surgery; Incontinence **Partial Cystectomy:** ➢ **Hospital Stay:** Approximately 1 week ➢ **Full Recovery:** 6 weeks, but no heavy lifting for 12 weeks. ➢ **Restrictions:** No heavy lifting or excessive stair climbing for 12 weeks. ➢ **Exercise:** Walking **Radical Cystectomy:** ➢ **Hospital Stay:** 8-9 days ➢ **Full Recovery: 6** weeks, but no heavy lifting for 12 weeks. ➢ **Restrictions**: No heavy lifting or excessive stair climbing for 12 weeks ➢ **Exercise:** Walking during recovery period for most patients – see MD protocol ➢ **Possible Side Effects:** Bowel Obstruction, Lower Extremity Lymphedema, Ureter Blockage, Urinary Tract Infection, Bleeding, Blood Clots (Legs), Declined Kidney Function, Incontinence, Vitamin B12 Deficiency, Dehydration, Electrolyte Imbalance

Exercise, Special Considerations & Precautions – Short and Long Term *Please follow MD/surgeon protocol, as every situation is unique.*	• Walking during recovery period for most patients– see MD protocol • Kegel exercises when cleared by MD • Avoid weightlifting, aerobic exercise, excessive stair climbing until cleared by MD • If lymph nodes removed or Radiation: See *Lymphedema* **Urostomy (Pouch):** • No lifting over 10 lbs. for about 4 weeks after surgery • Discuss swimming with MD • Start with low resistance and progress slowly

Sections from HEP portion of book		
Flex = Flexibility *Strength* - LE = Lower Extremity UE = Upper Extremity		
Examples of Exercises or Stretches after Surgery	**Section**	**Number**
Frog Stretch / Adductor	Flex	39
Diaphragmatic breathing	Components Of A Conditioning Program	Breathing Section
Pelvic Tilt	Core	3
Bridges	Core	5
Clamshells	LE	53

Kegel Exercises
Information from both Medline Plus and Bladder Cancer Canada

Kegel Exercises – *For Male specific see Below*

A Kegel exercise is like pretending you have to urinate and then holding it. You relax and tighten the muscles that control urine flow. It is important to find the right muscles to tighten. Next time you have to urinate, start to go and then stop. Feel the muscles in your vagina (for women), bladder, or anus get tight and move up. These are the pelvic floor muscles. If you feel them tighten, you have done the exercise right. Your thighs, buttock muscles, and abdomen should remain relaxed.

These exercises can be done in seated, supine or standing position.
In Supine:
- Make sure your bladder is empty.
- Lying on your back with legs hip width a part and knees bent with feet on the ground. Legs can be out straight if more comfortable.
- If required, place towel or pillow under head but not shoulders to help with any tightness felt in neck and upper back.
- Place fingers onto lower abdominals (between hip bones) and cough –this is the feeling you are looking for when you activate your pelvic floor (deep core) muscles.
- Engage these muscles independently by imagining you need to hold your urine.

Seated, supine or standing:
- Tighten your pelvic floor muscles and hold tight and count to 5-8 seconds and release.
- Relax the muscles and count to 10. Repeat 10 times, 3 times a day (morning, afternoon, and night).
- Breathe deeply and relax your body when you are doing these exercises.
- Make sure you are not tightening your stomach, thigh, buttock, or chest muscles.

If you still are not sure you are tightening the right muscles:
- Imagine that you are trying to keep yourself from passing gas.
- Women: Insert a finger into your vagina. Tighten the muscles as if you are holding in your urine, then let go. You should feel the muscles tighten and move up and down.
- Men: Insert a finger into your rectum. Tighten the muscles as if you are holding in your urine, then let go. You should feel the muscles tighten and move up and down. *(See Prostate Cancer for more information)*

Once you learn how to do them, do not practice Kegel exercises at the same time you are urinating more than twice a month. Doing the exercises while you are urinating can weaken your pelvic floor muscles over time or cause damage to bladder and kidneys.

In women, doing Kegel exercises incorrectly or with too much force may cause vaginal muscles to tighten too much. This can cause pain during sexual intercourse.

Kegel Exercises - Male Specific

- Tighten your rectum as if you are trying to control passing gas or pinching off a stool. Do not tense the muscles of your legs, buttocks, or abdomen. Do not hold your breath.
- You can also imagine that you are trying to stop the flow of urine. If you still cannot find these muscles, you might try actually urinating and then trying to slow or stop the flow of urine midstream without using leg, buttocks or abdominal muscles.
- When you find these muscles, you will feel the muscles pulling upward and inward. Your penis and testicles also will move up and down slightly as you contract and relax.
- If you still are unsure if you are using the proper muscles, or if symptoms are not improving, contact your physician for more help.

How to Do the Male Kegel Exercises
- Male Kegel exercise is best done after emptying your bladder.
- Tighten the muscles you located above and hold for 3 to 5 seconds, or as long as you can at first. As these muscles get stronger, you will able to hold them longer.
- Relax for 3 to 5 seconds or for as long as you tightened the muscles, then repeat.
- Breathe normally.
- Do 5 to 7 exercises at a time, 3 times a day minimum. As you get stronger, increase up to 15 exercises at a time, 4 times a day.
- In addition, for more advanced exercises, you might consider incorporating a series of quick flexes (1 second) into this routine of long flexes. For example, perform 30 quick (1 second flexes) rapidly. Then 1 long contraction for as long as you can. Then repeat. Add more repetitions as you get stronger.
- The key, as with any physical training, is to set up a consistent routine and to perform the exercise properly.

Things to Remember about Male Kegel Exercise
- Make sure you are ONLY using the pelvic muscles. When you are first beginning the male Kegel exercise, you may consider standing in front of a mirror with a hand or on your abdomen or buttocks to feel for movement. It is important that you do NOT use your abdominals, buttocks, or leg muscles.
- Remember to breathe normally while exercising. Kegel exercise does not involve holding your breath.
- Exercise takes time to strengthen these muscles, just as with any physical therapy. You should start noticing less leakage after 4-6 weeks of consistent daily exercise, and an even larger difference after 3 months. If you do not see an improvement, you may not be exercising the proper muscles. You should be keeping track of how many pads you use per day to monitor your own progress.
- Pelvic muscle exercises also improve orgasmic function thereby speeding your return to potency. Contracting these muscles can aid in squeezing more blood into the penis to improve erectile function.
- Be proactive, do your Kegel exercises faithfully and you will see results.

Ahlering, Thomas MD

References	Ahlering, Thomas MD – Kegel Exercises for Men - http://www.urology.uci.edu/prostate/kegel.html
Kegel	Medline Plus – Kegel Exercises - https://medlineplus.gov/ency/patientinstructions/000141.htm

Bone Cancer
Information and pictures from *National Cancer Institute* unless otherwise specified

What are Bone Tumors? *NCI – National Cancer Institute*	Several different kinds of tumors can grow in bones: primary bone tumors, which form from bone tissue and can be malignant (cancerous) or benign (not cancerous), and metastatic tumors (tumors that develop from cancer cells that formed elsewhere in the body and then spread to the bone). <ul><li>Malignant primary bone tumors (primary bone cancers) are less common than benign primary bone tumors.</li><li>Both types of primary bone tumors may grow and compress healthy bone tissue, but benign tumors usually do not spread or destroy bone tissue and are rarely a threat to life.</li><li>Primary bone cancers are included in the broader category of cancers called sarcomas. (Soft-tissue sarcomas—sarcomas that begin in muscle, fat, fibrous tissue, blood vessels, or other supporting tissue of the body, including synovial sarcoma—are not addressed in this fact sheet.)<ul><li>Primary bone cancer is rare. It accounts for much less than 1% of all new cancers diagnosed. In 2018, an estimated 3,450 new cases of primary bone cancer will be diagnosed in the United States.</li></ul></li><li>Cancer that metastasizes (spreads) to the bones from other parts of the body is called metastatic (or secondary) bone cancer and is referred to by the organ or tissue in which it began—for example, breast cancer that has metastasized to the bone.<ul><li>In adults, cancerous tumors that have metastasized to the bone are much more common than primary bone cancer. For example, at the end of 2008, an estimated 280,000 adults ages 18–64 years in the United States were living with metastatic cancer in bones.</li></ul></li><li>Although most types of cancer can spread to the bone, bone metastasis is particularly likely with certain cancers, including breast and prostate cancers.<ul><li>Metastatic tumors in the bone can cause fractures, pain, and abnormally high levels of calcium in the blood, a condition called hypercalcemia.</li></ul></li></ul>

Anatomy of the Spine

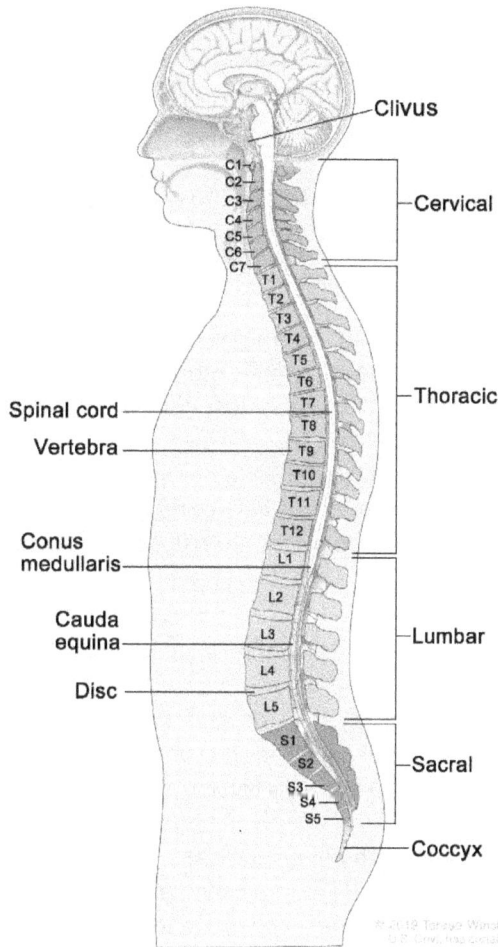

NCI – Picture of Spine

Anatomy of the spine. The spine is made up of bones, muscles, tendons, nerves, and other tissues that reach from the base of the skull near the spinal cord (clivus) to the coccyx (tailbone). The vertebrae (back bones) of the spine include the cervical spine (C1-C7), thoracic spine (T1-T12), lumbar spine (L1-L5), sacral spine (S1-S5), and the tailbone.

Each vertebra is separated by a disc. The vertebrae surround and protect the spinal cord. The spinal cord is divided into segments, each containing a pair of spinal nerves that send messages between the brain and the rest of the body.

Many spinal nerves extend beyond the conus medullaris (the end of the spinal cord) to form a bundle of nerves called the cauda equina.

Bone cancer

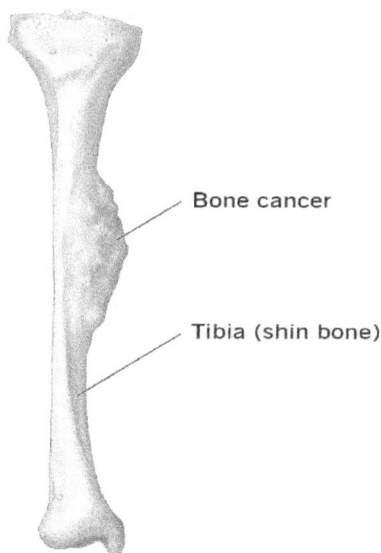

Although bone cancer can affect any bone, most tumors start in your leg bones, like your femur (thigh bone), tibia (shin bone) or your upper arm.

Cleveland Clinic – Bone Cancer

What are the different types of primary bone cancer?	Types of primary bone cancer are defined by which cells in the bone give rise to them. • **Osteosarcoma** Osteosarcoma arises from bone-forming cells called osteoblasts in osteoid tissue (immature bone tissue). This tumor typically occurs in the arm near the shoulder and in the leg near the knee in children, adolescents, and young adults, but can occur in any bone, especially in older adults. <ul><li>It often grows quickly and spreads to other parts of the body, including the lungs.</li><li>The risk of osteosarcoma is highest among children and adolescents ages 10 and 19.</li><li>Males are more likely than females to develop osteosarcoma.</li><li>Among children, osteosarcoma is more common in blacks and other racial/ethnic groups than in whites, but among adults it is more common in whites than in other racial/ethnic groups.</li><li>People who have Paget disease (a benign bone condition characterized by abnormal development of new bone cells) or a history of radiation to their bones also have an increased risk of developing osteosarcoma.</li></ul> • **Chondrosarcoma** Chondrosarcoma begins in cartilaginous tissue. Cartilage is a type of connective tissue that covers the ends of bones and lines the joints. <ul><li>Chondrosarcoma most often forms in the pelvis, upper leg, and shoulder and usually grows slowly, although sometimes it can grow quickly and spread to other parts of the body.</li><li>Chondrosarcoma occurs mainly in older adults (over age 40).</li><li>The risk increases with advancing age.</li><li>A rare type of chondrosarcoma called extra skeletal chondrosarcoma does not form in bone cartilage. Instead, it forms in the soft tissues of the upper part of the arms and legs.</li></ul>• **Ewing sarcoma** Ewing sarcoma usually arises in bone but may also rarely arise in soft tissue (muscle, fat, fibrous tissue, blood vessels, or other supporting tissue). <ul><li>Ewing sarcomas typically form in the pelvis, legs, or ribs, but can form in any bone.</li><li>This tumor often grows quickly and spreads to other parts of the body, including the lungs.</li><li>The risk of Ewing sarcoma is highest in children and adolescents younger than 19 years of age.</li><li>Boys are more likely to develop Ewing sarcoma than girls.</li><li>Ewing sarcoma is much more common in whites than in blacks or Asians.</li></ul>• **Chordoma** Chordoma is a very rare tumor that forms in bones of the spine. <ul><li>These tumors usually occur in older adults and typically form at the base of the spine (sacrum) and at the base of the skull.</li><li>About twice as many men as women are diagnosed with chordoma.</li><li>When they do occur in younger people and children, they are usually found at the base of the skull and in the cervical spine (neck).</li></ul>

What are the different types of primary bone cancer?
 	
Continued
	Giant cell tumor:
	Several types of benign bone tumors can, in rare cases, become malignant and spread to other parts of the body. These include giant cell tumor of bone (also called osteoclastoma) and osteoblastoma.
	• Giant cell tumor of bone mostly occurs at the ends of the long bones of the arms and legs, often close to the knee joint.
	   o These tumors, which typically occur in young and middle-aged adults, can be locally aggressive, causing destruction of bone.
	   o In rare cases they can spread (metastasize), often to the lungs.
	   o Osteoblastoma replaces normal hard bone tissue with a weaker form called osteoid.
	   o This tumor occurs mainly in the spine.
	   o It is slow-growing and occurs in young and middle-aged adults.
	   o Rare cases of this tumor becoming malignant have been reported.

What are the possible causes of bone cancer?	Although primary bone cancer does not have a clearly defined cause, researchers have identified several factors that increase the likelihood of developing these tumors.
	• **Previous cancer treatment with radiation, chemotherapy, or stem cell transplantation.**
	   o Osteosarcoma occurs more frequently in people who have had high-dose external radiation therapy (particularly at the location in the body where the radiation was given) or treatment with certain anticancer drugs, particularly alkylating agents; those treated during childhood are at particular risk.
	   o I n addition, osteosarcoma develops in a small percentage (approximately 5%) of children undergoing myeloablative hematopoietic stem cell transplantation.
	
	• **Certain inherited conditions.** A small number of bone cancers are due to hereditary condition. For example, children who have had hereditary retinoblastoma (an uncommon cancer of the eye) are at a higher risk of developing osteosarcoma, particularly if they are treated with radiation.
	   o Members of families with Li-Fraumeni syndrome are at increased risk of osteosarcoma and chondrosarcoma as well as other types of cancer.
	   o Additionally, people who have hereditary defects of bones have an increased lifetime risk of developing chondrosarcoma.
	   o Childhood chordoma is linked to tuberous sclerosis complex, a genetic disorder in which benign tumors form in the kidneys, brain, eyes, heart, lungs, and skin.
	   o Although Ewing sarcoma is not strongly associated with any heredity cancer syndromes or congenital childhood diseases, accumulating evidence suggests a strong inherited genetic component to Ewing sarcoma risk.
	
	• **Certain benign bone conditions.** People over the age of 40 who have Paget disease of bone (a benign condition characterized by abnormal development of new bone cells) are at an increased risk of developing osteosarcoma.

How is bone cancer diagnosed?	To help diagnose bone cancer, the doctor asks about the patient's personal and family medical history. The doctor also performs a physical examination and may order laboratory and other diagnostic tests. These tests may include the following:

- **X-rays**, which can show the location, size, and shape of a bone tumor. If x-rays suggest that an abnormal area may be cancer, the doctor is likely to recommend special imaging tests. Even if x-rays suggest that an abnormal area is benign, the doctor may want to do further tests, especially if the patient is experiencing unusual or persistent pain.
    - A **bone scan**, which is a test in which a small amount of radioactive material is injected into a blood vessel and travels through the bloodstream; it then collects in the bones and is detected by a scanner.
    - A **computed tomography (CT or CAT) scan**, which is a series of detailed pictures of areas inside the body, taken from different angles, that are created by a computer linked to an x-ray machine.
    - A **magnetic resonance imaging (MRI) procedure**, which uses a powerful magnet linked to a computer to create detailed pictures of areas inside the body without using x-rays.
    - A **positron emission tomography (PET) scan**, in which a small amount of radioactive glucose (sugar) is injected into a vein, and a scanner is used to make detailed, computerized pictures of areas inside the body where the glucose is used. Because cancer cells often use more glucose than normal cells, the pictures can be used to find cancer cells in the body.
    - An **angiogram**, which is an x-ray of blood vessels.
- **Biopsy** (removal of a tissue sample from the bone tumor) to determine whether cancer is present.
    - The surgeon may perform a needle biopsy, an excisional biopsy, or an incisional biopsy. During a needle biopsy, the surgeon makes a small hole in the bone and removes a sample of the tissue from the tumor with a needle-like instrument.
    - For **excisional biopsy**, the surgeon removes an entire lump or suspicious area for diagnosis.
    - In an **incisional biopsy**, the surgeon cuts into the tumor and removes a sample of tissue.
    - Biopsies are best done by an orthopedic oncologist (a doctor experienced in the treatment of bone cancer) because the placement of the biopsy incision can influence subsequent surgical options.
    - A pathologist (a doctor who identifies disease by studying cells and tissues under a microscope) examines the tissue to determine whether it is cancerous.
- **Blood tests** to determine the levels of two enzymes called alkaline phosphatase and lactate dehydrogenase.
    - Large amounts of these enzymes may be present in the blood of people with osteosarcoma or Ewing sarcoma.
    - High blood levels of alkaline phosphatase occur when the cells that form bone tissue are very active—when children are growing, when a broken bone is mending, or when a disease or tumor causes the production of abnormal bone tissue.
    - Because high levels of alkaline phosphatase are normal in growing children and adolescents, this test is not a reliable indicator of bone cancer.

How is primary bone cancer treated?	Treatment options depend on the type, size, location, and stage of the cancer, as well as the person's age and general health. Treatment options for bone cancer include surgery, chemotherapy, radiation therapy, cryosurgery, and targeted therapy. <ul><li>**Surgery** is the usual treatment for bone cancer.<ul><li>The surgeon removes the entire tumor with negative margins (that is, no cancer cells are found at the edge of the tissue removed during surgery).</li><li>The surgeon may also use special surgical techniques to minimize the amount of healthy tissue removed along with the tumor.</li><li>Dramatic improvements in surgical techniques and preoperative tumor treatment have made it possible for most patients with bone cancer in an arm or leg to avoid radical surgical procedures (that is, removal of the entire limb).</li><li>However, most patients who undergo limb-sparing surgery need reconstructive surgery to regain limb function.</li></ul></li></ul>

- **Chemotherapy** is the use of anticancer drugs to kill cancer cells.
    - Patients who have Ewing sarcoma (newly diagnosed and recurrent) or newly diagnosed osteosarcoma usually receive a combination of anticancer drugs before undergoing surgery.
    - Chemotherapy is not typically used to treat chondrosarcoma or chordoma.

- **Radiation therapy**, also called radiotherapy, involves the use of high-energy x-rays to kill cancer cells.
    - This treatment may be used in combination with surgery.
    - It is often used to treat Ewing sarcoma.
    - It may also be used with other treatments for osteosarcoma, chondrosarcoma, and chordoma, particularly when a small amount of cancer remains after surgery.
    - It may also be used for patients who are not having surgery.
    - A radioactive substance that collects in bone, called samarium, is an internal form of radiation therapy that can be used alone or with stem cell transplant to treat osteosarcoma that has come back after treatment in a different bone.

- **Cryosurgery** is the use of liquid nitrogen to freeze and kill cancer cells.
    - This technique can sometimes be used instead of conventional surgery to destroy tumors in bone.

- **Targeted therapy** is the use of a drug that is designed to interact with a specific molecule involved in the growth and spread of cancer cells.
    - The monoclonal antibody denosumab (Xgeva®) is a targeted therapy that is approved to treat adults and skeletally mature adolescents with giant cell tumor of bone that cannot be removed with surgery.
    - It prevents the destruction of bone caused by a type of bone cell called an osteoclast.

Rotationplasty
 	
Wikipedia
	Rotationplasty *(Wikipedia):* Rotationplasty, commonly known as a Van Nes rotation or Borggreve rotation, is a type of autograft wherein a portion of a limb is removed, while the remaining limb below the involved portion is rotated and reattached.
	• This procedure is used when a portion of an extremity is injured or involved with a disease, such as cancer.
	• The procedure is most commonly used to transfer the ankle joint to the knee joint following removal of a distal femoral bone tumor, such as osteosarcoma.
	• The limb is rotated because the ankle flexes in the opposite direction compared to the knee.
	• The benefit to the patient is that they have a functioning knee joint to which a prosthetic can be fitted, so that they can run and jump.
	Advantages
	• Rotationplasty allows the use of the knee joint, whereas amputation would result in loss of that joint. Therefore, it provides a better attachment point and range of motion for a prosthetic limb.
	   o As a result, children who have had rotationplasty can play sports, run, climb, and do more than would be possible with a jointless prosthetic.
	   o After the procedure, the leg is durable; patients do not typically have to undergo additional surgeries.
	Disadvantages
	• Rotationplasty can result in poor circulation throughout the leg, infection, nerve injuries, bone healing complications, and fracture of the leg.

What are the side effects of treatment for bone cancer?	**Side Effects:**
	People who have been treated for bone cancer have an increased likelihood of developing late effects of treatment as they age.
	• These late effects depend on the type of treatment and the patient's age at treatment and include physical problems involving the heart, lung, hearing, fertility, and bone; neurological problems; and second cancers (acute myeloid leukemia, myelodysplastic syndrome, and radiation-induced sarcoma).
	   o Treatment of bone tumors with cryosurgery may lead to the destruction of nearby bone tissue and result in fractures, but these effects may not be seen for some time after the initial treatment.
	• Bone cancer sometimes metastasizes, particularly to the lungs, or can recur (come back), either at the same location or in other bones in the body.
	   o People who have had bone cancer should see their doctor regularly and should report any unusual symptoms right away.
	   o Follow-up varies for different types and stages of bone cancer. Generally, patients are checked frequently by their doctor and have regular blood tests and x-rays.

References	Cancer Exercise Toolkit: Bony Metastases *https://cancerexercisetoolkit.trekeducation.org/screening-and-safety/bony-metastases/* CETI- Cancer Exercise Training Institute: *https://www.thecancerspecialist.com/* Cleveland Clinic Picture of Bone– Bone Cancer: *https://my.clevelandclinic.org/health/diseases/17745-bone-cancer* NIH – National Cancer Institute – "Primary Bone Cancer". *https://www.cancer.gov/types/bone/bone-fact-sheet* NIH – Picture of Spine – "Childhood Chordoma" *https://www.cancer.gov/types/bone/patient/child-chordoma-treatment-pdq* Physiopedia - Physical Activity in Metastatic Bone Disease - Physiotherapy Management *https://www.physio-pedia.com/Physical_Activity_in_Metastatic_Bone_Disease*Wikipedia: Rotationplasty - *https://en.wikipedia.org/wiki/Rotationplasty*

Exercise, Special Considerations & Precautions – Short and Long Term
 	
Physiopedia and *Cancer Exercise Toolkit*
 	
Please follow MD/surgeon protocol, as every situation is unique.
	Awareness of 'red flag' symptoms: *(Physiopedia)*
	• Bone pain in the vertebral column that worsens night: indicates high risk of spinal Metastatic Bone Disease, MBD and imminent fracture.
	• Bone pain on weight bearing (especially in the proximal femur): indicates high risk of MBD in the long bones and imminent fracture.
	• Worsening and intractable bone pain at any time.
	
	Awareness of symptoms that could indicate Metastatic Spinal Cord Compression (MSCC)
	  • Back or neck pain
	  • Progressive limb weakness
	  • Numbness or tingling sensation in toes, fingers or buttocks
	  • Bladder or bowel problems
	
	Evidence supports the use of aerobic and resistance exercises for MBD patients to improve physical function and mental health:
	  • Isometric exercises can be used in stable bone metastasis cases.
	  • Avoid overloading the affected areas.
	  • Avoid sheering or rotation forces at the affected area.
	  • Modalities increasing local blood flow, such as ultrasound therapy, heat, massage, or certain electrotherapies, should *not be performed* at the affected area.
	  • Seek medical advice if pain does not resolve quickly, there is a new onset of bone pain, or bone pain that has changed in nature or intensity, due to risk of fracture.
	  • Walking aids can be used to take the weight off affected lower limbs. *(Physiopedia)*
	
	Considerations for Exercise *(Cancer Exercise Toolkit)*
	It is still safe for people with bony metastases to exercise. However, some important adaptations will be required to ensure safe exercise participation:
	
	Adaptations and Considerations
	  • Consider location of bony metastases and limit loading of bone metastases site
	  • Avoid excessive spinal flexion, extension and rotation; clarify with medical team need for bracing
	  • Monitor for increasing functional pain – refer on for medical evaluation
	  • Consider if the exercise test is necessary and avoid manual muscle testing in affected limb
	  • Exercise as tolerated as limited by pain. Focus on postural alignment, controlled movement and technique
	  • Minimize fall or impact risk *(Cancer Exercise Toolkit)*

Exercise, Special Considerations & Precautions – Short and Long Term
 	
Information from CETI- Cancer Exercise Training Institute
 	
Please follow MD/surgeon protocol, as every situation is unique.
	• Avoid any exercise with risk of falling
	• Surgery – are they removing just bone or taking muscle
	• **Limb sparing surgery:** Usually involves high dose radiation, which increases the risk of lymphedema, which is higher than regular radiation.
	    ○ It may take up to a year to walk.
	• **Bone Graft:**
	    ○ Allograph (donor) has a greater chance of rejection but has a better outcome. Lasts longer / stronger and has a better probability of healing vs audiologist (self)
	    ○ Can be physically active – leg or arm. Avoid contact sport and risk of falling that can fracture the bone.
	• **Fusion or arthrodesis** – joint has limited mobility or ROM (to make if difficult for running, jumping, tennis, etc., depending on the affected joint.

BRAIN / ADULT CENTRAL NERVOUS SYSTEM
Information and pictures from *National Cancer Institute* unless otherwise specified

Description	An adult central nervous system tumor is a disease in which abnormal cells form in the tissues of the brain and/or spinal cord.

There are many types of brain and spinal cord tumors. The tumors are formed by the abnormal growth of cells and may begin in different parts of the brain or spinal cord. Together, the brain and spinal cord make up the central nervous system (CNS).

The brain controls many important body functions.
The brain has three major parts:

- *The cerebrum is the largest part of the brain. It is at the top of the head. The cerebrum controls thinking, learning, problem solving, emotions, speech, reading, writing, and voluntary movement.*
- *The cerebellum is in the lower back of the brain (near the middle of the back of the head). It controls movement, balance, and posture.*
- *The brain stem connects the brain to the spinal cord. It is in the lowest part of the brain (just above the back of the neck). The brain stem controls breathing, heart rate, and the nerves and muscles used to see, hear, walk, talk, and eat.*

The spinal cord connects the brain to nerves in most parts of the body.

- *The spinal cord is a column of nerve tissue that runs from the brain stem down the center of the back.*
- *It is covered by three thin layers of tissue called membranes. These membranes are surrounded by the vertebrae (back bones).*
- *Spinal cord nerves carry messages between the brain and the rest of the body, such as a message from the brain to cause muscles to move or a message from the skin to the brain to feel touch.*

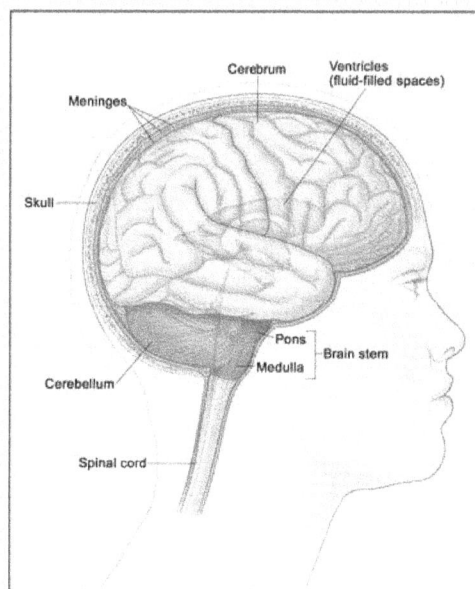

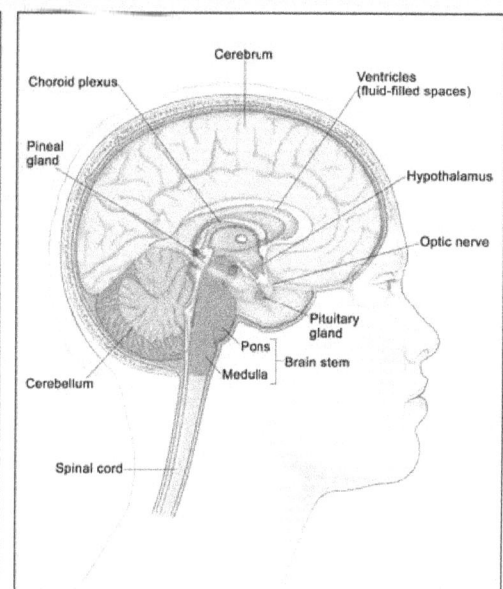

Description ***Continued***	The tumors may be either benign (not cancer) or malignant (cancer): • Benign brain and spinal cord tumors grow and press on nearby areas of the brain. They rarely spread into other tissues and may recur (come back). • Malignant brain and spinal cord tumors are likely to grow quickly and spread into other brain tissues. When a tumor grows into or presses on an area of the brain, it may stop that part of the brain from working the way it should. Both benign and malignant brain tumors cause signs and symptoms and need treatment. • A tumor that starts in another part of the body and spreads to the brain is called a metastatic brain tumor (or brain metastases). Metastatic brain tumors are more common than primary brain tumors. • Tumors that start in the brain are called primary brain tumors. Primary brain tumors may spread to other parts of the brain or to the spine. They rarely spread to other parts of the body. Up to half of metastatic brain tumors are from lung cancer. Other types of cancer that commonly spread to the brain include: • Melanoma. • Breast cancer. • Colon cancer. • Kidney cancer. • Nasopharyngeal cancer. • Cancer of unknown primary site. Cancer may spread to the leptomeninges (the two innermost membranes covering the brain and spinal cord). This is called leptomeningeal carcinomatosis. The most common cancers that spread to the leptomeninges include: • Breast cancer. • Lung cancer. • Leukemia. • Lymphoma. There are different types of brain and spinal cord tumors. • Brain and spinal cord tumors are named based on the type of cell they formed in and where the tumor first formed in the CNS. The grade of a tumor may be used to tell the difference between slow-growing and fast-growing types of the tumor. ○ The World Health Organization (WHO) tumor grades are based on how abnormal the cancer cells look under a microscope and how quickly the tumor is likely to grow and spread.

WHO Tumor Grading System	**WHO Tumor Grading System** • Grade I (low-grade) - The tumor cells look more like normal cells under a microscope and grow and spread more slowly than grade II, III, and IV tumor cells. They rarely spread into nearby tissues. Grade I brain tumors may be completely removed by surgery. • Grade II — The tumor cells grow and spread more slowly than grade III and IV tumor cells. They may spread into nearby tissue and may recur (come back). Some tumors may become a higher-grade tumor. • Grade III — The tumor cells look very different from normal cells under a microscope and grow more quickly than grade I and II tumor cells. They are likely to spread into nearby tissue. • Grade IV (high-grade) — The tumor cells do not look like normal cells under a microscope and grow and spread very quickly. There may be areas of dead cells in the tumor. Grade IV tumors usually cannot be completely removed by surgery.

Risk Factors	**Risk Factors:**
	• Being exposed to vinyl chloride may increase the risk of glioma.
	• Infection with the Epstein-Barr virus, having AIDS (acquired immunodeficiency syndrome), or receiving an organ transplant may increase the risk of primary CNS lymphoma.
	• Having certain genetic syndromes may increase the risk of brain tumors:
	   o Neurofibromatosis type 1 (NF1) or 2 (NF2).
	   o von Hippel-Lindau disease.
	   o Tuberous sclerosis.
	   o Li-Fraumeni syndrome.
	   o Turcot syndrome type 1 or 2.
	   o Nevoid basal cell carcinoma syndrome.

Treatments	Active surveillance Radiation therapy Supportive care is given to lessen the problems caused by the disease or its treatment **Surgery** • Surgery may be used to diagnose and treat adult brain and spinal cord tumors. Removing tumor tissue helps decrease the pressure of the tumor on nearby parts of the brain. • After the doctor removes all the cancer that can be seen at the time of the surgery, some patients may be given chemotherapy or radiation therapy after surgery to kill any cancer cells that are left. Treatment given after the surgery, to lower the risk that the cancer will come back, is called adjuvant therapy. **Chemotherapy** • To treat brain tumors, a wafer that dissolves may be used to deliver a chemotherapy drug directly to the brain tumor site after the tumor has been removed by surgery. The way chemotherapy is given depends on the type and grade of tumor and where it is in the brain. **Targeted therapy** • Other types of targeted therapies are being studied for adult brain tumors, including tyrosine kinase inhibitors and new VEGF inhibitors.

Treatments
 	
Continued
	Proton beam radiation therapy
	• A type of high-energy, external radiation therapy that uses streams of protons (tiny particles with a positive charge) to kill tumor cells.
	    ○ This type of treatment can lower the amount of radiation damage to healthy tissue near a tumor.
	    ○ It is used to treat cancers of the head, neck, and spine and organs such as the brain, eye, lung, and prostate.
	    ○ Proton beam radiation is different from x-ray radiation.
	
	Immunotherapy
	• Immunotherapy is being studied for the treatment of some types of brain tumors. Treatments may include the following:
	    ○ Dendritic cell vaccine therapy.
	    ○ Gene therapy.

Treatment of Primary Adult Brain Tumor by Type

ASTROCYTIC TUMORS	**ASTROCYTIC TUMORS** An astrocytic tumor begins in star-shaped brain cells called astrocytes, which help keep nerve cells healthy. An astrocyte is a type of glial cell. Glial cells sometimes form tumors called gliomas. Astrocytic tumors include the following: **Brain Stem Gliomas (usually high grade)** A tumor located in the part of the brain that connects to the spinal cord (the brain stem). It may grow rapidly or slowly, depending on the grade of the tumor. It is often a high-grade tumor, which spreads widely through the brain stem. Brain stem gliomas are rare in adults. Treatment of brain stem gliomas may include the following: • Radiation therapy. **Pineal Astrocytic Tumors (any grade)** A pineal astrocytic tumor forms in tissue around the pineal gland and may be any grade. The pineal gland is a tiny organ in the brain that makes melatonin, a hormone that helps control the sleeping and waking cycle. Treatment of pineal astrocytic tumors may include the following: • Surgery and radiation therapy. • For high-grade tumors, chemotherapy may also be given. **Pilocytic Astrocytomas (grade I)** A pilocytic astrocytoma grows slowly in the brain or spinal cord. It may be in the form of a cyst and rarely spread into nearby tissues. Treatment of pilocytic astrocytomas may include the following: • Surgery to remove the tumor. • Radiation therapy may also be given if the tumor remains after surgery.

ASTROCYTIC TUMORS *Continued*	**Diffuse Astrocytomas (grade II)** A diffuse astrocytoma grows slowly but often spreads into nearby tissues. The tumor cells look something like normal cells. It is also called a low-grade diffuse astrocytoma. Treatment of diffuse astrocytomas may include the following: • Surgery with or without radiation therapy. • Surgery followed by radiation therapy and chemotherapy. **Anaplastic Astrocytomas (grade III)** An anaplastic astrocytoma grows quickly and spreads into nearby tissues. The tumor cells look different from normal cells. An anaplastic astrocytoma is also called a malignant astrocytoma or high-grade astrocytoma. Treatment of anaplastic astrocytomas may include the following: • Surgery and radiation therapy. • Chemotherapy may also be given. • Surgery and chemotherapy. • A clinical trial of chemotherapy placed into the brain during surgery. • A clinical trial of a new treatment added to standard treatment. **Glioblastomas (grade IV)** A glioblastoma grows and spreads very quickly. The tumor cells look very different from normal cells. • A fast-growing type of central nervous system tumor that forms from glial (supportive) tissue of the brain and spinal cord and has cells that look very different from normal cells. • Glioblastoma usually occurs in adults and affects the brain more often than the spinal cord. • Also called GBM, glioblastoma multiforme, and grade IV astrocytoma. Treatment of glioblastomas may include the following: • Surgery followed by radiation therapy and chemotherapy given at the same time, followed by chemotherapy alone. • Surgery followed by radiation therapy. • Chemotherapy placed into the brain during surgery. • Radiation therapy and chemotherapy are given at the same time. • A clinical trial of a new treatment added to standard treatment.

OLIGODENDROGLIAL TUMORS	**OLIGODENDROGLIAL TUMORS** An oligodendroglial tumor begins in brain cells called oligodendrocytes, which help keep nerve cells healthy. An oligodendrocyte is a type of glial cell. Oligodendrocytes sometimes form tumors called oligodendrogliomas. Grades of oligodendroglial tumors include the following: • **Oligodendroglioma** (grade II): An oligodendroglioma grows slowly but often spreads into nearby tissues. The tumor cells look something like normal cells. • **Anaplastic** oligodendroglioma (grade III): An anaplastic oligodendroglioma grows quickly and spreads into nearby tissues. The tumor cells look different from normal cells. Treatment of *oligodendrogliomas* may include the following: • Surgery with or without radiation therapy. Chemotherapy may be given after radiation therapy. Treatment of *anaplastic* (a *term used to describe cancer cells that divide rapidly and have little or no resemblance to normal cells*) oligodendroglioma may include the following: • Surgery followed by radiation therapy with or without chemotherapy. • A clinical trial of a new treatment added to standard treatment.
MIXED GLIOMAS	**MIXED GLIOMAS** Mixed glioma is a brain tumor that has two types of tumor cells in it — **oligodendrocytes** and **astrocytes.** This type of mixed tumor is called oligoastrocytoma. • **Oligoastrocytoma (grade II)**: An oligoastrocytoma is a slow-growing tumor. The tumor cells look something like normal cells. . • **Anaplastic oligoastrocytoma (grade III)**: Anaplastic oligoastrocytoma grows quickly and spreads into nearby tissues. The tumor cells look different from normal cells. This type of tumor has a worse prognosis than oligoastrocytoma (grade II). Treatment of mixed gliomas may include the following: • Surgery and radiation therapy. • Sometimes chemotherapy is also given.
EPENDYMAL TUMORS	**EPENDYMAL TUMORS** An ependymal tumor usually begins in cells that line the fluid-filled spaces in the brain and around the spinal cord. An ependymal tumor may also be called an ependymoma. Grades of ependymomas include the following: • **Ependymoma (grade I or II)**: A grade I or II ependymoma grows slowly and has cells that look something like normal cells. There are two types of grade I ependymoma — myxopapillary ependymoma and subependymoma. A grade II ependymoma grows in a ventricle (fluid-filled space in the brain) and its connecting paths or in the spinal cord. • **Anaplastic ependymoma (grade III)**: An anaplastic ependymoma grows quickly and spreads into nearby tissues. The tumor cells look different from normal cells. This type of tumor usually has a worse prognosis than a grade I or II ependymoma. Treatment of *grade I and grade II* ependymomas may include the following: • Surgery to remove the tumor. • Radiation therapy may also be given if tumor remains after surgery. Treatment of *grade III* anaplastic ependymoma may include the following: • Surgery and radiation therapy.

MEDULLOBLASTOMAS	**MEDULLOBLASTOMAS** • A fast-growing type of cancer that forms in the cerebellum (the lower, back part of the brain). • Medulloblastomas tend to spread through the cerebrospinal fluid to the spinal cord or to other parts of the brain. They may also spread to other parts of the body, but this is rare. • Medulloblastomas are most common in children and young adults. They are a type of central nervous system embryonal tumor. Treatment of medulloblastomas may include the following: • Surgery and radiation therapy to the brain and spine. • A clinical trial of chemotherapy added to surgery and radiation therapy to the brain and spine
PINEAL PARENCHYMAL TUMORS	**PINEAL PARENCHYMAL TUMORS** A pineal parenchymal tumor forms in parenchymal cells or pineocytes, which are the cells that make up most of the pineal gland. These tumors are different from pineal astrocytic tumors. Grades of pineal parenchymal tumors include the following: • **Pineocytoma (grade II)**: A pineocytoma is a slow-growing pineal tumor. • **Pineoblastoma (grade IV)**: A pineoblastoma is a rare tumor that is very likely to spread. Treatment of pineal parenchymal tumors may include the following: • For pineocytomas, surgery and radiation therapy. • For pineoblastomas, surgery, radiation therapy, and chemotherapy.
MENINGEAL TUMORS	**MENINGEAL TUMORS** A meningeal tumor, also called a meningioma, forms in the meninges (thin layers of tissue that cover the brain and spinal cord). It can form from different types of brain or spinal cord cells. Meningiomas are most common in adults. Types of meningeal tumors include the following: • **Meningioma (grade I)**: A grade I meningioma is the most common type of meningeal tumor. A grade I meningioma is a slow-growing tumor. It forms most often in the dura mater. A grade I meningioma may be completely removed by surgery. • **Meningioma (grade II and III)**: This is a rare meningeal tumor. It grows quickly and is likely to spread within the brain and spinal cord. The prognosis is worse than a grade I meningioma because the tumor usually cannot be completely removed by surgery. A hemangiopericytoma is not a meningeal tumor but is treated like a grade II or III meningioma. A hemangiopericytoma usually forms in the dura mater. The prognosis is worse than a grade I meningioma because the tumor usually cannot be completely removed by surgery. Treatment of *grade I* meningiomas may include the following: • Active for tumors with no signs or symptoms. • Surgery to remove the tumor. Radiation therapy may also be given if tumor remains after surgery. • Stereotactic radiosurgery for tumors smaller than 3 centimeters. • Radiation therapy for tumors that cannot be removed by surgery. Treatment of *grade II* and III meningiomas and hemangiopericytomas may include the following: • Surgery and radiation therapy.

GERM CELL TUMORS	**GERM CELL TUMORS** A germ cell tumor forms in germ cells, which are the cells that develop into sperm in men or ova (eggs) in women. There are different types of germ cell tumors. These include germinomas, teratomas, embryonal yolk sac carcinomas, and choriocarcinomas. Germ cell tumors can be either benign or malignant. Treatment: • There is no standard treatment for germ cell tumors (germinoma, embryonal carcinoma, choriocarcinoma, and teratoma). • Treatment depends on what the tumor cells look like under a microscope, the tumor markers, where the tumor is in the brain, and whether it can be removed by surgery.
CRANIOPHARYNGIOMAS	**CRANIOPHARYNGIOMAS** A craniopharyngioma is a rare tumor that usually forms in the center of the brain just above the pituitary gland (a pea-sized organ at the bottom of the brain that controls other glands). Craniopharyngiomas can form from different types of brain or spinal cord cells. • Craniopharyngiomas are slow-growing and do not spread to other parts of the brain or to other parts of the body. However, they may grow and press on nearby parts of the brain, including the pituitary gland, hypothalamus, optic chiasm, optic nerves, and fluid-filled spaces in the brain. This may cause problems with growth, vision, and making certain hormones. • Craniopharyngiomas usually occur in children and young adults. Treatment of craniopharyngiomas may include the following: • Surgery to completely remove the tumor. • Surgery to remove as much of the tumor as possible, followed by radiation therapy.
Other Treatments	**Treatment of Primary Adult Spinal Cord Tumors** Treatment of spinal cord tumors may include the following: • Surgery to remove the tumor. • Radiation therapy. • A clinical trial of a new treatment. **Treatment of Recurrent Adult Central Nervous System Tumors** • There is no standard treatment for recurrent central nervous system (CNS) tumors. • Treatment depends on the patient's condition, the expected side effects of the treatment, where the tumor is in the CNS, and whether the tumor can be removed by surgery. Treatment may include the following: • Chemotherapy placed into the brain during surgery. • Chemotherapy with drugs not used to treat the original tumor. • Targeted therapy for recurrent glioblastoma. • Radiation therapy. • Surgery to remove the tumor. • A clinical trial of a new treatment.

Other Treatments *Continued*	**Treatment of Metastatic Adult Brain Tumors.** Treatment of one to four tumors that have spread to the brain from another part of the body may include the following: • Radiation therapy to the whole brain with or without surgery. • Radiation therapy to the whole brain with or without stereotactic radiosurgery. • Stereotactic radiosurgery. • Chemotherapy, if the primary tumor is one that responds to anticancer drugs. It may be combined with radiation therapy. Treatment of tumors that have spread to the leptomeninges may include the following: • Chemotherapy (systemic and/or intrathecal). • Radiation therapy may also be given. • Supportive care.
Potential Side Effects after Brain Surgery	**Side effects:** • Weakness. • Dizzy spells. • Poor balance or lack of coordination. • Personality or behavior changes. • Confusion. • Problems with your speech. **Other side effects:** • Infections • Bleeding • Seizures • Stoke • Headaches • Neck Stiffness • Brain Swelling • Coma • Brain Damage • Damage to healthy tissues
References	CETI- Cancer Exercise Training Institute: *https://www.thecancerspecialist.com/* National Cancer Institute – NCI - Adult Central Nervous System Tumors Treatment (PDQ®)–Patient Version - *https://www.cancer.gov/types/brain/patient/adult-brain-treatment-pdq#_134*

Recovery after Surgery *Information from CETI-* *Cancer Exercise Training Institute* ***Please follow MD/surgeon protocol, as every situation is unique.***	**Craniotomy** (removal of benign or malignant brain tumor) ➢ **Hospital Stay:** 3-4 days ➢ **Full Recovery:** 4-6 weeks or longer ➢ **Restrictions:** No heavy lifting over 10 lbs. and avoid activities that have a risk of falling for at least 6 weeks. ➢ **Exercise:** Walking **Possible Side Effects from Brain Surgery:** Blockage, infection, Headaches, Neck Stiffness, Vomiting, Brain Bleed, Damage to Healthy Brain Tissue, Memory Issues, Poor Concentration, Behavior or Personality Changes, Weakness, Difficulty Walking, Difficulty with Speech

Exercise, Special Considerations & Precautions – Short and Long Term ***Please follow MD/surgeon protocol, as every situation is unique.***	Depending on the surgery and / or treatment and the area of the brain affected, there may be a risk of **poor balance –** *(see Balance Section)* • Medical clearance – always follow the doctor's or surgeons' recommendations before starting any exercise program. • Start slow – see *balance f*or progression and more information. • Stability – be sure you have something stable nearby, such as the kitchen counter to hold or grab onto if needed • Solid surface – start your balance program on an even surface, such as the kitchen floor • No quick movements – avoid quick head turns, which can throw off your balance • Safety First – when you start your balance or any other type of exercise, if possible, have someone nearby until you feel confident.

COLON / COLORECTAL /RECTAL
Information and pictures from *National Cancer Institute* unless otherwise specified

Description *NCI (Colon & Rectal Cancer) and CDC*	Cancer that forms in the tissues of the colon (the longest part of the large intestine). Most colon cancers are adenocarcinomas (cancers that begin in cells that make and release mucus and other fluids). Rectal cancer is a disease in which malignant (cancer) cells form in the tissues of the rectum. (NCI) Colorectal cancer is a disease in which cells in the colon or rectum grow out of control. Sometimes it is called colon cancer, for short. The colon is the large intestine or large bowel. • The rectum is the passageway that connects the colon to the anus. • Sometimes abnormal growths, called polyps, form in the colon or rectum. Over time, some polyps may turn into cancer. • Screening tests can find polyps so they can be removed before turning into cancer. Screening also helps find colorectal cancer at an early stage when treatment works best. *(Colorectal Cancer – CDC)*

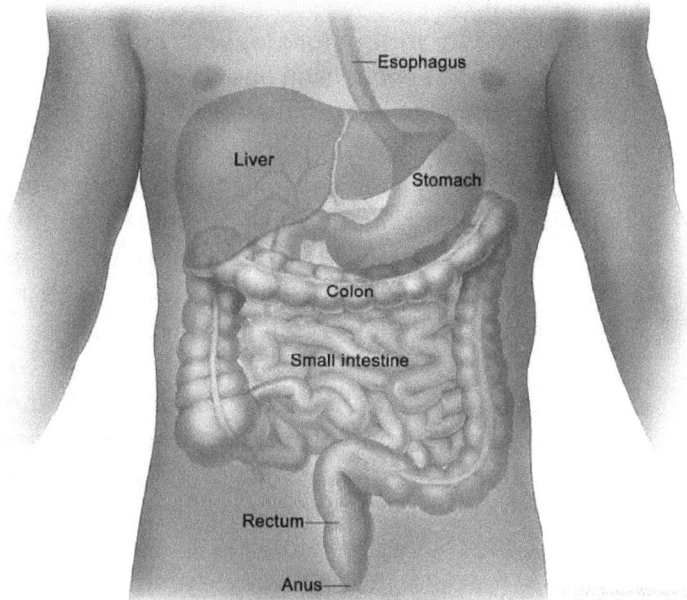

Lower Gastrointestinal Anatomy

The colon is part of the body's digestive system. The digestive system removes and processes nutrients (vitamins, minerals, carbohydrates, fats, proteins, and water) from foods and helps pass waste material out of the body. The digestive system is made up of the esophagus, stomach, and the small and large intestines.

The colon (large bowel) is the first part of the large intestine and is about 5 feet long. Together, the rectum and anal canal make up the last part of the large intestine and are about 6-8 inches long. The anal canal ends at the anus (the opening of the large intestine to the outside of the body). (NCI -colon cancer)

The rectum is part of the body's digestive system. The digestive system takes in nutrients (vitamins, minerals, carbohydrates, fats, proteins, and water) from foods and helps pass waste material out of the body. The digestive system is made up of the esophagus, stomach, and the small and large intestines. The colon (large bowel) is the first part of the large intestine and is about 5 feet long. Together, the rectum and anal canal make up the last part of the large intestine and are 6-8 inches long. The anal canal ends at the anus (the opening of the large intestine to the outside of the body). (NCI-rectal cancer)

COLORECTAL **Risk Factors** *CDC*	Your risk of getting colorectal cancer increases as you get older. Other risk factors include having: • Inflammatory bowel disease such as Crohn's disease or ulcerative colitis. • A personal or family history of colorectal cancer or colorectal polyps. • A genetic syndrome such as familial adenomatous polyposis (FAP)external icon or hereditary non-polyposis colorectal cancer (Lynch syndrome). Lifestyle factors that may contribute to an increased risk of colorectal cancer include— • Lack of regular physical activity. • A diet low in fruit and vegetables. • A low-fiber and high-fat diet, or a diet high in processed meats. • Overweight and obesity. • Alcohol consumption. • Tobacco use. *(Colorectal Cancer – CDC)*

COLORECTAL
 	
Treatment
 	
NCI - Colon Cancer Treatment
 	
Also see treatment for stages of colon cancer
	Surgery - *Also see treatment for stages of colon cancer*
	Surgery (removing the cancer in an operation) is the most common treatment for all stages of colon cancer. A doctor may remove the cancer using one of the following types of surgery:
	
	• **Local excision:** If the cancer is found at a very early stage, the doctor may remove it without cutting through the abdominal wall. Instead, the doctor may put a tube with a cutting tool through the rectum into the colon and cut the cancer out. This is called a local excision. If the cancer is found in a polyp (a small bulging area of tissue), the operation is called a polypectomy.
	
	• **Resection of the colon with anastomosis:** If the cancer is larger, the doctor will perform **a partial colectomy** (removing the cancer and a small amount of healthy tissue around it).
	   o The doctor may then perform an anastomosis (sewing the healthy parts of the colon together).
	   o The doctor will also usually remove lymph nodes near the colon and examine them under a microscope to see whether they contain cancer.
	
	• **Resection of the colon with colostomy:** If the doctor is not able to sew the 2 ends of the colon back together, a stoma (an opening) is made on the outside of the body for waste to pass through. This procedure is called a colostomy. A bag is placed around the stoma to collect the waste.
	   o Sometimes the colostomy is needed only until the lower colon has healed, and then it can be reversed.
	   o If the doctor needs to remove the entire lower colon, however, the colostomy may be permanent.
	
	• After the doctor removes all the cancer that can be seen at the time of the surgery, some patients may be given chemotherapy or radiation therapy after surgery to kill any cancer cells that are left.
	   o Treatment given after the surgery, to lower the risk that the cancer will come back, is called adjuvant therapy.

COLORECTAL **Treatment** *Continued*	**Radiofrequency ablation:** Radiofrequency ablation is the use of a special probe with tiny electrodes that kill cancer cells. • Sometimes the probe is inserted directly through the skin and only local anesthesia is needed. • In other cases, the probe is inserted through an incision in the abdomen. This is done in the hospital with general anesthesia. **Cryosurgery:** Cryosurgery is a treatment that uses an instrument to freeze and destroy abnormal tissue. • This type of treatment is also called cryotherapy. **Chemotherapy:** Chemoembolization of the hepatic artery may be used to treat cancer that has spread to the liver. • This involves blocking the hepatic artery (the main artery that supplies blood to the liver) and injecting anticancer drugs between the blockage and the liver. • The liver's arteries then deliver the drugs throughout the liver. • Only a small amount of the drug reaches other parts of the body. • The blockage may be temporary or permanent, depending on what is used to block the artery. • The liver continues to receive some blood from the hepatic portal vein, which carries blood from the stomach and intestine.

Treatment for stages of colon cancer
 	
Pictures and information from the **National Cancer Institute: Colon Cancer Treatment**
	Stage 0 (Carcinoma in Situ)
	Abnormal cells are found in the mucosa (innermost layer) of the colon and/or rectal wall. These abnormal cells may become cancer and spread into nearby normal tissue.
	
	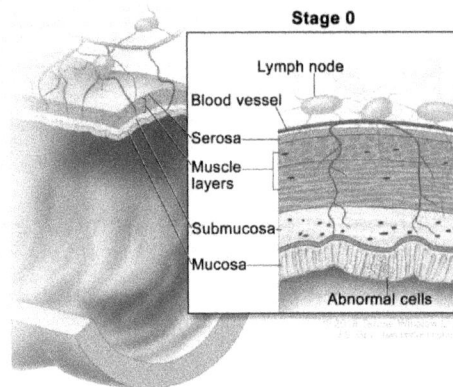
	
	Treatment of stage 0 (carcinoma in situ) may include the following types of surgery:
	• Local excision or simple polypectomy.
	  ○ **Local excision:** The removal of tissue from the body using a scalpel (a sharp knife), laser, or another cutting tool. A surgical excision is usually done to remove a lump or other suspicious growth. Some normal tissue around the lump is usually removed at the same time.
	  ○ **Simple polypectomy**: Surgery to remove a polyp
	• Resection and anastomosis. This is done when the tumor is too large to remove by local excision.
	  ○ **Resection:** Surgery to remove tissue or part or all of an organ.
	  ○ **Anastomosis:** A procedure to connect healthy sections of tubular structures in the body after the diseased portion has been surgically removed.
	
	Stage I Colon Cancer
	Cancer has formed in the mucosa (innermost layer) of the colon and/or rectum wall and has spread to the submucosa (layer of tissue next to the mucosa) or to the muscle layer of the colon and/or rectum wall. Also called Dukes A colorectal cancer.
	
	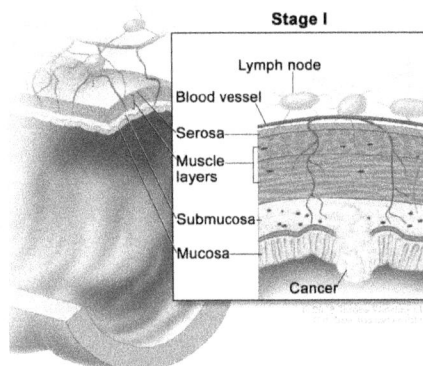
	
	Treatment of stage I colon cancer usually includes the following:
	• Resection and anastomosis. This is done when the tumor is too large to remove by local excision.
	  ○ **Resection:** Surgery to remove tissue or part or all of an organ.
	  ○ **Anastomosis:** A procedure to connect healthy sections of tubular structures in the body after the diseased portion has been surgically removed.

Treatment for stages of colon cancer
 	
Continued
	Stage II Colon Cancer
	Stage II colorectal cancer is divided into stages IIA, IIB, and IIC.
	• **In stage IIA,** cancer has spread through the muscle layer of the colon and/or rectum wall to the serosa (outermost layer) of the colon and/or rectum wall.
	• **In stage IIB,** cancer has spread through the serosa of the colon and/or rectum wall to the tissue that lines the organs in the abdomen (visceral peritoneum).
	• **In stage IIC,** cancer has spread through the serosa of the colon and/or rectum wall to nearby organs.
	
	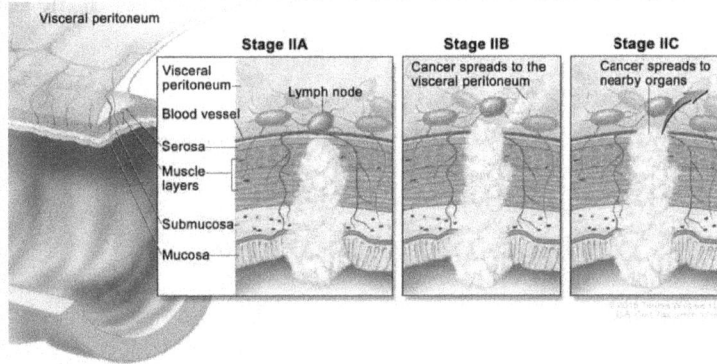
	
	Treatment of stage II colon cancer may include the following:
	• Resection and anastomosis. This is done when the tumor is too large to remove by local excision.
	    ○ **Resection:** Surgery to remove tissue or part or all of an organ.
	    ○ **Anastomosis:** A procedure to connect healthy sections of tubular structures in the body after the diseased portion has been surgically removed.
	
	Stage III Colon Cancer
	Stage III colorectal cancer is divided into stages IIIA, IIIB, and IIIC.
	
	In stage IIIA, cancer has spread:
	• Through the mucosa (innermost layer) of the colon wall to the submucosa (layer of tissue next to the mucosa) or to the muscle layer of the colon wall. Cancer has spread to one to three nearby lymph nodes or cancer cells have formed in tissue near the lymph nodes; or
	• Through the mucosa (innermost layer) of the colon wall to the submucosa (layer of tissue next to the mucosa). Cancer has spread to four to six nearby lymph nodes.
	
	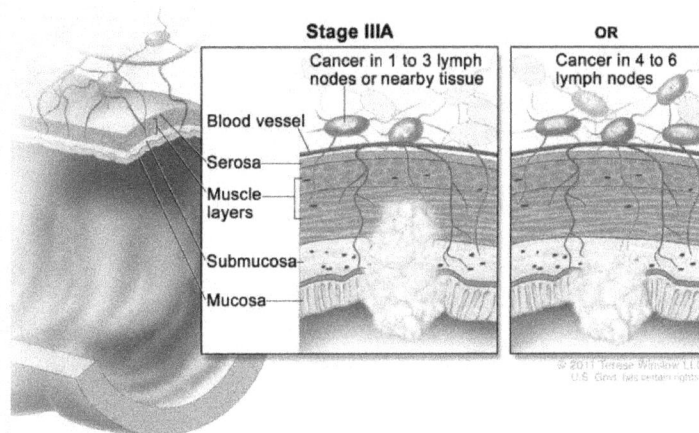

Treatment for stages of colon cancer *Continued*	*In stage IIIB, cancer has spread:* • Through the muscle layer of the colon wall to the serosa (outermost layer) of the colon wall or has spread through the serosa to the tissue that lines the organs in the abdomen (visceral peritoneum). Cancer has spread to one to three nearby lymph nodes or cancer cells have formed in tissue near the lymph nodes; **or** • To the muscle layer or to the serosa (outermost layer) of the colon wall. Cancer has spread to four to six nearby lymph nodes; **or** • Through the mucosa (innermost layer) of the colon wall to the submucosa (layer of tissue next to the mucosa) or to the muscle layer of the colon wall. Cancer has spread to seven or more nearby lymph nodes. 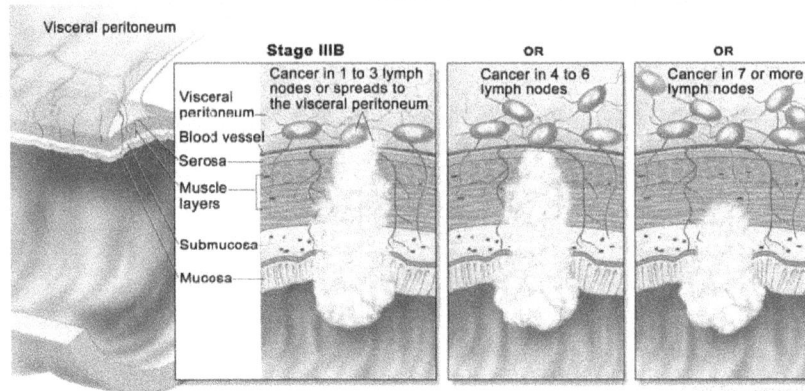 *In stage IIIC, cancer has spread:* • Through the serosa (outermost layer) of the colon wall to the tissue that lines the organs in the abdomen (visceral peritoneum). Cancer has spread to four to six nearby lymph nodes; **or** • Through the muscle layer of the colon wall to the serosa (outermost layer) of the colon wall or has spread through the serosa to the tissue that lines the organs in the abdomen (visceral peritoneum). Cancer has spread to seven or more nearby lymph nodes; **or** • Through the serosa (outermost layer) of the colon wall to nearby organs. Cancer has spread to one or more nearby lymph nodes or cancer cells have formed in tissue near the lymph nodes. 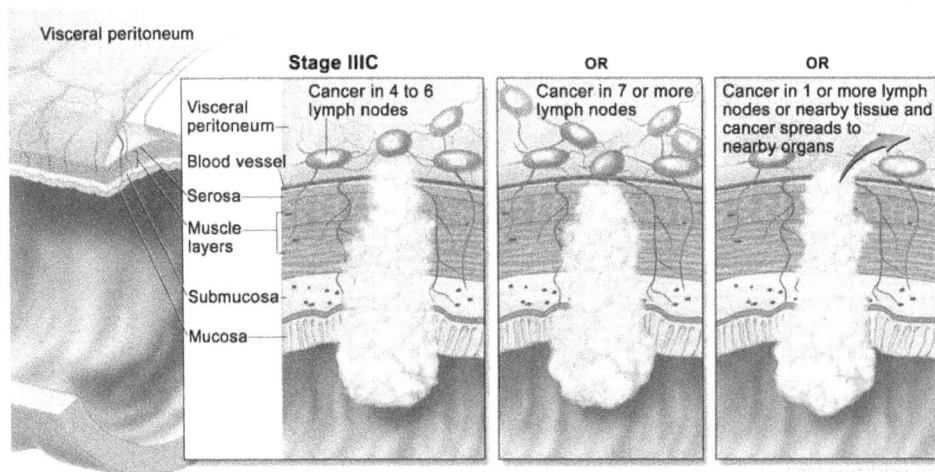

Treatment for stages of colon cancer
 	
Continued
	Treatment of **stage III** colon cancer may include the following:
	• Resection and anastomosis which may be followed by chemotherapy.
	    ○ **Resection:** Surgery to remove tissue or part or all of an organ.
	    ○ **Anastomosis:** A procedure to connect healthy sections of tubular structures in the body after the diseased portion has been surgically removed.
	    ○ **Chemotherapy:** Treatment that uses drugs to stop the growth of cancer cells, either by killing the cells or by stopping them from dividing.
	        ○ Chemotherapy may be given by mouth, injection, or infusion, or on the skin, depending on the type and stage of the cancer being treated.
	        ○ It may be given alone or with other treatments, such as surgery, radiation therapy, or biologic therapy.
	
	Stage IV and Recurrent Colon Cancer
	Stage IV colorectal cancer is divided into stages IVA, IVB, and IVC.
	• **In stage IVA**, cancer has spread to one area or organ that is not near the colon and/or rectum, such as the liver, lung, ovary, or a distant lymph node.
	• **In stage IVB**, cancer has spread to more than one area or organ that is not near the colon and/or rectum, such as the liver, lung, ovary, or a distant lymph node.
	• **In stage IVC,** cancer has spread to the tissue that lines the wall of the abdomen and may have spread to other areas or organs.
	
	Stage IV
	
	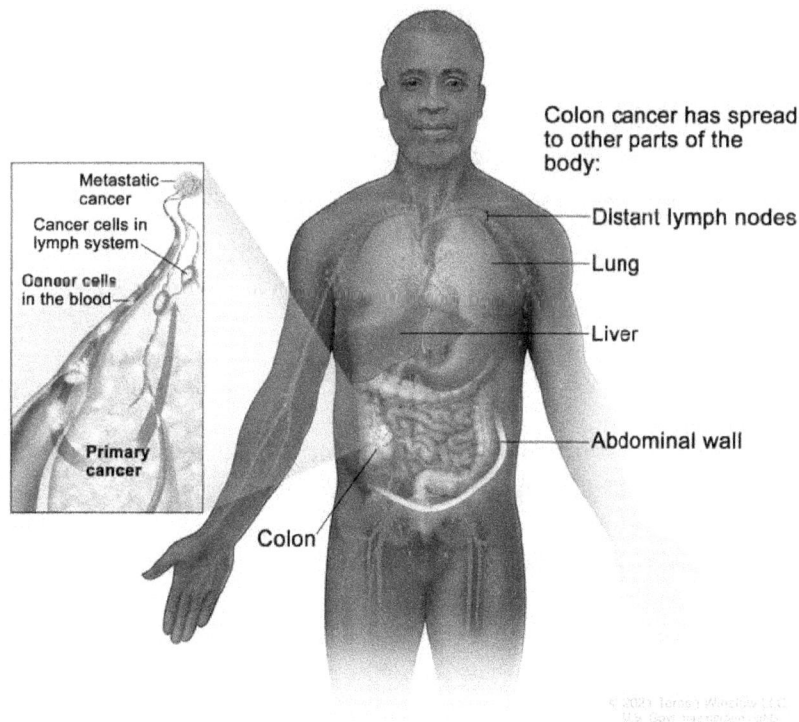

Treatment for stages of colon cancer
 	
Continued
	Treatment of **stage IV** and recurrent colon cancer may include the following:
	• **Local excision** for tumors that have recurred.
	• **Resection** with or without anastomosis.
	• **Surgery to remove parts of other organs**, such as the liver, lungs, and ovaries, where the cancer may have recurred or spread. Treatment of cancer that has spread to the liver may also include the following:
	    ○ Chemotherapy is given before surgery to shrink the tumor, after surgery, or both before and after.
	    ○ Radiofrequency ablation or cryosurgery, for patients who cannot have surgery.
	    ○ Chemoembolization of the hepatic artery.
	• **Radiation therapy** or chemotherapy may be offered to some patients as palliative therapy to relieve symptoms and improve quality of life.
	• **Chemotherapy** and/or targeted therapy with a monoclonal antibody or an angiogenesis inhibitor.
	• **Targeted therapy** with a protein kinase inhibitor and a monoclonal antibody in patients with a certain change in the BRAF gene.
	• **Immunotherapy.**
	• **Clinical trials** of chemotherapy and/or targeted therapy.

COLORECTAL **Possible Side Effects** *WebMD*	**Colostomy:** attaches the end of your colon to an opening in your belly, where waste will leave your body. Some people only need to use a pouch while they heal from surgery. • Once the colostomy is removed, you can use the bathroom normally again. **Ileostomy:** If there isn't enough colon left, the end of your small intestine will be attached to the opening. • You'll wear a pouch on the outside of your body to collect waste. **After surgery**, you might be in some pain. • Some people have bowel problems like constipation or diarrhea. These side effects often go away. • It might take a few weeks or months for your bowel habits to get back to normal after surgery. • If the **tumor blocks your colon**, the surgeon could put in a tube called a stent to keep the bowel open. ○ You'll get that stent put in during a colonoscopy. *(WebMD)*
RECTAL **Risk Factors** *NIH - Rectal Cancer Treatment* *Also see Colon/ Colorectal in previous section*	**Risk factors for colorectal cancer include the following:** • Having a family history of colon or rectal cancer in a first-degree relative (parent, sibling, or child). • Having a personal history of cancer of the colon, rectum, or ovary. • Having a personal history of high-risk adenomas (colorectal polyps that are 1 centimeter or larger in size or that have cells that look abnormal under a microscope). • Having inherited changes in certain genes that increase the risk of familial adenomatous polyposis (FAP) or Lynch syndrome (hereditary nonpolyposis colorectal cancer). • Having a personal history of chronic ulcerative colitis or Crohn disease for 8 years or more. • Having three or more alcoholic drinks per day. • Smoking cigarettes. • Being Black. • Being obese. • Older age is a main risk factor for most cancers. The chance of getting cancer increases as you get older. *(Rectal Cancer Treatment –NCI)*

RECTAL **Treatment** *NIH - Rectal Cancer Treatment*	Active surveillance Radiation therapy Targeted therapy **Surgery:** Surgery is the most common treatment for all stages of rectal cancer. The cancer is removed using one of the following types of surgery: <ul><li>**Polypectomy:** If the cancer is found in a polyp (a small piece of bulging tissue), the polyp is often removed during a colonoscopy.</li><li>**Local excision:** If the cancer is found on the inside surface of the rectum and has not spread into the wall of the rectum, the cancer and a small amount of surrounding healthy tissue is removed.</li><li>**Resection:** If the cancer has spread into the wall of the rectum, the section of the rectum with cancer and nearby healthy tissue is removed. Sometimes the tissue between the rectum and the abdominal wall is also removed. The lymph nodes near the rectum are removed and checked under a microscope for signs of cancer.</li><li>**Radiofrequency ablation:** The use of a special probe with tiny electrodes that kill cancer cells. Sometimes the probe is inserted directly through the skin and only local anesthesia is needed. In other cases, the probe is inserted through an incision in the abdomen. This is done in the hospital with general anesthesia.</li><li>**Cryosurgery:** A treatment that uses an instrument to freeze and destroy abnormal tissue. This type of treatment is also called cryotherapy.</li><li>**Pelvic exenteration:** If the cancer has spread to other organs near the rectum, the lower colon, rectum, and bladder are removed.<ul><li>In women, the cervix, vagina, ovaries, and nearby lymph nodes may be removed.</li><li>In men, the prostate may be removed.</li><li>Artificial openings (stoma) are made for urine and stool to flow from the body to a collection bag.</li></ul></li></ul>After the cancer is removed, the surgeon will either: <ul><li>Do an *anastomosis* (sew the healthy parts of the rectum together, sew the remaining rectum to the colon, or sew the colon to the anus)</li><li>Make a *stoma* (an opening) from the rectum to the outside of the body for waste to pass through.<ul><li>This procedure is done if the cancer is too close to the anus and is called a *colostomy*.</li><li>A bag is placed around the stoma to collect the waste.</li><li>Sometimes the colostomy is needed only until the rectum has healed, and then it can be reversed.</li><li>If the entire rectum is removed, however, the colostomy may be permanent.</li></ul></li></ul>**Chemotherapy:** Chemoembolization of the hepatic artery is a type of regional chemotherapy that may be used to treat cancer that has spread to the liver. <ul><li>This is done by blocking the hepatic artery (the main artery that supplies blood to the liver) and injecting anticancer drugs between the blockage and the liver.</li></ul>

RECTAL **Possible Side Effects** *American Cancer Society*	**Surgery:** • Rarely, the new connections between the ends of the colon may not hold together and may leak. • You may develop scar tissue in your abdomen that can cause organs or tissues to stick together. • Some people need a temporary or permanent colostomy (or ileostomy) **Radiation:** • Skin irritation at the site where radiation beams were aimed, which can range from redness to blistering and peeling • Problems with wound healing if radiation was given before surgery • Rectal irritation, which can cause diarrhea, painful bowel movements, or blood in the stool • Bowel incontinence (stool leakage) • Bladder irritation, which can cause problems like feeling like you have to go often, burning or pain while urinating, or blood in the urine • Sexual problems (erection issues in men and vaginal irritation in women) • Scarring, fibrosis (stiffening), and adhesions *(American Cancer Society)*
References	American Cancer Society – Rectal Cancer: *https://www.cancer.org/cancer/colon-rectal-cancer/treating/radiation-therapy.html* CDC – Center for Disease Control: Colorectal Cancer: *https://www.cdc.gov/cancer/colorectal/basic_info/what-is-colorectal-cancer.htm* CETI- Cancer Exercise Training Institute: *https://www.thecancerspecialist.com/* NCI - National Cancer Institute: Colon Cancer Treatment: *https://www.cancer.gov/types/colorectal/patient/colon-treatment-pdq#_320* NCI - National Cancer Institute Rectal Cancer Treatment *https://www.cancer.gov/types/colorectal/patient/rectal-treatment-pdq* WebMD – Colon/Rectal Cancer - *https://www.webmd.com/colorectal-cancer/colon-cancer-liver-metastasis-treatment#1*

Recovery after Surgery *Information from CETI-* *Cancer Exercise* *Training Institute* ***Please follow MD/surgeon protocol, as every situation is unique.***	**Total Colectomy:** ➢ **Hospital Stay:** A few days up to a week until bowel function is regained ➢ **Full Recovery:** Several weeks ➢ **Restrictions:** No heavy lifting over 10 lbs. for 1-2 months ➢ **Exercise:** Walking **Colostomy and Ileostomy:** ➢ **Hospital Stay:** 3-10 Days ➢ **Full Recovery:** 6-8 weeks ➢ **Restrictions:** No heavy lifting over 3 lbs., no strenuous exercises for 12 weeks ➢ **Exercise:** Walking **Proctectomy** (removal of the rectum): ➢ **Hospital Stay:** 4-7 days ➢ **Full Recovery:** May take 6-8 weeks ➢ **Restrictions:** No heavy lifting over 3 lbs., no strenuous exercises for 6 weeks ➢ **Exercise:** Walking **Low anterior resection:** ➢ **Hospital Stay:** 4-6 days ➢ **Full Recovery:** 3-6 weeks ➢ **Restrictions:** No heavy lifting over 10 lbs. or strenuous exercise for at least 6 weeks. ➢ **Exercise:** Walking and Kegel exercises soon after surgery (*see Kegel*) **Abdominoperineal resection:** ➢ **Hospital Stay:** Several Days ➢ **Full Recovery:** 3-6 weeks; women 6 months or more. ➢ **Restrictions:** No heavy lifting over 10 lbs. or strenuous exercise for at least 6 weeks. ➢ **Exercise:** Walking **Total meso-rectal excision (TME):** ➢ **Hospital Stay:** Several Days ➢ **Full Recovery:** 3-6 weeks ➢ **Exercise:** Pelvic floor muscle exercises 2-3 weeks after the stoma closes.

Recovery after Surgery
 	
Continued
	Pelvic exenteration (lower colon, rectum and bladder removed)**:**
	• **Women** – also cervix, ovaries, vagina & nearby lymph nodes may be removed – *also see endometrial cancer.*
	• **Men** – Prostate may be removed – *also see prostate cancer.*
	➢ **Hospital Stay:** (women) 7-10 days
	➢ **Full Recovery:** 3 months
	➢ **Restrictions:** No lifting over 10 lbs. for the first 6 weeks, bending, stretching.
	    o Women: According to CETI "If vaginal reconstruction is done, patients will only be able to lie on their back side or stand; they will be unable to sit for 6-8 weeks" or riding a bike.
	    o Avoid crunches, planks, sit-ups or high impact exercises
	➢ **Exercise:** Walking and Deep Breathing
	➢ **Possible Side Effects:** Lower Extremity Lymphedema, Blood Clots (Legs or Lungs), Deterioration of Muscle Flap, Injury to the Spleen, Instant Menopause in Women
	
	Proctectomy with Colo-Anal anastomosis:
	➢ **Hospital Stay:** Several Days
	➢ **Full Recovery:** 6-8 weeks
	➢ **Restrictions:** No heavy lifting over 3 lbs. or strenuous exercise for at least 6 weeks.
	➢ **Exercise:** Pelvic floor muscle exercises 2-3 weeks after the stoma closes.
	➢ **Possible Side Effects:** Obstruction, Peritonitis, Abscess, Sepsis, Parastomal Herniation, Anastomotic Leak

Exercise, Special Considerations & Precautions – Short and Long Term
 	
Please follow MD/surgeon protocol, as every situation is unique.
	• **Exercise**: Walking during recovery period for most patients – see MD protocol
	• Avoid weightlifting or sit ups until cleared by MD
	• **Ostomy** – Avoid contact sports and swimming – may need modifications.
	    o Avoid anything that causes intra-abdominal pressure or weightlifting due to risk of "blow" or hernia until cleared by MD
	• **Stoma** – To avoid hernia, start with low resistance and progress slowly
	• **Abdominoperineal resection:**
	    o If prostate removed – see Prostate Cancer
	    o If hysterectomy – see Endometrial Cancer
	• **Lymph Nodes removed or radiation** – See Lower Extremity lymphedema
	• **In what direction Is the incision** – For example, if it is vertical – avoid crunches, as you will most likely already be in a forward flexed position and need to work on stretches or extension.

ENDOMETRIAL
Information and pictures from *National Cancer Institute* unless otherwise specified

Description	Endometrial cancer is a disease in which malignant (cancer) cells form in the tissues of the endometrium. • *The endometrium is the lining of the uterus, a hollow, muscular organ in a woman's pelvis.* • *The uterus is where a fetus grows. In most nonpregnant women, the uterus is about 3 inches long.* • *The lower, narrow end of the uterus is the cervix, which leads to the vagina.* **Female Reproductive System** *The organs in the female reproductive system include the uterus, ovaries, fallopian tubes, cervix, and vagina. The uterus has a muscular outer layer called the myometrium and an inner lining called the endometrium.*

Risk Factors	• Taking tamoxifen for breast cancer or taking estrogen alone (without progesterone)
	 • Taking estrogen-only hormone replacement therapy (HRT) after menopause.
	 • Obesity.
	 • Having metabolic syndrome.
	 • Having type 2 diabetes.
	 • Exposure of endometrial tissue to estrogen made by the body. This may be caused by:
	     ○ Never giving birth.
	     ○ Menstruating at an early age.
	     ○ Starting menopause at a later age.
	 • Having polycystic ovarian syndrome.
	 • Having a family history of endometrial cancer in a first-degree relative (mother, sister, or daughter).
	 • Having certain genetic conditions, such as Lynch syndrome.
	 • Having endometrial hyperplasia.
	 • The chance of getting cancer increases as you get older.

Treatment	**Chemotherapy**
	Hormone therapy
	Radiation therapy
	Targeted therapy
	
	Surgery
	Surgery (removing the cancer in an operation) is the most common treatment for endometrial cancer. The following surgical procedures may be used:
	• **Total hysterectomy:** Surgery to remove the uterus, including the cervix.
	    o If the uterus and cervix are taken out through the vagina, the operation is called a **vaginal hysterectomy.**
	    o If the uterus and cervix are taken out through a large incision (cut) in the abdomen, the operation is called a total **abdominal hysterectomy**.
	    o If the uterus and cervix are taken out through a small incision (cut) in the abdomen using a laparoscope, the operation is called a total **laparoscopic hysterectomy.**
	• **Bilateral salpingo-oophorectomy:** Surgery to remove both ovaries and both fallopian tubes.
	• **Radical hysterectomy:** Surgery to remove the uterus, cervix, and part of the vagina. The ovaries, fallopian tubes, or nearby lymph nodes may also be removed.
	• **Lymph node dissection:** A surgical procedure in which the lymph nodes are removed from the pelvic area and a sample of tissue is checked under a microscope for signs of cancer. This procedure is also called **lymphadenectomy.**
	
	After the doctor removes all the cancer that can be seen at the time of the surgery, *some patients may be given radiation therapy or hormone treatment after surgery to kill any cancer cells that are left.*

Tumor Debulking *NCI (Tumor Debulking)* and *CETI*	**Tumor Debulking** – *NCI* Surgical removal of as much of a tumor as possible. Debulking may increase the chance that chemotherapy or radiation therapy will kill all the tumor cells. It may also be done to relieve symptoms or help the patient live longer. *(NCI –Tumor Debulking)* **Laparotomy / Tumor Debulking** - *CETI* This may include removal of the spleen, gallbladder, part of the stomach, liver and/or pancreas. If any of these organs are removed or damaged, please see side effects and recovery in addition to main surgery. **Side Effects:** *CETI* • Upper and Lower Extremity Lymphedema • Adhesions • Constipation and Bladder Issues ***If part or all of the following are removed or damaged:*** • Stomach – Digestive problems – see Stomach Cancer • Lung – Respiratory problems – see Lung Cancer • Liver – see Liver Cancer • Pancreas – Diabetes - see Pancreatic Cancer • Spleen – Immunocompromised • Ovaries – Menopause

Possible Side Effects *Cancer Support Community*	**Hysterectomy:** • Menstrual periods stop and can no longer get pregnant. • Menopause starts immediately if ovaries are removed. • Hot flashes and other symptoms of menopause may be worse than naturally occurring. • May affect sexual intimacy. **Lymph Node Dissection:** • Lower extremity lymphedema **Radiation Therapy** • May include fatigue, nausea, vomiting, diarrhea, or other problems with digestion. • Some women may have dryness, itching, tightening, and burning in the vagina. • Doctors may advise their patients not to have intercourse during radiation therapy. **Hormonal Therapy Progesterone:** • May retain fluid, have an increased appetite, and gain weight. • Women who are still menstruating may have changes in their periods. *Cancer Support Community*
References	Cancer Support Commun6ity – Endometrial Cancer: *https://www.cancersupportcommunity.org/endometrial-cancer* CETI- Cancer Exercise Training Institute: *https://www.thecancerspecialist.com/* NCI - National Cancer Institute - Endometrial Cancer: *https://www.cancer.gov/types/uterine* NCI – National Cancer Institute - Tumor Debulking – Definition: *https://www.cancer.gov/search/results?swKeyword=debulking*

Recovery after Surgery
 	
Information from **CETI-** *Cancer Exercise Training Institute*
 	
Please follow MD/surgeon protocol, as every situation is unique.
	Laparoscopic hysterectomy:
	➢ **Hospital Stay:** Same day
	➢ **Full Recovery:** 1-2 weeks
	  Restrictions: No heavy lifting over 10 lbs. for 6- 8 weeks.
	    o No intercourse for 8-12 weeks.
	➢ **Exercise:** Walking
	
	Vaginal hysterectomy:
	➢ **Hospital Stay:** 3-7 days
	➢ **Full Recovery:** 6-8 weeks
	➢ **Restrictions:** 6-8 weeks
	    o No heavy lifting over 10 lbs.
	    o Avoid sit-ups, crunches, planks and high impact activities
	    o No intercourse for 8-12 weeks.
	➢ **Exercise:** Walking and pelvic floor exercises *(see Kegel under Bladder)*
	
	Abdominal Radical hysterectomy:
	➢ **Hospital Stay:** 5-7 days
	➢ **Full Recovery:** 6-8 weeks
	➢ **Restrictions:** 6-8 weeks
	    o No heavy lifting over 10 lbs.
	    o Avoid sit-ups, crunches, planks and high impact activities
	    o No intercourse for 8-12 weeks.
	➢ **Exercise:** Walking and pelvic floor exercises *(see Kegel under Bladder)*
	➢ **Potential Side Effects of Hysterectomy:** Unusual Bleeding, Wound Infection, Damage to Urinary/Intestinal System, Pelvic Pain, Lower Extremity Edema
	
	Laparotomy / Tumor Debulking:
	➢ **Hospital Stay:** 3-7 days
	➢ **Full Recovery:** 10-12 weeks
	➢ **Restrictions:** 6-8 weeks
	    o No heavy lifting over 10 lbs.
	    o Avoid sit-ups, crunches, planks and high impact activities
	➢ **Exercise:** Walking and pelvic floor exercises *(see Kegel under Bladder)*

Exercise, Special Considerations & Precautions – Short and Long Term
 	
Please follow MD/surgeon protocol, as every situation is unique.
	• Walk and stretch as soon as your doctor says it is OK.
	• Don't lift anything heavier than 5-10 pounds for the full recovery period.
	• Engage in abdominal exercises only after the *full recovery period*.
	• Lymph Node Removal – Risk of Lower Extremity lymphedema. *(See Lymphedema)*
	• Swelling of the abdomen is from fluid retention and abdominal gas and can last sometimes up to six months after the hysterectomy.
	• Menopausal Women – Increased risk of Osteoporosis
	• Avoid the following cleared from MD
	    o High impact exercises such as running, jumping, burpees. High impact activities may also cause pelvic organ prolapse when the pelvic muscles have not been able to regain most of their pre- operative strength.
	    o Abdominal exercises such as sit ups, crunches, planks
	    o Heavily loaded resistance exercises that require you to hold your breath or grunt to lift.
	        ▪ This includes intense abdominal exertion, stretching or putting extra pressure on the pelvic floor for at least 6 to 8 weeks after your surgery.
	        ▪ Heavy lifting will increase the pressure in the abdominal area and put extra tension on the healing wound.

	Examples of Exercise or Stretches after Hysterectomy – IF allowed – follow MD protocol
Pelvic Floor Elevator	• Start by lying on your back, with knees bent and feet flat. Take a gentle inhaled breath for 3-4 seconds, breathing into your ribcage and tummy,and gently exhale through pursed lips for 5 seconds. • Think of your pelvic floor like an elevator, withclosing doors and a G floor, and 1st floor. • Start your pelvic floor contraction by 'closing the elevator doors' (squeeze around anus and urethra like you are trying to stop the flow of urine) • Then, feel a gentle lift of the pelvic floor elevator up • to the 1st floor.
Point Tummy Vacuum	• Get on your hands and knees. • Position your shoulders right above your hands and your hips above the knees. • While you take a deep breath, you let your belly hang to the ground. Next, you exhale and pull your stomach in as far as you can. • Hold this position for 10 seconds and relax for 5 seconds. you can start with 6 to 8 repetitions.
Head sit-up	• Lie down with your knees bent and your arms crossed over your stomach or folded in back of your head. • Use your hands to gently pull your abdominal muscles together and raise your head and point your chin toward your chest. • Hold the position for 3 to 5 seconds and slowly return your head to the starting position. • Relax and repeat the movement.
Targeted Breathing Exercises	Take long, slow breaths, completely filling the lungs, belly and rib cage before slowly exhaling.
Kegel	See Kegel
Lymphedema	If lymph nodes were removed or had radiation, please see lymphedema section.

KIDNEY - Renal Cell
Information and pictures from *National Cancer Institute* unless otherwise specified

Description	Renal cell cancer is the most common type of kidney cancer. Renal cell cancer (also called kidney cancer or renal cell adenocarcinoma) is a disease in which malignant (cancer) cells are found in the lining of tubules (very small tubes) in the kidney It begins in the lining of the renal tubules in the kidney. The renal tubules filter the blood and produce urine. Also called hypernephroma, renal cell adenocarcinoma, and renal cell carcinoma. *There are 2 kidneys, one on each side of the backbone, above the waist. Tiny tubules in the kidneys filter and clean the blood. They take out waste products and make urine. The urine passes from each kidney through a long tube called a ureter into the bladder. The bladder holds the urine until it passes through the urethra and leaves the body.*
Risk Factors	**Risk Factors for Kidney Cancer:** • Smoking. • Misusing certain pain medicines, including over-the-counter pain medicines, for a long time. • Being overweight. • Having high blood pressure. • Having a family history of renal cell cancer. • Having certain genetic conditions, such as von Hippel-Lindau disease or hereditary papillary renal cell carcinoma.

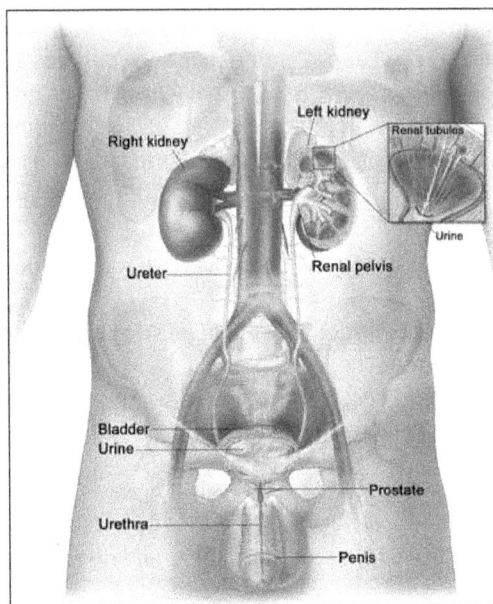

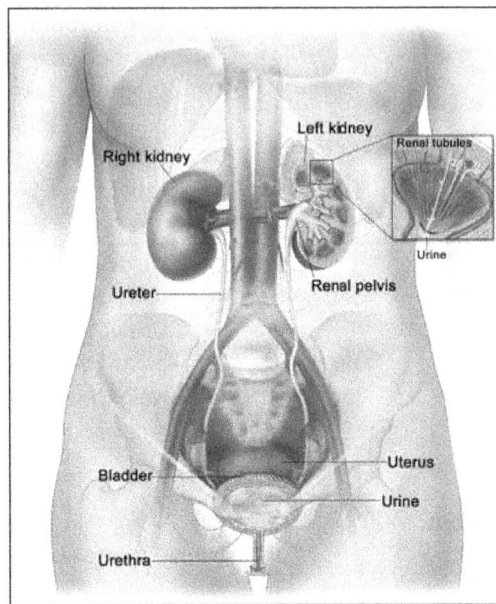

Treatment	Chemotherapy Radiation therapy Targeted therapy **Surgery:** Surgery to remove part or all of the kidney is often used to treat renal cell cancer. The following types of surgery may be used: • **Partial nephrectomy**: A surgical procedure to remove the cancer within the kidney and some of the tissue around it. 　○ A partial nephrectomy may be done to prevent loss of kidney function when the other kidney is damaged or has already been removed. • **Simple nephrectomy:** A surgical procedure to remove the kidney only. • **Radical nephrectomy:** A surgical procedure to remove the kidney, the adrenal gland, surrounding tissue, and, usually, nearby lymph nodes. **Arterial embolization:** When surgery to remove the cancer is not possible, a treatment called arterial embolization may be used to shrink the tumor. • A small incision is made, and a catheter (thin tube) is inserted into the main blood vessel that flows to the kidney. Small pieces of a special gelatin sponge are injected through the catheter into the blood vessel. • The sponges block the blood flow to the kidney and prevent the cancer cells from getting oxygen and other substances they need to grow. After the doctor removes all the cancer that can be seen at the time of the surgery, *some patients may be given chemotherapy or radiation therapy after surgery to kill any cancer cells that are left*. Treatment given after the surgery, to lower the risk that the cancer will come back, is called adjuvant therapy. **Biologic therapy:** The following types of biologic therapy are being used or studied in the treatment of renal cell cancer: • **Nivolumab:** Nivolumab is a monoclonal antibody that boosts the body's immune response against renal cell cancer cells. • **Interferon:** Interferon affects the division of cancer cells and can slow tumor growth. • **Interleukin-2 (IL-2):** IL-2 boosts the growth and activity of many immune cells, especially lymphocytes (a type of white blood cell). Lymphocytes can attack and kill cancer cells.

Possible Side Effects	**Possible Side Effects** A person can live with part of one working kidney, but if both kidneys are removed or not working, the person will need dialysis (a procedure to clean the blood using a machine outside of the body – *see below*)) or a *kidney transplant* (replacement with a healthy donated kidney). **Kidney transplant:** This may be done when the disease is in the kidney only and a donated kidney can be found. If the patient must wait for a donated kidney, other treatment is given as needed. **Dialysis:** The process of removing blood from an artery (as of a patient affected with kidney failure), purifying it by dialysis, adding vital substances, and returning it to a vein — also called hemodialysis. **Surgery:** • Infection • Pain • Bleeding • Potential Kidney failure **Biological therapy:** • Fluid buildup in the lungs • Difficulty breathing • Kidney damage • Intestinal bleeding • Rapid heartbeat
References	CETI- Cancer Exercise Training Institute: *https://www.thecancerspecialist.com/* National Cancer Institute – Kidney Cancer: *https://www.cancer.gov/types/kidney* National Cancer Institute - Renal Cell Cancer Treatment *https://www.cancer.gov/types/kidney/patient/kidney-treatment-pdq*

Recovery after Surgery
 	
Information from **CETI-** *Cancer Exercise Training Institute*
 	
Please follow MD/surgeon protocol, as every situation is unique.
	Open Nephrectomy:
	➤ **Hospital Stay:** Up to one week
	➤ **Full Recovery:** 3-6 weeks
	➤ **Restrictions:** No heavy lifting or strenuous activities for 6 weeks.
	➤ **Permanent Contraindications**: Those with *one* kidney should avoid high impact sports such as:
	    ○ Hockey, football, martial arts, boxing/sparring, skiing, soccer, wrestling, etc.
	    ○ If participating use extra protective padding.
	➤ **Exercise:** Walking
	➤ **Possible Side Effects:** Bleeding, Infection, Pneumonia, Incisional Hernia, Kidney Failure
	  • Lymphedema if lymph nodes are removed
	  • Damage to internal organs, such as:
	    ○ Spleen – Immunocompromised
	    ○ Pancreas – See Pancreatic Cancer
	    ○ Bowels, Aorta or Vena Cava
	  • Radical Nephrectomy: Removal of the adrenal gland (fight or flight) resulting in low energy.

Exercise, Special Considerations & Precautions – Short and Long Term ***Please follow MD/surgeon protocol, as every situation is unique.***	• Avoid exercises that use your abdominal muscles and strenuous activities such as bicycle riding, jogging, weightlifting, or aerobic exercise until your doctor says it is okay. • For at least 6 weeks, avoid lifting anything that would make you strain. • Hold a pillow over the cuts the doctor made (incisions) when you cough or take deep breaths. This will support your belly and decrease your pain. • Do breathing exercises at home as instructed by your doctor. This will help prevent pneumonia. • Absolutely no heavy lifting or exercising (jogging, swimming, treadmill, biking) for six weeks or until instructed by your doctor. • Transplant recipients can engage in virtually any type of exercise or sport. ○ ***Those sports that regularly involve direct blows to the kidney are discouraged.***

LEUKEMIA (CLL & AML)

Information and pictures from *National Cancer Institute* unless otherwise specified

Description	**CLL** - Chronic lymphocytic leukemia is a type of cancer in which the bone marrow makes too many lymphocytes (a type of white blood cell).

- Chronic lymphocytic leukemia (also called CLL) is a cancer of the blood and bone marrow that usually gets worse slowly. CLL is one of the most common types of leukemia in adults. It often occurs during or after middle age; it rarely occurs in children.

AML - Adult acute myeloid leukemia (AML) is a type of cancer in which the bone marrow makes a large number of abnormal blood cells.

- Acute myeloid leukemia (AML) is a cancer of the blood and bone marrow. It is the most common type of acute leukemia in adults. This type of cancer usually gets worse quickly if it is not treated. AML is also called acute myelogenous leukemia and acute nonlymphocytic leukemia.

ALL - Adult acute lymphoblastic leukemia (ALL) is a type of cancer in which the bone marrow makes too many lymphocytes (a type of white blood cell).

- Adult acute lymphoblastic leukemia (ALL; also called acute lymphocytic leukemia) is a cancer of the blood and bone marrow. This type of cancer usually gets worse quickly if it is not treated.

CML - Chronic myelogenous leukemia is a disease in which the bone marrow makes too many white blood cells.

- Chronic myelogenous leukemia (also called CML or chronic granulocytic leukemia) is a slowly progressing blood and bone marrow disease that usually occurs during or after middle age and rarely occurs in children.

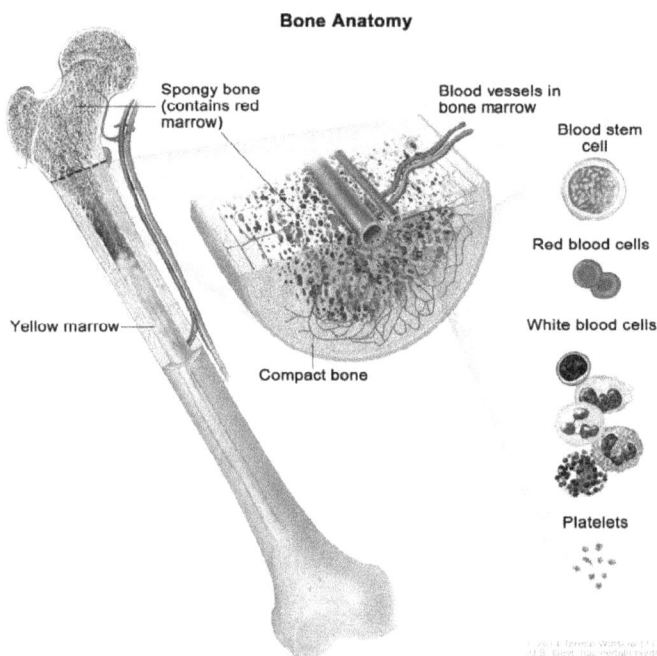

Bone Anatomy

Spongy bone (contains red marrow)

Blood vessels in bone marrow

Blood stem cell

Red blood cells

White blood cells

Yellow marrow

Compact bone

Platelets

The bone is made up of compact bone, spongy bone, and bone marrow. Compact bone makes up the outer layer of the bone. Spongy bone is found mostly at the ends of bones and contains red marrow. Bone marrow is found in the center of most bones and has many blood vessels. There are two types of bone marrow: red and yellow. Red marrow contains blood stem cells that can become red blood cells, white blood cells, or platelets. Yellow marrow is made mostly of fat.

Risk Factors	**Risk Factors for Leukemia:** • Being male. • Older age. • Smoking. • Having had treatment with chemotherapy or radiation therapy in the past. • Being exposed to radiation in the environment (such as nuclear radiation) or to the chemical benzene. • Having a personal history of a blood disorder such as myelodysplastic syndrome. • Having certain syndromes or inherited disorders.
CLL **Chronic Lymphocytic Leukemia**	Chronic lymphocytic leukemia is a type of cancer in which the bone marrow makes too many lymphocytes (a type of white blood cell). • Chronic lymphocytic leukemia (also called CLL) is a blood and bone marrow disease that usually gets worse slowly. • CLL is one of the most common types of leukemia in adults. It often occurs during or after middle age; it rarely occurs in children. Leukemia may affect red blood cells, white blood cells, and platelets. Normally, the body makes blood stem cells (immature cells) that become mature blood cells over time. A blood stem cell may become a myeloid stem cell or a lymphoid stem cell. A **myeloid stem cell** becomes one of three types of mature blood cells: • Red blood cells that carry oxygen and other substances to all tissues of the body. • White blood cells that fight infection and disease. • Platelets that form blood clots to stop bleeding. A **lymphoid stem cell** becomes a lymphoblast cell and then one of three types of lymphocytes (white blood cells): • B lymphocytes that make antibodies to help fight infection. • T lymphocytes that help B lymphocytes make antibodies to fight infection. • Natural killer cells that attack cancer cells and viruses. In CLL, too many blood stem cells become abnormal lymphocytes and do not become healthy white blood cells. • The abnormal lymphocytes may also be called leukemia cells. • The lymphocytes are not able to fight infection very well. • Also, as the number of lymphocytes increases in the blood and bone marrow, there is less room for healthy white blood cells, red blood cells, and platelets. This may cause infection, anemia, and easy bleeding.

Treatment	Chemotherapy
	Clinical trial of bone marrow or peripheral stem cell transplantation.
	Radiation therapy
	Watchful waiting
	
	Targeted therapy with any of the following drugs:
	• Ibrutinib with or without rituximab or Obinutuzumab.
	• Venetoclax with or without rituximab or Obinutuzumab.
	• Acalabrutinib with or without rituximab or Obinutuzumab.
	• Chemotherapy and rituximab.
	
	Immunotherapy
	Immunotherapy is a treatment that uses the patient's immune system to fight cancer. Substances made by the body or made in a laboratory are used to boost, direct, or restore the body's natural defenses against cancer. This cancer treatment is a type of biologic therapy.
	
	Immunomodulating agent:
	• Lenalidomide stimulates T cells to kill leukemia cells. It may be used alone or with rituximab in patients with symptomatic or progressive, recurrent, or refractory CLL.
	• CAR T-cell therapy: This treatment changes the patient's T cells (a type of immune system cell) so they will attack certain proteins on the surface of cancer cells.
	    o T cells are taken from the patient and special receptors are added to their surface in the laboratory. The changed cells are called chimeric antigen receptor (CAR) T cells.
	    o The CAR T cells are grown in the laboratory and given to the patient by infusion. The CAR T cells multiply in the patient's blood and attack cancer cells.
	    o CAR T-cell therapy is being studied in the treatment of recurrent or refractory CLL.
	
	Chemotherapy with bone marrow or peripheral stem cell transplant
	• Chemotherapy is given to kill cancer cells. Healthy cells, including blood-forming cells, are destroyed by the cancer treatment.
	    o A bone marrow or peripheral stem cell transplant are treatments to replace the blood-forming cells.
	    o Stem cells (immature blood cells) are removed from the blood or bone marrow of the patient or a donor and are frozen and stored.
	    o After the patient completes chemotherapy, the stored stem cells are thawed and given back to the patient through an infusion.
	    o These reinfused stem cells grow into (and restore) the body's blood cells.

AML **Adult Acute Myeloid Leukemia**	Adult acute myeloid leukemia (AML) is a type of cancer in which the bone marrow makes abnormal myeloblasts (a type of white blood cell), red blood cells, or platelets. This is a cancer of the blood and bone marrow. • This type of cancer usually gets worse quickly if it is not treated. • It is the most common type of acute leukemia in adults. • AML is also called acute myelogenous leukemia, acute myeloblastic leukemia, acute granulocytic leukemia, and acute nonlymphocytic leukemia. ***See CLL for myeloid stem cell types.*** In AML, the myeloid stem cells usually become a type of immature white blood cell called myeloblasts (or myeloid blasts). The myeloblasts in AML are abnormal and do not become healthy white blood cells. • Sometimes in AML, too many stem cells become abnormal red blood cells or platelets. These abnormal white blood cells, red blood cells, or platelets are also called leukemia cells or blasts. • Leukemia cells can build up in the bone marrow and blood so there is less room for healthy white blood cells, red blood cells, and platelets. When this happens, infection, anemia, or easy bleeding may occur. • The leukemia cells can spread outside the blood to other parts of the body, including the central nervous system (brain and spinal cord), skin, and gums. There are different subtypes of AML. Most AML subtypes are based on how mature (developed) the cancer cells are at the time of diagnosis and how different they are from normal cells. • **Acute promyelocytic leukemia (APL)** is a subtype of AML that occurs when parts of two genes stick together. APL usually occurs in middle-aged adults. Signs of APL may include both bleeding and forming blood clots.

Treatment	**Chemotherapy**
	Radiation therapy
	
	The treatment of adult AML usually has 2 phases.
	• **Remission induction therapy:** This is the first phase of treatment.
	    o The goal is to kill the leukemia cells in the blood and bone marrow. This puts the leukemia into remission.
	• **Post-remission therapy:** This is the second phase of treatment. Itbegins after the leukemia is in remission.
	    o The goal of post- remission therapy is to kill any remaining leukemia cells that maynot be active but could begin to regrow and cause a relapse.
	    o This phase is also called *remission continuation therapy*.

Treatment
 	
Continued
	Stem Cell Transplant:
	• A procedure in which a patient receives healthy stem cells (blood-forming cells) to replace their own stem cells that have been destroyed by treatment with radiation or high doses of chemotherapy.
	    ○ The healthy stem cells may come from the blood or bone marrow of the patient or from a related or unrelated donor.
	    ○ A stem cell transplant may be autologous (using a patient's own stem cells that were collected and saved before treatment), allogeneic (using stem cells from a related or unrelated donor), syngeneic (using stem cells donated by an identical twin), or cord blood (using umbilical cord blood donated after a baby is born).
	
	Chemotherapy with stem cell transplant:
	• Chemotherapy is given to kill cancer cells. Healthy cells, including blood-forming cells, are also destroyed by the cancer treatment.
	    ○ Stem cell transplant is a treatment to replace the blood-forming cells. Stem cells (immature blood cells) are removed from the blood or bone marrow of the patient or a donor and are frozen and stored.
	    ○ After the patient completes chemotherapy and/or total-body irradiation, the stored stem cells are thawed and given back to the patient through an infusion.
	    ○ These reinfused stem cells grow into (and restore) the body's blood cells.
	
	Targeted therapy:
	Targeted therapy is a type of treatment that uses drugs or other substances to identify and attack specific cancer cells. Targeted therapies usually cause less harm to normal cells than chemotherapy or radiation therapy do. There are different types of targeted therapy:
	• *Monoclonal antibodies*: Monoclonal antibodies are immune system proteins made in the laboratory to treat many diseases, including cancer. Gemtuzumab ozogamicin is a type of antibody-drug conjugate used to treat patients with newly diagnosed or relapsed AML. It contains a monoclonal antibody that binds to CD33, which is found on some leukemia cells, and also contains a toxic substance, which may help kill cancer cells.
	• **Midostaurin**, a protein kinase inhibitor used with certain types of chemotherapy to treat newly diagnosed patients with AML that has a mutation in the FLT3 gene.
	• *Gilteritinib*, a tyrosine kinase inhibitor that may be used to treat patients with AML that has come back or did not get better with other treatment and has a mutation in the FLT3 gene.
	• *Glasdegib, ivosidenib,* and *enasidenib*, which may be used as a less intensive treatment in older or frail patients who cannot receive standard treatment.
	
	Other drug therapy:
	• *Arsenic trioxide* and *all-trans retinoic acid (ATRA)* are anticancer drugs that kill leukemia cells, stop the leukemia cells from dividing, or help the leukemia cells mature into white blood cells.
	    ○ These drugs are used in the treatment of a subtype of AML called acute promyelocytic leukemia.

References	**NCI – National Cancer Institute:** Acute Myeloid Leukemia Treatment - *https://www.cancer.gov/types/leukemia/patient/adult-aml-treatment-pdq* Adult Acute Lymphoblastic Leukemia Treatment - *https://www.cancer.gov/types/leukemia/patient/adult-all-treatment-pdq* Chronic Lymphocytic Leukemia Treatment - *https://www.cancer.gov/types/leukemia/patient/cll-treatment-pdq* Chronic Myelogenous Leukemia Treatment - *https://www.cancer.gov/types/leukemia/patient/cml-treatment-pdq* Leukemia Overview - *https://www.cancer.gov/types/leukemia*

LIVER (Adult Primary Liver Cancer)
Information and pictures from *National Cancer Institute* unless otherwise specified

Description	Adult primary liver cancer is a disease in which malignant (cancer) cells form in the tissues of the liver. *The liver is one of the largest organs in the body. It has two lobes and fills the upper right side of the abdomen inside the rib cage.* *Three of the many important functions of the liver are:* • *To filter harmful substances from the blood so they can be passed from the body in stools and urine.* • *To make bile to help digest fat that comes from food.* • *To store glycogen (sugar), which the body uses for energy.* 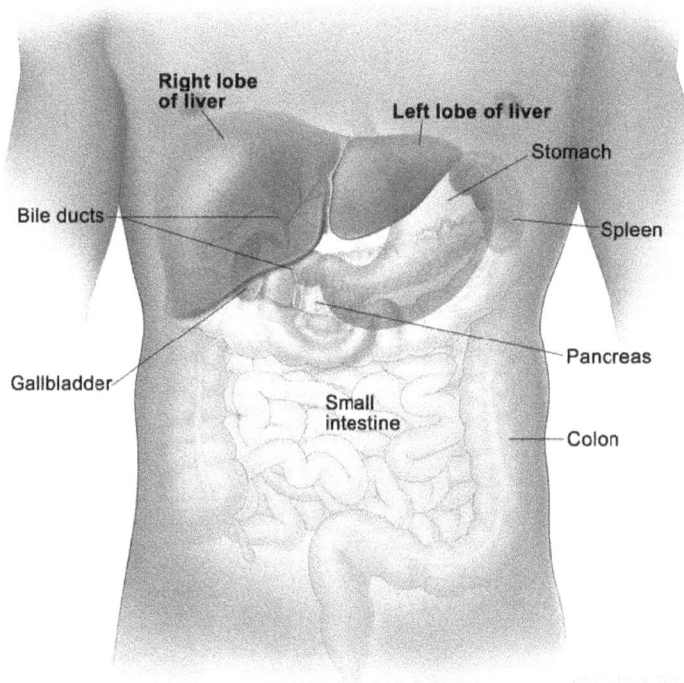 There are two types of adult primary liver cancer. • Hepatocellular carcinoma – Most common • Cholangiocarcinoma (bile duct cancer).
Risk Factors	**Risk factors of Liver Cancer:** • Having hepatitis B or hepatitis C. • Having cirrhosis, which can be caused by: hepatitis (especially hepatitis C) • Drinking large amounts of alcohol for many years or being an alcoholic. • Having metabolic syndrome, • Having liver injury that is long-lasting • Having hemochromatosis • Eating foods tainted with aflatoxin (poison from a fungus that can grow on foods)

Treatment	**Radiation therapy**
	Targeted therapy
	
	Surgery:
	• **A partial hepatectomy** (surgery to remove the part of the liver where cancer is found) may be done.
	    ○ A wedge of tissue, an entire lobe, or a larger part of the liver, along with some of the healthy tissue around it is removed.
	    ○ The remaining liver tissue takes over the functions of the liver and may re-grow.
	• **Total Hepatectomy with Liver transplant:** In a liver transplant, the entire liver is removed and replaced with a healthy donated liver. A liver transplant may be done when the disease is in the liver only and a donated liver can be found. If the patient has to wait for a donated liver, other treatment is given as needed.
	    ○ Possible side effect is rejection of the liver.
	    ○ Other side effects may be specific to drugs given.
	    ○ Immediately call your doctor if you experience a fever, redness or pus at your surgery site, bleeding or signs of liver failure - yellowing of the skin or whites of the eyes, dark urine or confusion - after surgery.
	
	Ablation therapy removes or destroys tissue. Different types of ablation therapy are used for liver cancer:
	• **Radiofrequency ablation:** The use of special needles that are inserted directly through the skin or through an incision in the abdomen to reach the tumor.
	    ○ High-energy radio waves heat the needles and tumor which kills cancer cells.
	• **Microwave therapy:** A type of treatment in which the tumor is exposed to high temperatures created by microwaves.
	    ○ This can damage and kill cancer cells or make them more sensitive to the effects of radiation and certain anticancer drugs.
	• **Percutaneous ethanol injection:** A cancer treatment in which a small needle is used to inject ethanol (pure alcohol) directly into a tumor to kill cancer cells.
	    ○ Several treatments may be needed. Usually local anesthesia is used, but if the patient has many tumors in the liver, general anesthesia may be used.
	• **Cryoablation:** A treatment that uses an instrument to freeze and destroy cancer cells. This type of treatment is also called cryotherapy and cryosurgery.
	    ○ The doctor may use ultrasound to guide the instrument.
	• **Electroporation therapy:** A treatment that sends electrical pulses through an electrode placed in a tumor to kill cancer cells.
	    ○ Electroporation therapy is being studied in clinical trials.
	
	Embolization therapy:
	• The use of substances to block or decrease the flow of blood through the hepatic artery to the tumor.
	• When the tumor does not get the oxygen and nutrients it needs, it will not continue to grow. Embolization therapy is used for patients who cannot have surgery to remove the tumor or ablation therapy and whose tumor has not spread outside the liver.
	• The liver receives blood from the hepatic portal vein and the hepatic artery.
	    ○ Blood that comes into the liver from the hepatic portal vein usually goes to the healthy liver tissue.
	    ○ Blood that comes from the hepatic artery usually goes to the tumor.
	    ○ When the hepatic artery is blocked during embolization therapy, the healthy liver tissue continues to receive blood from the hepatic portal vein.

Treatment *Continued*	There are two main types of embolization therapy: • **Transarterial embolization (TAE):** A small incision (cut) is made in the inner thigh and a catheter (thin, flexible tube) is inserted and threaded up into the hepatic artery. Once the catheter is in place, a substance that blocks the hepatic artery and stops blood flow to the tumor is injected. • **Transarterial chemoembolization (TACE):** This procedure is like TAE except an anticancer drug is also given. The procedure can be done by attaching the anticancer drug to small beads that are injected into the hepatic artery or by injecting the anticancer drug through the catheter into the hepatic artery and then injecting the substance to block the hepatic artery. Most of the anticancer drug is trapped near the tumor and only a small amount of the drug reaches other parts of the body. This type of treatment is also called ***chemoembolization.*** **Targeted therapy** Targeted therapy is a type of treatment that uses drugs or other substances to identify and attack specific cancer cells. • Targeted therapies usually cause less harm to normal cells than chemotherapy or radiation therapy do. Tyrosine kinase inhibitors are a type of targeted therapy used in the treatment of adult primary liver cancer. • Tyrosine kinase inhibitors are small-molecule drugs that go through the cell membrane and work inside cancer cells to block signals that cancer cells need to grow and divide. • Some tyrosine kinase inhibitors also have angiogenesis inhibitor effects. Sorafenib, Lenvatinib, regorafenib, and Cabozantinib are types of tyrosine kinase inhibitors used to treat advanced liver cancer. **Immunotherapy** Immunotherapy is a treatment that uses the patient's immune system to fight cancer. • Substances made by the body or made in a laboratory are used to boost, direct, or restore the body's natural defenses against cancer. This cancer treatment is a type of biologic therapy. • Immune checkpoint inhibitor therapy is a type of immunotherapy. • PD-1 and PD-L1 inhibitor therapy: PD-1 is a protein on the surface of T cells that helps keep the body's immune responses in check. PD-L1 is a protein found on some types of cancer cells. ○ When PD-1 attaches to PD-L1, it stops the T cell from killing the cancer cell. PD-1 and PD-L1 inhibitors keep PD-1 and PD-L1 proteins from attaching to each other. This allows the T cells to kill cancer cells. Pembrolizumab is a type of PD-1 inhibitor. 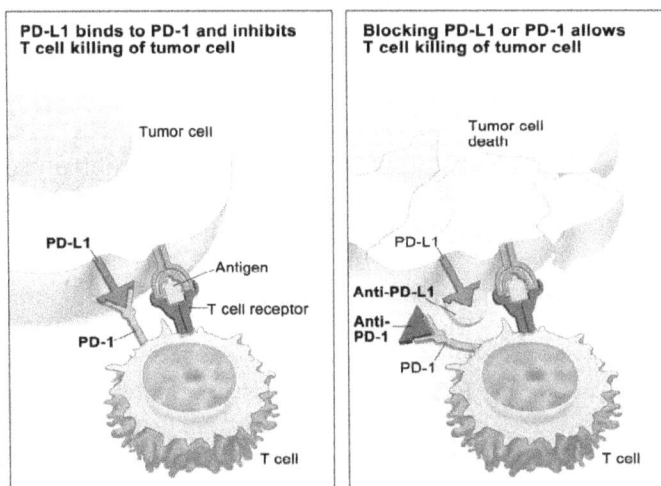

Treatment **by Type**	**Localized Adult Primary Liver Cancer** Treatment of localized adult primary liver cancer may include the following: • Surveillance for lesions smaller than 1 centimeter. • Partial hepatectomy. • Total hepatectomy and liver transplant. • Ablation of the tumor using one of the following methods: • Radiofrequency ablation. • Microwave therapy. • Percutaneous ethanol injection. • Cryoablation. • A clinical trial of electroporation therapy. **Locally Advanced or Metastatic Adult Primary Liver Cancer** Treatment of locally advanced or metastatic adult primary liver cancer that cannot be treated with surgery may include the following: • Embolization therapy using Transarterial embolization (TAE) or Transarterial chemoembolization (TACE). • Targeted therapy with sorafenib, Lenvatinib, Regorafenib, or Cabozantinib. • Immune checkpoint inhibitor therapy with pembrolizumab. • Radiation therapy. • A clinical trial of targeted therapy after chemoembolization or combined with chemotherapy. • A clinical trial of new targeted therapy drugs. • A clinical trial of immunotherapy. • A clinical trial of immunotherapy combined with targeted therapy. • A clinical trial of stereotactic body radiation therapy or proton-beam radiation therapy. **Recurrent Adult Primary Liver Cancer** Treatment options for recurrent adult primary liver cancer may include the following: • Total hepatectomy and liver transplant. • Partial hepatectomy. • Ablation. • Transarterial chemoembolization and targeted therapy with sorafenib, as palliative therapy to relieve symptoms and improve quality of life.

Possible Specific Side Effects or Complications *Mayo Clinic*	**Liver transplant surgery** carries a risk of significant complications. There are risks associated with the procedure itself as well as with the drugs necessary to prevent rejection of the donor liver after the transplant. **Risks associated with the procedure include:** • Bile duct complications, including bile duct leaks or shrinking of the bile ducts • Bleeding or Blood clots • Failure of donated liver • Infection • Rejection of donated liver • Mental confusion or seizures • Long-term complications may also include recurrence of liver disease in the transplanted liver. **Anti-rejection medication side effects** After a liver transplant, you'll take medications for the rest of your life to help prevent your body from rejecting the donated liver. These anti-rejection medications can cause a variety of side effects, including: • Bone thinning • Diabetes • Diarrhea • Headaches • High blood pressure • High cholesterol • Because anti-rejection drugs work by suppressing the immune system, they also increase your risk of infection. Your doctor may give you medications to help you fight infections. (*Liver Transplant – Mayo Clinic*)
Graft vs. Host Disease *NIH - National Center for Biotechnology Information*	**Graft vs. Host Disease -** (GVHD) Graft-versus-host disease (GVHD) is a severe complication that can occur following hematopoietic stem cell transplantation. • This condition arises when immunocompetent T lymphocytes from the donor graft recognize the recipient's tissues as foreign due to histocompatibility differences and initiate an immune response against them. • This attack typically occurs within the first 100 days post-transplant, leading to tissue damage in various organs, including the skin, gastrointestinal tract, liver, and lungs. • GVHD can manifest as acute or chronic forms, each with distinct clinical presentations and management strategies
References	CETI- Cancer Exercise Training Institute: *https://www.thecancerspecialist.com/* In Tech – "Physiotherapy in Liver Transplantation" Meriç Şenduran1 and S. Ufuk Yurdalan *https://www.intechopen.com/chapters/28298* Mayo Clinic - Liver Transplant: *https://www.mayoclinic.org/tests-procedures/liver-transplant/about/pac-20384842#:~:text=Your%20transplant%20team%20includes%20a%20nutrition%20specialist%20%28dietitian%29,your%20new%20liver%2C%20it%27s%20important%20to%20avoid%20alcohol* NCI - National Cancer Institute Adult Primary Liver Cancer Treatment (PDQ®)–Patient Version: *https://www.cancer.gov/types/liver/patient/adult-liver-treatment-pdq#_27* NIH – National Center for Biotechnology Information - Graft-Versus-Host Disease Angel A. Justiz Vaillant; Pranav Modi; Oranus Mohammadi. Last Update: June 7, 2024. *https://www.ncbi.nlm.nih.gov/books/NBK538235/*

Recovery after Surgery
 	
Information from CETI-
Cancer Exercise Training Institute
 	
Please follow MD/surgeon protocol, as every situation is unique.
	Partial Hepatectomy:
	➢ **Hospital Stay:** 5-10 days (Laparoscopy may be shorter length)
	➢ **Full Recovery:** 6-8 weeks
	➢ **Restrictions:** No heavy lifting over 5 lbs. or strenuous exercise for at least 8 weeks.
	➢ **Exercise:** Walking
	➢ **Possible Side Effects:** Pain, Weakness, Fatigue, Bleeding, Infection, Temporary Liver Failure, Pleural Effusion, Pulmonary Infection, Ascites (fluid buildup in stomach), Urinary Tract Infection, G.I. Bleeding, Biliary Tract Hemorrhage, Bile Leakage, Subphrenic Infection
	    o Gall Bladder is usually removed
	    o May have damage to Diaphragm
	
	Total Hepatectomy with Liver Transplant:
	➢ **Hospital Stay:** Intensive care for several days and then 8-10 days
	➢ **Full Recovery:** 6 months or more
	➢ **Restrictions:** No heavy lifting over 5 lbs. or strenuous exercise for at least 8 weeks.
	➢ **Exercise:** Walking
	➢ **Possible Side Effects:** Infection, Hemorrhage, Hepatic Artery U Portal Vein Thrombosis, Immunocompromise, Mental Confusion, Seizures, Post Transplant Lymphoproliferative Disorder (PTLD), Leaks or Shrinkage of the Bile Ducts
	    o Graft Rejection – Graft vs. Host Disease (*see above for more information*)
	    o May have damage to Diaphragm

Exercise and Sports Participation
 	
Excerpt from In Tech, *"Physiotherapy in Liver Transplantation"*
 	
Please follow MD/surgeon protocol, as every situation is unique.
	4.3 Sports Participation - *Physiotherapy in Liver Transplantation*
	
	Long Term After 3 Months
	• Sports participation after solid organ transplantation is the final objection of the long-term rehabilitation process for maximizing quality of life. It is recommended to encourage the patients to participate in a sports activity three months after the surgery.
	  ○ This time is required to achieve optimal flexibility, muscular strength, muscular endurance and aerobic capacity and to provide proper post-operative wound healing and graft stabilization so that the patient can do sports without any deterioration.
	• Patients should start with light activities such as walking, stair climbing, golf, bowling, darts, archery and fishing.
	  ○ Table tennis and volleyball can be suggested as medium intensity activities.
	  ○ Swimming, athletics, badminton, cycling, rowing, squashes, tennis, mini marathons are recommended after getting used to light and moderate activities.
	• However, swimming in community pools or lakes is not recommended because of the high risk of infectious organisms.
	  ○ High impact and contact sports such as football, basketball, horse riding and bungee jumping are not preferable as they may cause serious trauma and lead to organ damage.
	  ○ Patients usually have a fear of organ damage or severe pain avoiding them to participate in sports.
	• Contact sports also have an additional fracture risk for weight bearing bones due to long term osteoporotic effects of corticosteroids.
	• As liver transplantation surgery induces a denervation of the liver and intrahepatic vascular system strenuous exercises may carry a high risk for reduction in portal blood flow due to increased demands of contracting muscles (Ersoz&Ersoz, 2003).
	• Selected and well-prepared liver transplant recipients were able to participate in mountain trek and tolerate exposure to high altitude similar to healthy subjects after a 6-month aerobic training and a hypercaloric diet including sugars, proteins and abundant hydration (Pirenne et al., 2004).
	• Feeling of distress, muscle and joint pain, incisional pain and fatigue are the complaints of transplant recipients during or after exercises.
	  ○ Running, skiing, bike riding and tennis, shotput and bodybuilding were reported as the most popular sports among a group of patients with liver and kidney transplantation (Pupkal et al., 2008).
	• Patients may participate in a sport not only for leisure time activities but also for professional competitions.
	  ○ The World Transplant Games Federation, officially recognized by the International Olympic Committee, is a world-wide organization staging international sporting events for transplant athletes for over 20 years in order to demonstrate the ability of sports participation after organ transplantation and to raise awareness of the vitality of organ donation.
	
	Physiotherapy in Liver Transplantation

LUNG
Information and pictures from *National Cancer Institute* unless otherwise specified

Non- Small Cell

Non-small cell lung cancer is a diseasein which malignant (cancer) cells form in the tissues of the lung. A group of lung cancers named for the kinds of cells found in the cancer and how the cells look under a microscope.

- The three main types of non-small cell lung cancer are adenocarcinoma (most common), squamous cell carcinoma, and large cell carcinoma.

Non-small cell lung cancer is the most common of the two main types of lung cancer (non-small cell lung cancer and small cell lung cancer).

The lungs are a pair of cone-shaped breathing organs in the chest. The lungs bring oxygen into the body as you breathe in. They release carbon dioxide, a waste product of the body'scells, as you breathe out. Each lung has sections called lobes. The left lunghas two lobes. The right lung is slightly larger and has three lobes.

- *Two tubes called bronchi lead from the trachea (windpipe) to the right and left lungs. The bronchi are sometimes also involved in lung cancer.*
- *Tiny air sacs called alveoli and small tubes called bronchioles make up the inside of the lungs.*
- *A thin membrane called the pleura covers the outside of each lung and lines the inside wall of the chest cavity. This creates a sac called the pleural cavity. The pleural cavity normally contains a small amount of fluid that helps the lungs move smoothly in the chest when you breathe.*

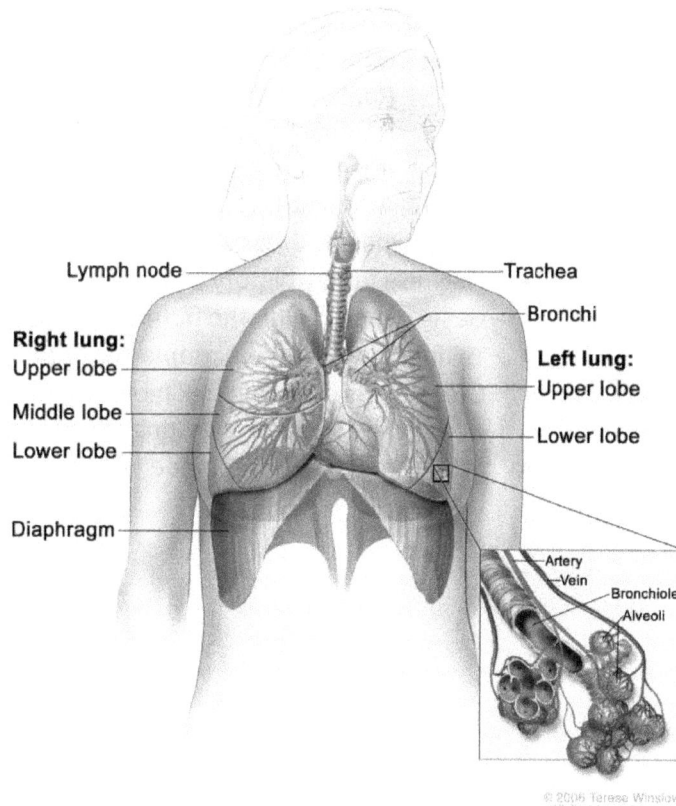

National Cancer Institute
Non-Small Cell Lung Cancer Treatment (PDQ®)–Patient Version

Non-Small Cell *Continued*	Each type of non-small cell lung cancerhas different kinds of cancer cells. The cancer cells of each type grow and spread in different ways. The types of non-small cell lung cancer are named for the kinds of cells found in the cancer and how the cells look under a microscope: • **Squamous cell carcinoma:** Cancer thatbegins in squamous cells, which are thin, flat cells that look like fish scales. This is also called epidermoid carcinoma. • **Large cell carcinoma:** Cancer that maybegin in several types of large cells. • **Adenocarcinoma:** Cancer that begins in the cells that line the alveoli and make substances such as mucus. Other less common types of non-smallcell lung cancer are pleomorphic, carcinoid tumor, salivary gland carcinoma, and unclassified carcinoma.

Risk Factors	**Risk factors of Lung Cancer:**
	• Smoking cigarettes, pipes, or cigars, now or in the past. This is the most important risk factor for lung cancer.
	    o The earlier in life a person starts smoking, the more often a person smokes, and the more years a person smokes, the greater the risk of lung cancer.
	• Being exposed to secondhand smoke.
	• Being exposed to asbestos, arsenic, chromium, beryllium, nickel, soot, or tar in the workplace.
	• Being exposed to radiation from any of the following:
	    o Radiation therapy to the breast or chest.
	    o Radon in the home or workplace.
	    o Imaging tests such as CT scans.
	    o Atomic bomb radiation.
	• Living where there is air pollution.
	• Having a family history of lung cancer.
	• Being infected with the human immunodeficiency virus (HIV).
	• Taking beta carotene supplements and being a heavy smoker.
	• Older age is the main risk factor for most cancers.
	    o The chance of getting cancer increases as you get older.
	• When smoking is combined with other risk factors, the risk of lung cancer is increased.

Treatment *Pictures and section from Non-Small Cell Lung Cancer Treatment (PDQ®)–Patient Version*	Chemotherapy Immunotherapy Radiation therapy **Surgery** Four types of surgery are used to treat lung cancer: • **Wedge resection:** Surgery to remove a tumor and some of the normal tissue around it. When a slightly larger amount of tissue is taken, it is called a segmental resection. 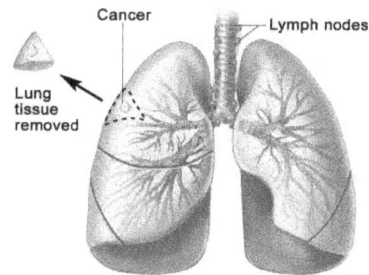 • **Lobectomy:** Surgery to remove a whole lobe (section) of the lung. 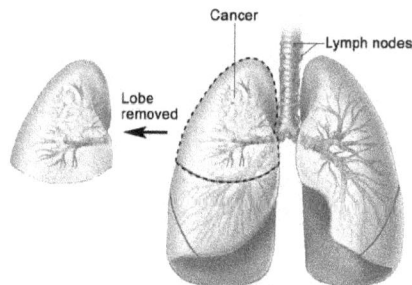 • **Pneumonectomy:** Surgery to remove one whole lung. • **Sleeve resection:** Surgery to remove part of the bronchus. 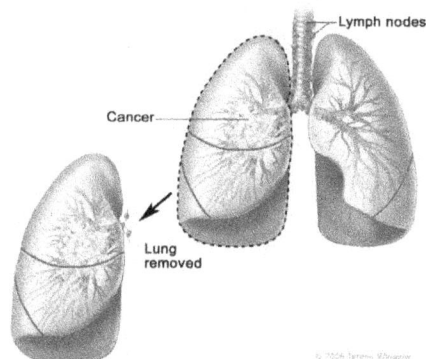

Treatment
 	
Continued
	Targeted therapy:
	• **Monoclonal antibodies** - Monoclonal antibodies are immune system proteins made in the laboratory to treat many diseases, including cancer.
	   ○ As a cancer treatment, these antibodies can attach to a specific target on cancer cells or other cells that may help cancer cells grow. The antibodies are able to then kill the cancer cells, block their growth, or keep them from spreading.
	   ○ Monoclonal antibodies are given by infusion. They may be used alone or to carry drugs, toxins, or radioactive material directly to cancer cells.
	• **Tyrosine kinase inhibitors** - Tyrosine kinase inhibitors are small-molecule drugs that go through the cell membrane and work inside cancer cells to block signals that cancer cells need to grow and divide.
	   ○ Some tyrosine kinase inhibitors also have angiogenesis inhibitor effects.
	• **Mammalian target of rapamycin inhibitors** block a protein called mTOR, which may keep cancer cells from growing and prevent the growth of new blood vessels that tumors need to grow. Everolimus is a type of mTOR inhibitor.
	
	Laser therapy is a cancer treatment that uses a laser beam (a narrow beam of intense light) to kill cancer cells.
	
	Photodynamic therapy (PDT) is a cancer treatment that uses a drug and a certain type of laser light to kill cancer cells.
	• A drug that is not active until it is exposed to light is injected into a vein. The drug collects more in cancer cells than in normal cells.
	   ○ Fiberoptic tubes are then used to carry the laser light to the cancer cells, where the drug becomes active and kills the cells.
	• Photodynamic therapy causes little damage to healthy tissue. It is used mainly to treat tumors on or just under the skin or in the lining of internal organs.
	   ○ When the tumor is in the airways, PDT is given directly to the tumor through an endoscope.
	
	Cryosurgery is a treatment that uses an instrument to freeze and destroy abnormal tissue, such as carcinoma in situ. This type of treatment is also called cryotherapy.
	• For tumors in the airways, cryosurgery is done through an endoscope.
	
	Electrocautery is a treatment that uses a probe or needle heated by an electric current to destroy abnormal tissue.
	• For tumors in the airways, electrocautery is done through an endoscope.
	
	Watchful waiting is closely monitoring a patient's condition without giving any treatment until signs or symptoms appear or change.
	• This may be done in certain rare cases of non-small cell lung cancer.
	
	New types of treatment are being tested in clinical trials.
	• **Chemoprevention**
	• **Radiosensitizers**
	• **New combinations**

Possible Side Effects	**Possible Side Effects:** • May need to be on oxygen • Surgery: Side effects are very specific to particular surgery done.
Small Cell *See non-small cell for description of lungs risk factors and side effects*	Small cell lung cancer is a disease in which malignant (cancer) cells form in the tissues of the lung. • An aggressive (fast-growing) cancer that forms in tissues of the lung and can spread to other parts of the body. • The cancer cells look small and oval-shaped when looked at under a microscope. There are two main types of small cell lung cancer. • These two types include many different types of cells. • The cancer cells of each type grow and spread in different ways. The types of small cell lung cancer are named for the kinds of cells found in the cancer and how the cells look when viewed under a microscope: • **Small cell carcinoma (oat cell cancer).** • **Combined small cell carcinoma.** The following stages are used for small cell lung cancer: • **Limited-Stage Small Cell Lung Cancer** In limited-stage, cancer is in the lung where it started and may have spread to the area between the lungs or to the lymph nodes above the collarbone. • **Extensive-Stage Small Cell Lung Cancer** In extensive-stage, cancer has spread beyond the lung or the area between the lungs or the lymph nodes above the collarbone to other places in the body. • **Small cell lung cancer can recur (come back) after it has been treated.** The cancer may come back in the chest, central nervous system, or in other parts of the body.

Treatment	Chemotherapy Immunotherapy Laser therapy Radiation therapy Targeted therapy **Surgery:** • Surgery may be used if the cancer is found in one lung and in nearby lymph nodes only. • Because this type of lung cancer is usually found in both lungs, surgery alone is not often used. • During surgery, the doctor will also remove lymph nodes to find out if they have cancer in them. • Sometimes, surgery may be used to remove a sample of lung tissue to find out the exact type of lung cancer. After the doctor removes all the cancer that can be seen at the time of the surgery, *some patients may be given chemotherapy or radiation therapy after surgery to kill any cancer cells that are left.* Treatment given after the surgery, to lower the risk that the cancer will come back, is called adjuvant therapy. **Endoscopic stent placement:** • An endoscope is a thin, tube-like instrument used to look at tissues inside the body. An endoscope has a light and a lens for viewing and may be used to place a stent in a body structure to keep the structure open. • An endoscopic stent can be used to open an airway blocked by abnormal tissue.
References	CETI- Cancer Exercise Training Institute: *https://www.thecancerspecialist.com/* National Cancer Institute – NCI – **Lung Cancer**: *https://www.cancer.gov/types/lung* National Cancer Institute – NCI - **Non-Small Cell** Lung Cancer Treatment (PDQ®)– Patient Version: *https://www.cancer.gov/types/lung/patient/non-small-cell-lung-treatment-pdq* National Cancer Institute – NCI - **Small Cell** Lung Cancer Treatment:*https://www.cancer.gov/types/lung/patient/small-cell-lung-treatment-pdq*

Recovery after Surgery *Information from CETI- Cancer Exercise Training Institute* ***Please follow MD/surgeon protocol, as every situation is unique.***	**Video Assisted Thoracotomy (VATS)** ➢ **Hospital Stay:** 4-5 days ➢ **Full Recovery:** 1-2 months. ➢ **Restrictions:** No heavy lifting over 10 lbs. or straining for 2 weeks. Be cautious when using upper body/back and arms for 6 weeks. ➢ **Exercise:** Walking. **Thoracotomy (must spread ribs to get to the lungs)** ➢ **Hospital Stay:** 5-7 days ➢ **Full Recovery:** 3 months or more ➢ **Restrictions:** Avoid strenuous activity, such as heavy lifting over 10 lbs. for 8 weeks. Be cautious when using upper body/back and arms for 6 weeks. ➢ **Exercise:** Walking. **Possible Side Effects of Surgery:** Pneumonia, Infection/Bleeding at Incision Site, Hemorrhage, Blood Clots (legs or lungs), Lung Collapse/Pneumothorax or Air/Fluid Leaking into Surgical Area (bronchopleural fistula), Accumulation of Fluid (chest), Chronic Pain, Abnormal Heart Rhythm, Difficulty Breathing (extended stay on breathing machine).

Exercise, Special Considerations & Precautions – Short and Long Term
 	
Please follow MD/surgeon protocol, as every situation is unique.
	Symptoms may be variable depending on surgery and how they accessed the lungs (ex. cutting through ribs, etc.)
	• Improve your posture.
	   o Work on keeping your shoulders and chin back and opening your body to encourage deep breathing.
	• After clearance from MD: Upper body stretching to increase lung capacity.
	• Purse lip breathing and diaphragmatic breathing techniques
	   o Deep diaphragmatic breathing can be painful or uncomfortable.
	   o Avoid overexpanding the chest until healed
	• Do not apply pressure to chest lying on your stomach or against equipment
	• Progress to pulmonary rehab

LYMPHOMA (Non-Hodgkin and Hodgkin)
Information and pictures from *National Cancer Institute* unless otherwise specified

Description *Also see Lymph Nodes / Lymphedema*	Lymphoma is a disease in which malignant (cancer) cells form in the lymph system. It is a type of cancer that forms in the lymph system, which is part of the body's immune system. Types: • **Non-Hodgkin lymphoma** can be indolent or aggressive. It can begin in B lymphocytes, T lymphocytes, or natural killer cells. Lymphocytes can also be found in the blood and also collect in the lymph nodes, spleen, and thymus. • **Hodgkin lymphoma:** The two main types of Hodgkin lymphoma are classic and nodular lymphocyte predominant.

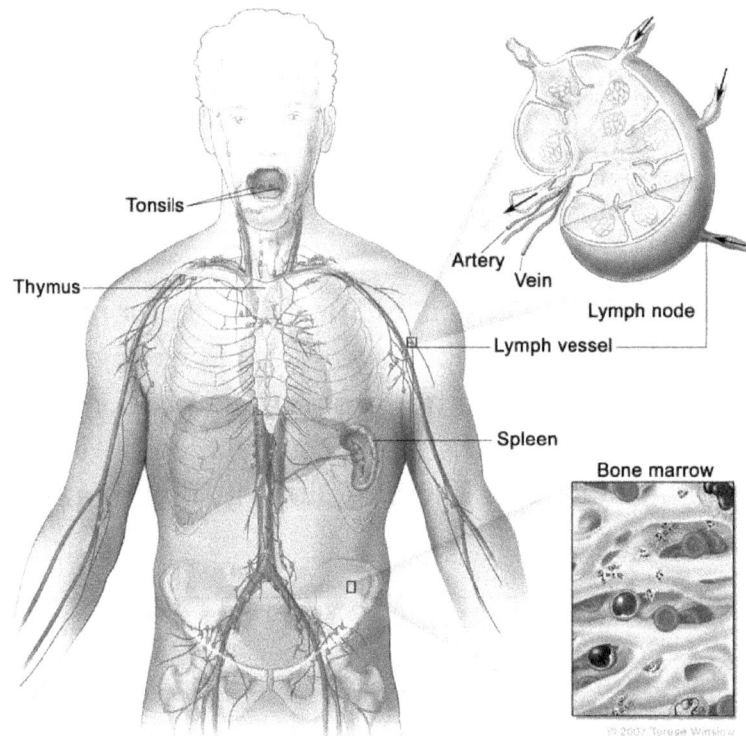

The immune system protects the body from foreign substances, infection, and diseases. The lymph system is made up of the following:

- *Lymph: Colorless, watery fluid that carries white blood cells called lymphocytes through the lymph system. Lymphocytes protect the body against infection and the growth of tumors. There are three types of lymphocytes:*
    - *B lymphocytes that make antibodies to help fight infection. Also called B cells. Most types of non- Hodgkin lymphoma begin in B lymphocytes.*
    - *T lymphocytes that help B lymphocytes make the antibodies that help fight infection. Also called T cells.*
    - *Natural killer cells that attack cancer cells and viruses. Also called NK cells.*

Anatomy of the lymph system, showing the lymph vessels and lymph organs including lymph nodes, tonsils, thymus, spleen, and bone marrow. Lymph (clear fluid) and lymphocytes travel through the lymph vessels and into the lymph nodes where the lymphocytes destroy harmful substances. The lymph enters the blood through a large vein near the heart.

Description *Continued*	• **Lymph vessels**: A network of thin tubes that collect lymph from different parts of the body and return it to the bloodstream. • **Lymph nodes**: Small, bean-shaped structures that filter lymph and store white blood cells that help fight infection and disease. Lymph nodes are located along the network of lymph vessels found throughout the body. Clusters of lymph nodes are found in the neck, underarm, abdomen, pelvis, and groin. • **Spleen**: An organ that makes lymphocytes, filters the blood, stores blood cells, and destroys old blood cells. Thymus: An organ in which lymphocytes grow and multiply • **Tonsils:** Two small masses of lymph tissue at the back of the throat. The tonsils make lymphocytes. • **Bone marrow:** The soft, spongy tissue in the center of large bones. Bone marrow makes white blood cells, red blood cells, and platelets. • **Lymph tissue is** also found in other parts of the body such as the stomach, thyroid gland, brain, and skin. Cancer can spread to the liver and lungs.
Non-Hodgkin Lymphoma	**Non-Hodgkin lymphoma** grows and spreads at different rates and can be indolent or aggressive. The treatments for indolent and aggressive lymphoma are different. • **Indolent lymphoma** tends to grow and spread slowly and has few signs and symptoms. • **Aggressive lymphoma** grows and spreads quickly and has signs and symptoms that can be severe. The treatments for indolent and aggressive lymphoma are different

Indolent and Aggressive Non-Hodgkin Lymphomas	**Indolent Non-Hodgkin Lymphomas:**
	• **Follicular lymphoma.** Follicular lymphoma is the most common type of indolent non-Hodgkin lymphoma. It is a very slow-growing type of non-Hodgkin lymphoma that begins in B lymphocytes.
	• **Lymphoplasmacytic lymphoma.** In most cases of lymphoplasmacytic lymphoma, B lymphocytes that are turning Into plasma cells make large amounts of a protein called monoclonal immunoglobulin M (IgM) antibody.
	• **Marginal zone lymphoma.** This type of non-Hodgkin lymphoma begins in B lymphocytes in a part of lymph tissue called the marginal zone. The prognosis may be worse for patients aged 70 years or older, those with stage III or stage IV disease, and those with high lactate dehydrogenase (LDH) levels. There are five different types of marginal zone lymphoma. They are grouped by the type of tissue where the lymphoma formed:
	   ○ *Nodal marginal zone lymphoma.* Nodal marginal zone lymphoma forms in lymph nodes. This type of non-Hodgkin lymphoma is rare. It is also called monocytoid B-cell lymphoma.
	   ○ *Gastric mucosa-associated lymphoid tissue (MALT) lymphoma.* Gastric MALT lymphoma usually begins in the stomach. This type of marginal zone lymphoma forms in cells in the mucosa that help make antibodies.
	   ○ *Extragastric MALT lymphoma.* This begins outside of the stomach in almost every part of the body including other parts of the gastrointestinal tract, salivary glands, thyroid, lung, skin, & around the eye.
	   ○ *Mediterranean abdominal lymphoma.* This is a type of MALT lymphoma that occurs in young adults in eastern Mediterranean countries. It often forms in the abdomen and patients may also be infected with bacteria called Campylobacter jejuni.

Indolent and Aggressive Non-Hodgkin Lymphomas
 	
Continued
	○ **Splenic marginal zone lymphoma.** This type of marginal zone lymphoma begins in the spleen and may spread to the peripheral blood and bone marrow. The most common sign of this type of splenic marginal zone lymphoma is a spleen that is larger than normal.
	• **Primary cutaneous anaplastic large cell lymphoma.** This type of non-Hodgkin lymphoma is in the skin only. It can be a benign (not cancer) nodule that may go away on its own or it can spread to many places on the skin and need treatment.
	
	Aggressive Non-Hodgkin lymphomas:
	• **Diffuse large B-cell lymphoma.** Diffuse large B-cell lymphoma is the most common type of non-Hodgkin lymphoma. It grows quickly in the lymph nodes and often the spleen, liver, bone marrow, or other organs are also affected. Signs and symptoms of diffuse large B-cell lymphoma may include fever, drenching night sweats, and weight loss. These are also called B symptoms.
	    ○ **Primary mediastinal large B-cell lymphoma.** This type of non-Hodgkin lymphoma is a type of diffuse large B-cell lymphoma. It is marked by the overgrowth of fibrous (scar-like) lymph tissue. A tumor most often forms behind the breastbone. It may press on the airways and cause coughing and trouble breathing.
	• **Follicular large cell lymphoma, stage III.** This is a very rare type of non-Hodgkin lymphoma. Treatment of this type of follicular lymphoma is more like treatment of aggressive NHL than of indolent NHL.
	• **Anaplastic large cell lymphoma.** Anaplastic large cell lymphoma is a type of non-Hodgkin lymphoma that usually begins in T lymphocytes. The cancer cells also have a marker called CD30 on the surface of the cell.
	There are two types of anaplastic large cell lymphoma:
	    ○ *Cutaneous anaplastic large cell lymphoma.* This type of anaplastic large cell lymphoma mostly affects the skin, but other parts of the body may also be affected. Signs of cutaneous anaplastic large cell lymphoma include one or more bumps or ulcers on the skin. This type of lymphoma is rare and indolent.
	    ○ *Systemic anaplastic large cell lymphoma.* This type of anaplastic large cell lymphoma begins in the lymph nodes and may affect other parts of the body. This type of lymphoma is more aggressive.
	• **Extranodal NK-/T-cell lymphoma.** Extranodal NK-/T-cell lymphoma usually begins in the area around the nose. It may also affect the paranasal sinus (hollow spaces in the bones around the nose), roof of the mouth, trachea, skin, stomach, and intestines.
	• **Lymphomatoid granulomatosis.** This mostly affects the lungs. It may also affect the paranasal sinuses (hollow spaces in the bones around the nose), skin, kidneys, and central nervous system.
	• **Angioimmunoblastic T-cell lymphoma.** This type of non-Hodgkin lymphoma begins in T cells. Swollen lymph nodes are a common sign. Other signs may include a skin rash, fever, weight loss, or drenching night sweats.
	• **Peripheral T-cell lymphoma.** Peripheral T-cell lymphoma begins in mature T lymphocytes. This type of T lymphocyte matures in the thymus gland and travels to other lymphatic sites in the body such as the lymph nodes, bone marrow, and spleen. There are three subtypes of peripheral T-cell lymphoma:
	    ○ *Hepatosplenic T-cell lymphoma.* This is an uncommon type of peripheral T-cell lymphoma that occurs mostly in young men. It begins in the liver and spleen and the cancer cells also have a T-cell receptor called gamma/delta on the surface of the cell.

Indolent and Aggressive Non-Hodgkin Lymphomas *Continued*	<ul><li>○ ***Subcutaneous panniculitis-like T-cell lymphoma.*** Subcutaneous panniculitis-like T-cell lymphoma begins in the skin or mucosa.</li><li>○ ***Enteropathy-type intestinal T-cell lymphoma.*** This type of peripheral T-cell lymphoma occurs in the small bowel of patients with untreated celiac disease (an immune response to gluten that causes malnutrition). P</li></ul><ul><li>**Intravascular large B-cell lymphoma.** This type of non-Hodgkin lymphoma affects blood vessels, especially the small blood vessels in the brain, kidney, lung, and skin. Signs and symptoms of intravascular large B-cell lymphoma are caused by blocked blood vessels. It is also called intravascular lymphomatosis.</li><li>**Burkitt lymphoma.** This is a type of B-cell non-Hodgkin lymphoma that grows and spreads very quickly. It may affect the jaw, bones of the face, bowel, kidneys, ovaries, or other organs. There are three main types of Burkitt lymphoma (endemic, sporadic, and immunodeficiency related). Endemic</li><li>**Lymphoblastic lymphoma.** This may begin in T cells or B cells, but it usually begins in T cells. In this type of non-Hodgkin lymphoma, there are too many lymphoblasts (immature white blood cells) in the lymph nodes and the thymus gland. These lymphoblasts may spread to other places in the body, such as the bone marrow, brain, and spinal cord. L</li><li>**T-cell leukemia/lymphoma.** This is caused by the human T-cell leukemia virus type 1 (HTLV-1). Signs include bone and skin lesions, high blood calcium levels, and lymph nodes, spleen, and liver that are larger than normal.</li><li>**Mantle cell lymphoma.** This is a type of B-cell non-Hodgkin lymphoma that usually occurs in middle-aged or older adults. It begins in the lymph nodes and spreads to the spleen, bone marrow, blood, and sometimes the esophagus, stomach, and intestines.</li><li>**Posttransplantation lymphoproliferative disorder**. This disease occurs in patients who have had a heart, lung, liver, kidney, or pancreas transplant and need lifelong immunosuppressive therapy. Most posttransplant lymphoproliferative disorders affect the B cells and have Epstein-Barr virus in the cells.</li><li>**True histiocytic lymphoma.** This is a rare, very aggressive type of lymphoma. It is not known whether it begins in B cells or T cells.</li><li>**Primary effusion lymphoma.** This begins in B cells that are found in an area where there is a large build-up of fluid, such as the areas between the lining of the lung and chest wall (pleural effusion), the sac around the heart and the heart (pericardial effusion), or in the abdominal cavity.</li><li>**Plasmablastic lymphoma.** This is a type of large B-cell non-Hodgkin lymphoma that is very aggressive. It is most often seen in patients with HIV infection.</li></ul>
Risk Factors Non-Hodgkin Lymphoma	<ul><li>Being older, male, or White.</li><li>Having one of the following medical conditions that weakens the immune system:<ul><li>○ An inherited immune disorder (such as hypogammaglobulinemia or Wiskott-Aldrich syndrome).</li><li>○ An autoimmune disease (such as rheumatoid arthritis, psoriasis, or Sjögren syndrome).</li><li>○ HIV/AIDS.</li><li>○ Human T-lymphotrophic virus type I or Epstein-Barr virus infection.</li><li>○ Helicobacter pylori infection.</li></ul></li><li>Taking immunosuppressant drugs after an organ transplant.</li></ul>

Treatment
 	
Non-Hodgkin Lymphoma
	General Treatment of Non-Hodgkin Lymphoma – *(see references for more specific information)*:
	
	Antibiotic therapy
	Chemotherapy
	Immunotherapy
	Immunotherapy
	Radiation therapy
	Stem cell transplant
	Targeted therapy
	Watchful waiting
	
	Intrathecal chemotherapy may also be used in the treatment of lymphoma that first forms in the testicles or sinuses (hollow areas) around the nose, diffuse large B-cell lymphoma, Burkitt lymphoma, lymphoblastic lymphoma, and some aggressive T-cell lymphomas.
	  • It is given to lessen the chance that lymphoma cells will spread to the brain and spinal cord.
	  • This is called CNS prophylaxis.
	
	Surgery
	The type of surgery used depends on where the lymphoma formed in the body:
	  • Local excision for certain patients with mucosa-associated lymphoid tissue (MALT) lymphoma, PTLD, and small bowel T-cell lymphoma.
	  • Splenectomy for patients with marginal zone lymphoma of the spleen.
	  • Small bowel surgery is often needed to diagnose celiac disease in adults who develop a type of T-cell lymphoma.
	
	Plasmapheresis
	  • If the blood becomes thick with extra antibody proteins and affects circulation, plasmapheresis is done to remove extra plasma and antibody proteins from the blood.
	     o In this procedure, blood is removed from the patient and sent through a machine that separates the plasma (the liquid part of the blood) from the blood cells.
	  • The patient's plasma contains the unneeded antibodies and is not returned to the patient. The normal blood cells are returned to the bloodstream along with donated plasma or a plasma replacement.
	     o Plasmapheresis does not keep new antibodies from forming.
	
	Vaccine therapy
	  • Vaccine therapy is a cancer treatment that uses a substance or group of substances to stimulate the immune system to find the tumor and kill it.
	
	'

Possible Side Effects / Late Side Effects
 	
Non-Hodgkin Lymphoma
	Possible Side Effects / Late Side Effects:
	• Heart problems.
	• Infertility
	• Loss of bone density.
	• Neuropathy (nerve damage that causes numbness or trouble walking).
	• Patients who have a heart, lung, liver, kidney, or pancreas transplant usually need to take drugs to suppress their immune system for the rest of their lives.
	• Long-term immunosuppression after an organ transplant can cause a certain type of non-Hodgkin lymphoma called post-transplant lymphoproliferative disorder (PLTD).
	• A second cancer, such as:
	    o Lung cancer.
	    o Brain cancer.
	    o Kidney cancer.
	    o Bladder cancer.
	    o Melanoma.
	    o Hodgkin lymphoma.
	    o Myelodysplastic syndrome.
	    o Acute myeloid leukemia.

Hodgkin Lymphoma	The two main types of Hodgkin lymphoma are *classic* and *nodular* lymphocyte predominant. • Most Hodgkin lymphomas are the classic type. • When a sample of lymph node tissue is looked at under a microscope, Hodgkin lymphoma cancer cells, called Reed-Sternberg cells, may be seen. The *classic type* is broken down into the following four subtypes: • Nodular sclerosing Hodgkin lymphoma. • Mixed cellularity Hodgkin lymphoma. • Lymphocyte-depleted Hodgkin lymphoma. • Lymphocyte-rich classic Hodgkin lymphoma. *Nodular* lymphocyte-predominant Hodgkin lymphoma (NLPHL) is rare and tends to grow slower than classic Hodgkin lymphoma. • NLPHL often presents as a swollen lymph node in the neck, chest, armpit, or groin. • Most people do not have any other signs or symptoms of cancer at diagnosis. • Treatment is often different from classic Hodgkin lymphoma.

Hodgkin Lymphomas
 	
Continued
	Hodgkin lymphoma may be grouped for treatment as follows:
	• *Early Favorable*
	   ○ Early favorable Hodgkin lymphoma is stage I or stage II, without risk factors that increase the chance that the cancer will come back after it is treated.
	• *Early Unfavorable*
	   ○ Early unfavorable Hodgkin lymphoma is stage I or stage II with one or more of the following risk factors that increase the chance that the cancer will come back after it is treated:
	      ▪ Having a tumor in the chest that is larger than 1/3 of the width of the chest or is at least 10 centimeters.
	      ▪ Having cancer in an organ other than the lymph nodes.
	      ▪ Having a high sedimentation rate (in a sample of blood, the red blood cells settle to the bottom of the test tube more quickly than normal).
	      ▪ Having three or more lymph nodes with cancer.
	      ▪ Having B symptoms (fever for no known reason, weight loss for no known reason, or drenching night sweats).
	• *Advanced*
	   ○ Advanced Hodgkin lymphoma is stage III or stage IV.
	   ○ *Advanced favorable* Hodgkin lymphoma means that the patient has 0–3 of the risk factors below.
	   ○ *Advanced unfavorable* Hodgkin lymphoma means that the patient has 4 or more of the risk factors below.
	   ○ The more risk factors a patient has, the more likely it is that the cancer will come back after it is treated:
	      ▪ Having a low blood albumin level (below 4).
	      ▪ Having a low hemoglobin level (below 10.5).
	      ▪ Being male.
	      ▪ Being 45 years or older.
	      ▪ Having stage IV disease.
	      ▪ Having a high white blood cell count (15,000 or higher).
	      ▪ Having a low lymphocyte count (below 600 or less than 8% of the white blood cell count).
	      ▪ Hodgkin lymphoma can recur (come back) after it has been treated.
	      ▪ The cancer may come back in the lymph system or in other parts of the body.

Risk Factors **Hodgkin Lymphoma**	**Risk factors for Hodgkin lymphoma include the following:** Not every person with one or more of these risk factors will develop Hodgkin lymphoma, and it can develop in people who don't have any known risk factors. • **Age.** Hodgkin lymphoma is most common in early adulthood (age 20–39 years) and in late adulthood (age 65 years and older). • **Being male.** The risk of Hodgkin lymphoma is slightly higher in males than in females. • **Past Epstein-Barr virus infection.** Having an infection with the Epstein-Barr virus in the teenage years or early childhood increases the risk of Hodgkin lymphoma. • **A family history of Hodgkin lymphoma.** Having a parent, brother, or sister with Hodgkin lymphoma increases the risk of developing Hodgkin lymphoma. **Hodgkin lymphoma can recur (come back) after it has been treated.** • The cancer may come back in the lymph system or in other parts of the body.

Treatment **Hodgkin Lymphoma**	**Treatment for Hodgkin Lymphoma include:** **Active surveillance** **Chemotherapy** **Immunotherapy** **Radiation therapy** **Stem cell transplant** **Steroid therapy** **Targeted therapy** **Watchful waiting** **Chemotherapy with stem cell transplant** High doses of chemotherapy are given to kill cancer cells. Healthy cells, including blood-forming cells, are also destroyed by the cancer treatment. <ul><li>Stem cell transplant is a treatment to replace the blood-forming cells. Stem cells (immature blood cells) are removed from the blood or bone marrow of the patient or a donor and are frozen and stored.</li><li>After the patient completes chemotherapy and radiation therapy, the stored stem cells are thawed and given back to the patient through an infusion.</li><li>These reinfused stem cells grow into (and restore) the body's blood cells.</li></ul> **Treatment of Early *Favorable* Classic Hodgkin Lymphoma** Treatment of early favorable classic Hodgkin lymphoma in adults may include the following: <ul><li>Combination chemotherapy.</li><li>Combination chemotherapy with radiation therapy to the areas of the body with cancer.</li><li>Radiation therapy alone in patients who cannot be treated with combination chemotherapy.</li></ul> **Treatment of Early *Unfavorable* Classic Hodgkin Lymphoma** Treatment of early unfavorable classic Hodgkin lymphoma in adults may include the following: <ul><li>Combination chemotherapy with radiation therapy to the areas of the body with cancer.</li><li>Combination chemotherapy.</li><li>Targeted therapy with a monoclonal antibody (brentuximab vedotin) and combination chemotherapy with or without radiation therapy.</li></ul> **Treatment of *Advanced* Classic Hodgkin Lymphoma** Treatment of advanced classic Hodgkin lymphoma in adults may include the following: <ul><li>Combination chemotherapy.</li></ul>

Treatment Hodgkin Lymphoma *Continued*	**Treatment of *Recurrent* Classic Hodgkin Lymphoma:** Treatment of recurrent classic Hodgkin lymphoma in adults may include the following: • Immunotherapy with an immune checkpoint inhibitor (pembrolizumab or nivolumab alone), targeted therapy with a monoclonal antibody (brentuximab vedotin) alone, or a combination. This may be followed by stem cell transplant. • Combination chemotherapy, which may be followed by pembrolizumab or nivolumab. Stem cell transplant may be considered. • Combination chemotherapy with radiation therapy to the areas of the body with cancer for patients older than 60 years. • Radiation therapy with or without chemotherapy, for patients whose cancer came back only in the lymph nodes. • Chemotherapy as palliative therapy to relieve symptoms and improve quality of life. **Treatment of *Nodular Lymphocyte–Predominant* Hodgkin Lymphoma (NLPHL)** Treatment of NLPHL in adults may include the following: • Watchful waiting or active surveillance. • Radiation therapy to the areas of the body with cancer, for patients with early-stage NLPHL. • Chemotherapy, for patients with advanced-stage NLPHL. • Targeted therapy with a monoclonal antibody (rituximab).
Possible Side Effects / Late Side Effects **Hodgkin Lymphoma**	**Treatment for Hodgkin lymphoma may cause side effects.** Side effects from cancer treatment that begin after treatment and continue for months or years are called *late effects*. These late effects depend on the type of treatment and the patient's age when treated, and may include the following: • Second cancers. • Solid tumors, such as mesothelioma and cancer of the lung, breast, thyroid, bone, soft tissue, stomach, esophagus, colon, rectum, cervix, and head and neck. • Acute myelogenous leukemia. • Infertility. • Hypothyroidism (too little thyroid hormone in the blood). • Heart disease, such as heart attack. • Lung problems, such as trouble breathing. • Avascular necrosis of bone (death of bone cells caused by lack of blood flow). • Severe infection. • Chronic fatigue. • Cognitive impairment. • Regular follow-up by doctors who are experts in finding and treating late effects is important for the long-term health of patients treated for Hodgkin lymphoma.
References	National Cancer Institute (NCI) - **Hodgkin** Lymphoma: *https://www.cancer.gov/types/lymphoma/patient/adult-hodgkin-treatment-pdq* National Cancer Institute (NCI) - Adult **Non-Hodgkin** Lymphoma Treatment: *https://www.cancer.gov/types/lymphoma/patient/adult-nhl-treatment-pdq* National Cancer Institute (NCI) - **Non-Hodgkin** Lymphoma: *https://www.cancer.gov/types/lymphoma*

MELANOMA

Information and pictures from *National Cancer Institute* unless otherwise specified

Description	Melanoma is a disease in which malignant (cancer) cells form in melanocytes (cells that color the skin).

The skin is the body's largest organ. It protects against heat, sunlight, injury, and infection. Skin also helps control body temperature and stores water, fat, and vitamin D. The skin has several layers, but the two main layers are the epidermis (upper or outer layer) and the dermis (lower or inner layer).

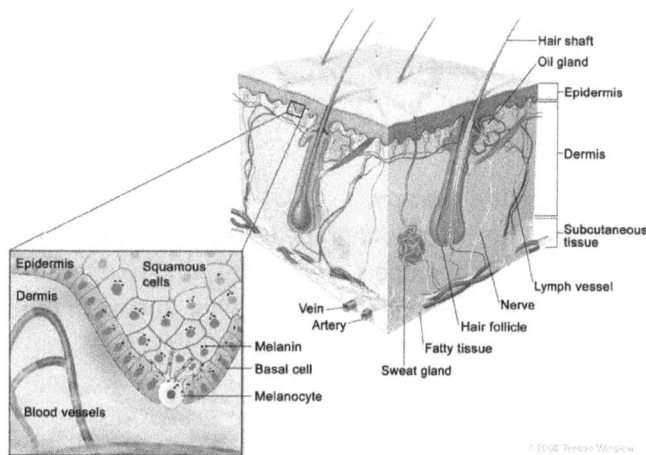

Skin cancer begins in the epidermis, which is made up of three kinds of cells:
- **Squamous cells:** Thin, flat cells that form the top layer of the epidermis.
- **Basal cells:** Round cells under the squamous cells.
- **Melanocytes:** Cells that make melanin and are found in the lower part of the epidermis.
  - Melanin is the pigment that gives skin its natural color. When skin is exposed to the sun or artificial light, melanocytes make more pigment and cause the skin to darken.

There are different types of cancer that start in the skin. There are two forms of skin cancer: melanoma and nonmelanoma.
- **Melanoma** is a rare form of skin cancer. It is more likely to invade nearby tissues and spread to other parts of the body than other types of skin cancer.
  - When melanoma starts in the skin, it is called cutaneous melanoma.
  - Melanoma may also occur in mucous membranes (thin, moist layers of tissue that cover surfaces such as the lips).
- **Nonmelanoma:** The most common types of skin cancer are basal cell carcinoma and squamous cell carcinoma. They are nonmelanoma skin cancers.
  - Nonmelanoma skin cancers rarely spread to other parts of the body.

Melanoma can occur anywhere on the skin.
- ***In men***, melanoma is often found on the trunk (the area from the shoulders to the hips) or the head and neck.
- ***In women***, melanoma forms most often on the arms and legs.
- When melanoma occurs in the eye, it is called intraocular or ocular melanoma.

Risk Factors	**Risk Factors for Skin Cancer:** • Ultraviolet (UV) light exposure • Fair / Light Skin • Moles • Family history of melanoma • Personal history of melanoma or other skin cancers • Weakened Immune system • Older • Males
Treatment	**Chemotherapy** **Immunotherapy** **Radiation therapy** **Targeted therapy** **Vaccine therapy** • Vaccine therapy uses a substance or group of substances meant to cause the immune system to respond to a tumor and kill it. • Vaccine therapy is being studied in the treatment of stage III melanoma that can beremoved by surgery. **Surgery** • Surgery to remove the tumor is the primary treatment of all stages of melanoma. ○ A wide local excision is used to remove the melanoma and some of the normal tissue around it. • Skin grafting (taking skin from another part of the body to replace the skin that is removed) may be done to cover the wound caused by surgery. • After the doctor removes all the melanomathat can be seen at the time of the surgery,some patients may be given chemotherapy after surgery to kill any cancer cells that are left. • Surgery to remove cancer that has spread to the lymph nodes, lung, gastrointestinal (GI) tract, bone, or brain may be done to improvethe patient's quality of life by controlling symptoms.
Lymph Nodes/ Lymphadenectomy *(Also See Section on Lymph Nodes)*	**Lymph Nodes/ Lymphadenectomy** It is important to know whether cancer has spread to the lymph nodes. • Lymph node mapping and sentinel lymph node biopsy are done to check for cancer in the sentinel lymphnode during surgery. *(See Lymph Nodes)*. • A pathologist views the tissue under a microscope to look for cancer cells. • If cancer cells are found, more lymph nodes will be removed, and tissue samples will be checked for signs of cancer. • This is called a lymphadenectomy.

Possible Side Effects	**Possible Side Effects:** • Vitiligo (loss of pigment) • Skin rash • Lymphedema • Thyroid issues • Colitis • Itching • Joint pain
References	National Cancer Institute - (NCI) - Melanoma Treatment (PDQ®): *https://www.cancer.gov/types/skin/patient/melanoma-treatment-pdq* National Cancer Institute - (NCI) Skin Cancer Treatment: *https://www.cancer.gov/types/skin/patient/skin-treatment-pdq*

PANCREATIC
Information and pictures from *National Cancer Institute* unless otherwise specified

Description	Pancreatic cancer is a disease in which malignant (cancer) cells form in the tissues of the pancreas.

The pancreas is a gland about 6 inches long that is shaped like a thin pear lying on its side. The wider end of the pancreas is called the head, the middle section is called the body, and the narrow end is called the tail. The pancreas lies between the stomach and the spine.

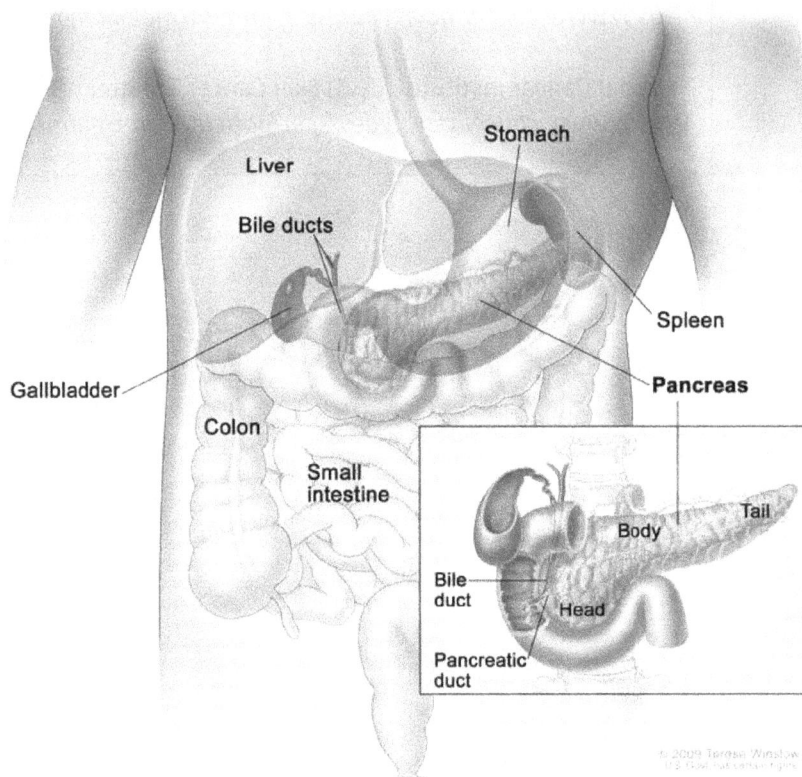

The pancreas has three areas: head, body, and tail. It is found in the abdomen near the stomach, intestines, and other organs.

The pancreas has two main jobs in the body:
- To make juices that help digest (break down) food.
- To make hormones, such as insulin and glucagon, that help control blood sugar levels.
  - Both of these hormones help the body use and store the energy it gets from food.
  - The digestive juices are made by exocrine

Risk Factors	**Risk factors for pancreatic cancer include the following:**
	• Smoking.
	• Being very overweight.
	• Having a personal history of diabetes or chronic pancreatitis.
	• Having a family history of pancreatic cancer or pancreatitis.
	• Having certain hereditary conditions, such as:
	    o Multiple endocrine neoplasia type 1 (MEN1) syndrome.
	    o Hereditary nonpolyposis colon cancer (HNPCC; Lynch syndrome).
	    o von Hippel-Lindau syndrome.
	    o Peutz-Jeghers syndrome.
	    o Hereditary breast and ovarian cancer syndrome.
	    o Familial atypical multiple mole melanoma (FAMMM) syndrome.
	    o Ataxia-telangiectasia.

Treatment	**Chemoradiation therapy**
	Chemotherapy
	Radiation therapy
	Targeted therapy
	
	Surgery
	One of the following types of surgery may be used to take out the tumor:
	• **Whipple procedure**: A surgical procedure in which the head of the pancreas, the gallbladder, part of the stomach, part of the small intestine, and the bile duct are removed. Enough of the pancreas is left to produce digestive juices and insulin.
	• **Total pancreatectomy:** This operation removes the whole pancreas, part of the stomach, part of the small intestine, the common bile duct, the gallbladder, the spleen, and nearby lymph nodes.
	• **Distal pancreatectomy:** Surgery to remove the body and the tail of the pancreas. The spleen may also be removed if cancer has spread to the spleen.
	
	If the cancer has spread and cannot be removed, the following types of palliative surgery may be done to relieve symptoms and improve quality of life:
	• **Biliary bypass:** If cancer is blocking the bile duct and bile is building up in the gallbladder, a biliary bypass may be done.
	    o During this operation, the doctor will cut the gallbladder or bile duct in the area before the blockage and sew it to the small intestine to create a new pathway around the blocked area.
	• **Endoscopic stent placement:** If the tumor is blocking the bile duct, surgery may be done to put in a stent (a thin tube) to drain bile that has built up in the area.
	    o The doctor may place the stent through a catheter that drains the bile into a bag on the outside of the body or the stent may go around the blocked area and drain the bile into the small intestine.
	• **Gastric bypass:** If the tumor is blocking the flow of food from the stomach, the stomach may be sewn directly to the small intestine so the patient can continue to eat normally

Treatment for 'Types' of Pancreatic Cancers	**Resectable or Borderline Resectable Pancreatic Cancer** Treatment of resectable or borderline resectable pancreatic cancer may include the following: • Chemotherapy with or without radiation therapy followed by surgery. • Surgery. • Surgery followed by chemotherapy. • Surgery followed by chemoradiation. • A clinical trial of chemotherapy and/or radiation therapy before surgery. • A clinical trial of different ways of giving radiation therapy. • Surgery to remove the tumor may include Whipple procedure, total pancreatectomy, or distal pancreatectomy. • Palliative therapy can be started at any stage of disease. See the Palliative Therapy section for information about treatments that may improve quality of life or relieve symptoms in patients with pancreatic cancer. **Locally Advanced Pancreatic Cancer** Treatment of pancreatic cancer that is locally advanced may include the following: • Chemotherapy with or without targeted therapy. • Chemotherapy and chemoradiation. • Surgery (Whipple procedure, total pancreatectomy, or distal pancreatectomy). • Palliative surgery or stent placement to bypass blocked areas in ducts or the small intestine. Some patients may also receive chemotherapy and chemoradiation to shrink the tumor to allow for surgery. • A clinical trial of new anticancer therapies together with chemotherapy or chemoradiation. • A clinical trial of radiation therapy given during surgery or internal radiation therapy. • Palliative therapy can be started at any stage of disease. See the Palliative Therapy section for information about treatments that may improve quality of life or relieve symptoms in patients with pancreatic cancer. **Metastatic or Recurrent Pancreatic Cancer** Treatment of pancreatic cancer that has metastasized or recurred may include the following: • Chemotherapy with or without targeted therapy. • Clinical trials of new anticancer agents with or without chemotherapy. • Palliative therapy can be started at any stage of disease. See the Palliative Therapy section for information about treatments that may improve quality of life or relieve symptoms in patients with pancreatic cancer. **Palliative Therapy** Palliative therapy can improve the patient's quality of life by controlling the symptoms and complications of pancreatic cancer. Palliative therapy for pancreatic cancer includes the following: • Palliative surgery or stent placement to bypass blocked areas in ducts or the small intestine. • Palliative radiation therapy to help relieve pain by shrinking the tumor. • An injection of medicine to help relieve pain by blocking nerves in the abdomen. • Other palliative medical care alone.

Possible Specific Side Effects	**Possible Specific Side Effects:**
	• Patients with pancreatic cancer have special nutritional needs.
	  ○ Surgery to remove the pancreas may affect its ability to make pancreatic enzymes that help to digest food. As a result, patients may have problems digesting food and absorbing nutrients into the body.
	  ○ To prevent malnutrition, the doctor may prescribe medicines that replace these enzymes.
	• Pain can occur when the tumor presses on nerves or other organs near the pancreas.
	  ○ When pain medicine is not enough, there are treatments that act on nerves in the abdomen to relieve the pain. The doctor may inject medicine into the area around affected nerves or may cut the nerves to block the feeling of pain.
	  ○ Radiation therapy with or without chemotherapy can also help relieve pain by shrinking the tumor.

References	CETI- Cancer Exercise Training Institute: *https://www.thecancerspecialist.com/* CDC - Diabetes – Get Active: *https://www.cdc.gov/diabetes/managing/active.html* National Cancer Institute *(NCI)* Pancreatic Cancer - Treatment: *https://www.cancer.gov/types/pancreatic/patient/pancreatic-treatment-pdq* National Cancer Institute *(NCI)* Pancreatic Cancer - Types: *https://www.cancer.gov/types/pancreatic* University Hospitals of Leicester - Exercise Advice for People after Liver and Pancreas Surgery: *https://yourhealth.leicestershospitals.nhs.uk/library/chuggs/hepatobiliary/418-exercise-advice-for-people-following-liver-and-pancreas-surgery/file*

Recovery after Surgery
 	
*Information from **CETI**- Cancer Exercise Training Institute*
 	
Please follow MD/surgeon protocol, as every situation is unique.
	Whipple Procedure
	➤ **Hospital Stay:** 1-2 weeks (first night in intensive care)
	➤ **Full Recovery:** Several months
	➤ **Restrictions:** No heavy lifting over a few lbs. for 6 weeks
	➤ **Exercise:** Walking during recovery period for most patients – see MD protocol
	➤ **Possible Side Effects:** Infections, Bleeding, Trouble Emptying Stomach after Eating, Weight Loss, Trouble Digesting, Change in Bowel Habits, Diabetes
	
	Total Pancreatectomy:
	➤ **Hospital Stay:** *Laparoscopic* 3-5 days; *Open:* 10 days
	➤ **Full Recovery:** 2 months
	➤ **Restrictions:** No heavy lifting over 10 lbs. for 8 weeks
	➤ **Exercise:** Walking during recovery period for most patients – see MD protocol
	➤ **Possible Side Effects:** Constipation, Pain, Post-operative Bleeding, Fatigue, Cramping, Diarrhea, Weight Loss, Fistula or Pancreatic Anastomotic Leak, Osteopenia, Liver Disease, Immune System Compromised, Delayed Gastric Emptying
	    ○ **Lymphedema** if lymph nodes are removed *(see Lymphedema)*
	    ○ **Diabetes** – Insulin Dependence. *(See Special Considerations below)*

Exercise Recommen-dations
 	
University Hospitals of Leicester
 	
Please follow MD/surgeon protocol, as every situation is unique.
	Day 1
	Glute squeezes and ankle pumps
	
	Day 2
	• Walking
	• Trunk rotation / knee rolling – this will also help release trapped gas
	• Pelvic tilt
	
	Day 3 or per MD protocol
	• Lying down
	   o Ankle pumps
	   o SAQ
	   o Pelvic tilt > bridging
	• Sitting:
	   o Arms:
	      - Shoulder flexion.
	      - Arm punches (alternating hands reaching up towards the ceiling.
	      - Bicep curls with hand weights or soup cans as tolerated
	   o Legs: SLAQ
	• Standing: Marching in place holding onto chair or stable surface
	
	Weeks 6-12
	Six to eight weeks after your operation you can start to do low-impact exercise such as jogging and cycling (on a flat surface).
	• Swimming is another good form of exercise, but please note that your wound must be healed before swimming.
	• Start these activities gradually. Common sense will guide you as to how much exercise your body can take.
	
	University Hospitals of Leicester

Exercise Recommendations after Pancreatic Surgery per MD protocol
(see above for timetable)

Sections from HEP portion of book

Flex = Flexibility   *Strength* - LE = Lower Extremity   UE = Upper Extremity

Exercise	Section	Number
Trunk rotation	Flex	60
Pelvic tilts	Core	3
Ankle Pumps	LE	6
Bridging	Core	5
SAQ	LE	15
LAQ	LE	21
Standing Marching	Balance	49
Shoulder flexion	UE	39 No Resistance
Arm punches above head or forward	x	x

Special Considerations for People with Diabetes *CDC* ***Please follow MD/surgeon protocol, as every situation is unique.***	One of the "side effects" of pancreatic cancer/surgery is diabetes. It is important to understand the correlation between blood sugar and exercise. Before starting any physical activity, check with your health care provider to talk about the best physical activities for you. Be sure to discuss which activities you like, how to prepare, and what you should avoid. <ul><li>Drink plenty of fluids while being physically active to prevent dehydration (harmful loss of water in the body).</li><li>Make sure to check your blood sugar before being physically active, especially if you take insulin.</li><li>If it's **below 100 mg/dL,** you may need to eat a small snack containing 15-30 grams of carbohydrates, such as 2 tablespoons of raisins or ½ cup of fruit juice or regular soda (not diet), or glucose tablets so your blood sugar doesn't fall too low while being physically active.<ul><li>Low blood sugar (hypoglycemia) can be very serious.</li></ul></li><li>If it's **above 240 mg/dL,** your blood sugar may be too high (hyperglycemia) to be active safely.<ul><li>Test your urine for ketones – substances made when your body breaks down fat for energy. The presence of ketones indicates that your body doesn't have enough insulin to control your blood sugar.</li><li>If you are physically active when you have high ketone levels, you risk ketoacidosis – a serious diabetes complication that needs immediate treatment.</li></ul></li><li>When you're physically active, wear cotton socks and athletic shoes that fit well and are comfortable.</li><li>After your activity, check to see how it has affected your blood glucose level.</li><li>After being physically active, check your feet for sores, blisters, irritation, cuts, or other injuries.</li><li>*Call your health care provider if an injury doesn't begin to heal after 2 days.*</li></ul> *CDC – Diabetes – Get Active*

PROSTATE
Information and pictures from *National Cancer Institute* unless otherwise specified

Description	Prostate cancer is a disease in which malignant (cancer) cells form in the tissues of the prostate. *The prostate is a gland in the male reproductive system. It lies just below the bladder (the organ that collects and empties urine) and in front of the rectum (the lower part of the intestine). It is about the size of a walnut and surrounds part of the urethra (the tube that empties urine from the bladder). The prostate gland makes fluid that is part of the semen* Normal prostate and benign prostatic hyperplasia (BPH). 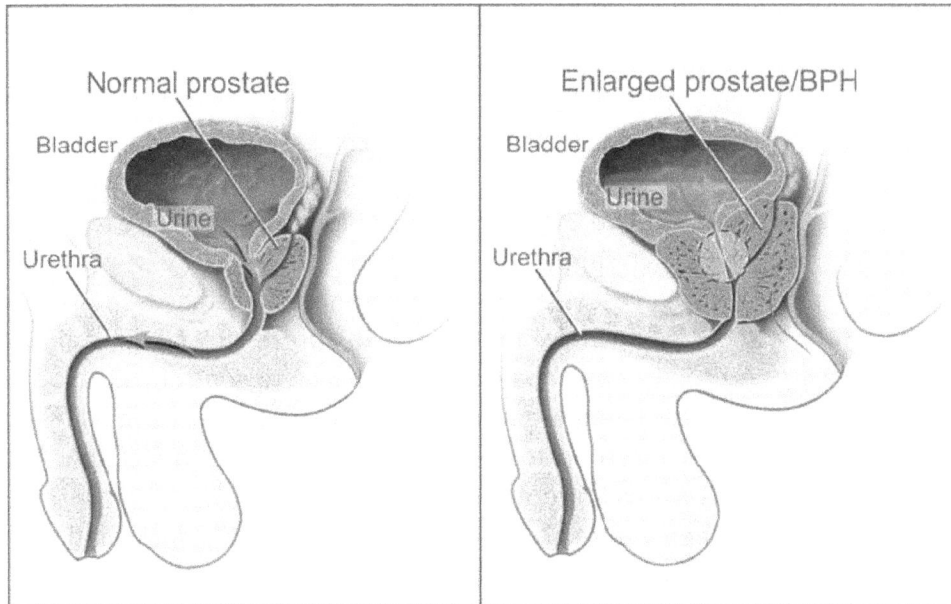 • A normal prostate does not block the flow of urine from the bladder. • An enlarged prostate presses on the bladder and urethra and blocks the flow of urine.

Risk Factors	**Age**
	• Age is an important risk factor for prostate cancer. Prostate cancer is rarely seen in men younger than 40 years; the incidence rises rapidly with each decade thereafter.
	    ○ For example, the probability of being diagnosed with prostate cancer is 1 in 456 for men 49 years or younger, 1 in 54 for men aged 50 through 59 years, 1 in 19 for men aged 60 through 69 years, and 1 in 11 for men aged 70 years and older, with an overall lifetime risk of developing prostate cancer of 1 in 8.
	
	Ancestry
	• The risk of developing and dying from prostate cancer is higher among Black men, is of intermediate levels among White men, and is lowest among native Japanese.
	    ○ Conflicting data have been published regarding the etiology of these outcomes, but some evidence is available that access to health care may play a role in disease outcomes.
	    ○ According to the Surveillance, Epidemiology, and End Results (SEER) Program, incidence of prostate cancer in African American men exceeds those of White men at all ages.

Risk Factors *Continued*	**Family History** • Approximately 15% of men with a diagnosis of prostate cancer will be found to have a first-degree relative (e.g., brother, father) with prostate cancer, compared with approximately 8% of the U.S. population. ○ Approximately 9% of all prostate cancers may result from heritable susceptibility genes. **Other Risks:** • Hormones • Dietary Fat, Dairy and Calcium Intake, Multivitamin Use, Folate • Cadmium Exposure, Dioxin Exposure • Prostatitis *See Prostate Cancer Prevention (PDQ®)–Health Professional Version AND Genetics of Prostate Cancer (PDQ®)–Health Professional Version for more information.*
Treatment	**Biologic therapy** **Bisphosphonate therapy** **Chemotherapy** **Hormone therapy** **Radiation therapy** **Targeted therapy** **Watchful waiting or Active surveillance** **Internal radiation therapy** uses a radioactive substance sealed in needles, seeds, wires, or catheters that are placed directly into or near the cancer. • In early-stage prostate cancer, the radioactive seeds are placed in the prostate using needles that are inserted through the skin between the scrotum and rectum. • The placement of the radioactive seeds in the prostate is guided by images from transrectal ultrasound or computed tomography (CT). The needles are removed after the radioactive seeds are placed in the prostate. **Radiopharmaceutical therapy** uses a radioactive substance to treat cancer including **Alpha emitter radiation therapy**, which uses a radioactive substance to treat prostate cancer that has spread to the bone. **Surgery** Patients in good health whose tumor is in the prostate gland only may be treated with surgery to remove the tumor. The following types of surgery are used: • **Radical prostatectomy**: A surgical procedure to remove the prostate, surrounding tissue, and seminal vesicles. There are two types of radical prostatectomy: ○ **Retropubic prostatectomy:** A surgical procedure to remove the prostate through an incision (cut) in the abdominal wall. ▪ Removal of nearby lymph nodes may be done at the same time. ○ **Perineal prostatectomy:** A surgical procedure to remove the prostate through an incision (cut) made in the perineum (area between the scrotum and anus). Nearby lymph nodes may also be removed through a separate incision in the abdomen. • **Pelvic lymphadenectomy:** A surgical procedure to remove the lymph nodes in the pelvis. A pathologist views the tissue under a microscope to look for cancer cells. If the lymph nodes contain cancer, the doctor will not remove the prostate and may recommend other treatment.

Treatment *Continued*	• **Transurethral resection of the prostate (TURP):** A surgical procedure to remove tissue from the prostate using a resectoscope (a thin, lighted tube with a cutting tool) inserted through the urethra. 　○ This procedure is done to treat benign prostatic hypertrophy, and it is sometimes done to relieve symptoms caused by a tumor before other cancer treatment is given. 　○ TURP may also be done in men whose tumor is in the prostate only and who cannot have a radical prostatectomy. **Cryosurgery** is a treatment that uses an instrument to freeze and destroy prostate cancer cells. Ultrasound is used to find the area that will be treated. • *Cryosurgery can cause impotence and leakage of urine from the bladder or stool from the rectum.* **High-intensity–focused ultrasound therapy** is a treatment that uses ultrasound (high-energy sound waves) to destroy cancer cells. To treat prostate cancer, an endorectal probe is used to make the sound waves. **Proton beam radiation therapy** is a type of high-energy, external radiation therapy that targets tumors with streams of protons (small, positively charged particles). This type of radiation therapy is being studied in the treatment of prostate cancer. **Hormone therapy** Hormone therapy is a cancer treatment that removes hormones or blocks their action and stops cancer cells from growing. Hormones are substances made by glands in the body and circulated in the bloodstream. • In prostate cancer, male sex hormones can cause prostate cancer to grow. • Drugs, surgery, or other hormones are used to reduce the amount of male hormones or block them from working. This is called androgen deprivation therapy (ADT). Hormone therapy for prostate cancer may include the following: • *Abiraterone acetate* can prevent prostate cancer cells from making androgens. It is used in men with advanced prostate cancer that has not gotten better with other hormone therapy. It is also used in men with high-risk prostate cancer that has improved with treatments that lower hormone levels. • *Orchiectomy* is a surgical procedure to remove one or both testicles, the main source of male hormones, such as testosterone, to decrease the amount of hormone being made. • *Estrogens* (hormones that promote female sex characteristics) can prevent the testicles from making testosterone. However, estrogens are seldom used today in the treatment of prostate cancer because of the risk of serious side effects. • *Luteinizing hormone-releasing hormone* agonists can stop the testicles from making testosterone. Examples are leuprolide, goserelin, and buserelin. • *Antiandrogens* can block the action of androgens (hormones that promote male sex characteristics), such as testosterone. Examples are flutamide, bicalutamide, enzalutamide, apalutamide, nilutamide, and darolutamide. • *Drugs that can prevent the adrenal glands from making androgens* include ketoconazole, aminoglutethimide, hydrocortisone, and progesterone.

Possible Side Effects	**Surgery:**
	
	Transurethral resection of the prostate (TURP)
	• Recurring urinary tract infections
	• Kidney or bladder damage
	• Inability to control urination or an inability to urinate at all
	• Bladder stones
	• Blood in your urine *(Mayo)*
	
	Radical prostatectomy
	• Impotence
	• Heart attack / stroke
	• Bladder spasms
	• Blood clot in the legs
	• Leakage of urine from the bladder or stool from the rectum.
	• Shortening of the penis (1 to 2 centimeters). The exact reason for this is not known.
	• Inguinal hernia (bulging of fat or part of the small intestine through weak muscles into the groin).
	    ○ Inguinal hernia may occur more often in men treated with radical prostatectomy than in men who have some other types of prostate surgery, radiation therapy, or prostate biopsy alone.
	    ○ It is most likely to occur within the first 2 years after radical prostatectomy.
	
	Pelvic lymphadenectomy: If lymph nodes are removed, there may be additional side effects:
	• Lymphedema
	• Seroma
	• Infection
	• Nerve damage
	
	Bone Pain: Prostate cancer that has spread to the bone and certain types of hormone therapy can weaken bones and lead to bone pain.
	    Treatments for bone pain include the following:
	    ○ Pain medicine.
	    ○ External radiation therapy.
	    ○ Strontium-89 (a radioisotope).
	    ○ Targeted therapy with a monoclonal antibody, such as denosumab.
	    ○ Bisphosphonate therapy.
	    ○ Corticosteroids.
	
	Radiation therapy: Increased risk of bladder and/or gastrointestinal cancer. This can also cause impotence and urinary problems that may get worse with age.
	
	Hormone therapy: Hot flashes, impaired sexual function, loss of desire for sex, and weakened bones
	
	Cryosurgery: Can cause impotence and leakage of urine from the bladder or stool from the rectum

References	CETI- Cancer Exercise Training Institute: *https://www.thecancerspecialist.com/* Mayo Clinic - Transurethral resection of the prostate (TURP): *https://www.mayoclinic.org/tests-procedures/turp/about/pac-20384880)* National Cancer Institute - NCI - **Genetics of Prostate Cancer (**PDQ®)–Health Professional Version: *https://www.cancer.gov/types/prostate/hp/prostate-genetics-pdq* National Cancer Institute - NCI - **Prostate Cancer:** *https://www.cancer.gov/types/prostate* National Cancer Institute - NCI - **Prostate Cancer Prevention** (PDQ®)–Health Professional Version: *https://www.cancer.gov/types/prostate/hp/prostate-prevention-pdq*

Recovery after Surgery
 	
 *Information from **CETI-**Cancer Exercise Training Institute*
 	
 Please follow MD/surgeon protocol, as every situation is unique.
	Radical prostatectomy
	 ➢ **Hospital Stay:** 2-3 days
	 ➢ **Full Recovery:** 3 months
	 ➢ **Other:** May have a catheter for up to 3 weeks after surgery.
	     ○ Can use a leg bag for walking during this time.
	 ➢ **Restrictions:** No heavy lifting or straining for one month or bicycle for 12 weeks.
	 ➢ **Exercise:** Walking.
	     ○ Pelvic floor exercise after catheter is removed. *(See Kegel under Bladder)*
	 ➢ **Possible Side Effects**: Bladder Spasms, Heart Attack, Stroke, Inguinal Hernia, Lower Extremity Blood Clots, Incontinence and/or Long-Term Stress Incontinence, Infertility, Impotence, Shorting of Penis by 1-2cm
	
	 Transurethral resection of the prostate (TURP)
	 ➢ **Hospital Stay:** 1-2 days
	 ➢ **Full Recovery:** 1-2 weeks
	 ➢ **Other:** Catheter for 1-3 days.
	 ➢ **Restrictions:** Avoid strenuous activity, such as heavy lifting, for four to six weeks or until your doctor says it's OK. Hold off on sex for four to six weeks. (*Mayo Clinic - Transurethral resection of the prostate (TURP)*
	 ➢ **Exercise:** Walking. Pelvic floor exercise after catheter is removed. *(See Kegel)*
	 ➢ **Possible Side Effects:** Recurrent Urinary Tract Infections, Partial Impotence or Incontinence, Retrograde Ejaculation, Difficulty Urinating, Blood in Urine (after surgery), Low Sodium

Exercise, Special Considerations & Precautions – Short and Long Term
 	
Information from CETI- Cancer Exercise Training Institute
 	
Please follow MD/surgeon protocol, as every situation is unique.
	Radical prostatectomy
	• **First Week:** Walk inside: 6-8 x for 5-10 min
	• **First Month Restrictions:**
	   o Strenuous exercise
	   o Lifting
	   o Straining
	   o Bike
	• **3 Month / 12 Week Restrictions or until cleared by surgeon:**
	   o Bike
	
	Retropubic Incision: Vertical incision through the lower abdomen
	• **Avoid – 12 weeks or until cleared by surgeon:**
	   o Crunches until able to stand erect (exercises should stretch the abdomen). *(Strengthen lower back)*
	   o Planks
	
	Perineal Prostatectomy: Incision in the perineum between the anus and scrotum.
	• **Avoid – 12 weeks or until cleared by surgeon:**
	   o Jumping / high impact
	   o Riding a bicycle
	   o Squats
	   o Lunges Exercise
	
	Pelvic lymph node dissection through retropubic approach:
	• **Potential side effects:**
	   o Lower extremity lymphedema
	   o Infection
	   o Seroma
	   o Nerve damage
	• **Recommendations:**
	   o 5 min low aerobic exercise as warm up
	   o Lymphatic drainage exercises
	   o No restrictions on the upper body
	   o Lower extremity range of motion exercises

STOMACH

Information and pictures from *National Cancer Institute* unless otherwise specified

| Description | Gastric cancer is a disease in which malignant (cancer) cells form in the lining of the stomach. |

The stomach is a J-shaped organ in the upper abdomen. It is part of the digestive system, which processes nutrients (vitamins, minerals, carbohydrates, fats, proteins, and water) in foods that are eaten and helps pass waste material out of the body. Food moves from the throat to the stomach through a hollow, muscular tube called the esophagus. After leaving the stomach, partly digested food passes into the small intestine and then into the large intestine.

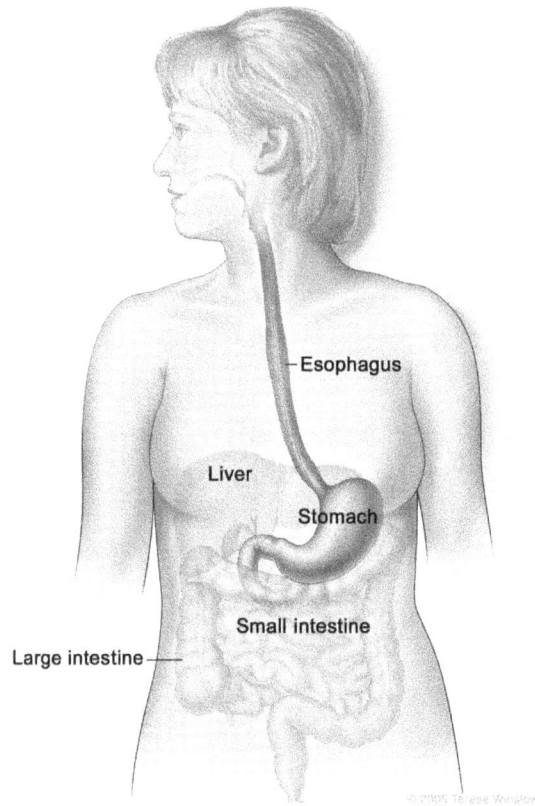

- After gastric cancer has been diagnosed, tests are done to find out if cancer cells have spread within the stomach or to other parts of the body.
- Cancer may spread from where it began to other parts of the body.
- The following stages are used for gastric cancer:
  - Stage 0 (Carcinoma in Situ)
  - Stage I
  - Stage II
  - Stage III
  - Stage IV
- Gastric cancer can recur (come back) after it has been treated.

Risk Factors	**Risk Factors for Stomach Cancer:**
	• Having any of the following medical conditions:
	    ○ Helicobacter pylori (H. pylori) infection of the stomach.
	    ○ Chronic gastritis (inflammation of the stomach).
	    ○ Pernicious anemia.
	    ○ Intestinal metaplasia (a condition in which the normal stomach lining is replaced with the cells that line the intestines).
	    ○ Gastric polyps.
	    ○ Epstein-Barr virus infection.
	    ○ Familial syndromes (including familial adenomatous polyposis).
	• Eating a diet high in salted, smoked foods and low in fruits and vegetables.
	• Eating foods that have not been prepared or stored properly.
	• Being older or male.
	• Smoking cigarettes.
	• Having a mother, father, sister, or brother who has had stomach cancer.
	• *BRCA 1 and BRCA2 may increase the chances of stomach cancer. (CETI)*

Treatments	**Immunotherapy** **Radiation therapy** **Targeted therapy** **Surgery** Surgery is a common treatment of all stages of gastric cancer. The following types of surgery may be used: • **Subtotal gastrectomy**: Removal of the part of the stomach that contains cancer, nearby lymph nodes, and parts of other tissues and organs near the tumor. The spleen may be removed. The spleen is an organ that makes lymphocytes, stores red blood cells and lymphocytes, filters the blood, and destroys old blood cells. The spleen is on the left side of the abdomen near the stomach. • **Total gastrectomy:** Removal of the entire stomach, nearby lymph nodes, and parts of the esophagus, small intestine, and other tissues near the tumor. The spleen may be removed. The esophagus is connected to the small intestine so the patient can continue to eat and swallow. If the tumor is blocking the stomach but the cancer cannot be completely removed by standard surgery, the following procedures may be used: • **Endoluminal stent placement:** A procedure to insert a stent (a thin, expandable tube) in order to keep a passage (such as arteries or the esophagus) open. For tumors blocking the passage into or out of the stomach, surgery may be done to place a stent from the esophagus to the stomach or from the stomach to the small intestine to allow the patient to eat normally. • **Endoluminal laser therapy:** A procedure in which an endoscope (a thin, lighted tube) with a laser attached is inserted into the body. A laser is an intense beam of light that can be used as a knife. • **Gastrojejunostomy:** Surgery to remove the part of the stomach with cancer that is blocking the opening into the small intestine. The stomach is connected to the jejunum (a part of the small intestine) to allow food and medicine to pass from the stomach into the small intestine. **Endoscopic mucosal resection** • Endoscopic mucosal resection is a procedure that uses an endoscope to remove early-stage cancer and precancerous growths from the lining of the digestive tract without surgery. An endoscope is a thin, tube-like instrument with a light and a lens for viewing. It may also include tools to remove growths from the lining of the digestive tract.

Treatments *Continued*	**Chemotherapy** • Chemotherapy is a cancer treatment that uses drugs to stop the growth of cancer cells, either by killing the cells or by stopping them from dividing. When chemotherapy is taken by mouth or injected into a vein or muscle, the drugs enter the bloodstream and can reach cancer cells throughout the body (systemic chemotherapy). *(See Chemotherapy for more information)* • A type of regional chemotherapy being studied to treat gastric cancer is intraperitoneal (IP) chemotherapy. In IP chemotherapy, the anticancer drugs are carried directly into the peritoneal cavity (the space that contains the abdominal organs) through a thin tube. • Hyperthermic intraperitoneal chemotherapy (HIPEC) is a treatment used during surgery that is being studied for gastric cancer. After the surgeon has removed as much tumor tissue as possible, warmed chemotherapy is sent directly into the peritoneal cavity. **Chemoradiation** • Chemoradiation therapy combines chemotherapy and radiation therapy to increase the effects of both. Chemoradiation given after surgery, to lower the risk that the cancer will come back, is called adjuvant therapy. Chemoradiation given before surgery, to shrink the tumor (neoadjuvant therapy), is being studied.
Treatment by Stages	**Treatment of stage I gastric cancer** may include the following: • Surgery (total or subtotal gastrectomy). • Endoscopic mucosal resection for certain patients with stage IA gastric cancer. • Surgery (total or subtotal gastrectomy) followed by chemoradiation therapy. • Surgery and chemotherapy. • A clinical trial of chemoradiation therapy given before surgery. **Treatment of stage II gastric cancer and stage III gastric cancer** may include the following: • Surgery (total or subtotal gastrectomy). • Surgery and chemotherapy. • Surgery (total or subtotal gastrectomy) followed by chemoradiation therapy or chemotherapy. • A clinical trial of chemoradiation therapy given before surgery. • A clinical trial of chemotherapy given before surgery. **Treatment of stage IV gastric cancer, gastric cancer that cannot be removed by surgery, or recurrent gastric cancer** may include the following: • Chemotherapy as palliative therapy to relieve symptoms and improve the quality of life. • Targeted therapy with a monoclonal antibody with or without chemotherapy. • Immunotherapy with pembrolizumab. • Endoluminal laser therapy or endoluminal stent placement to relieve a blockage in the stomach, or gastrojejunostomy to bypass the blockage. • Radiation therapy as palliative therapy to stop bleeding, relieve pain, or shrink a tumor that is blocking the stomach. • Surgery as palliative therapy to stop bleeding or shrink a tumor that is blocking the stomach. • Clinical trials of combinations of immunotherapy and chemotherapy. • A clinical trial of targeted therapy with regorafenib and nivolumab. • A clinical trial of surgery and hyperthermic intraperitoneal chemotherapy (HIPEC).

Post Gastrectomy and Side Effects
 	
Web MD
	Your hospital stay will depend on the type of gastrectomy performed.
	
	• For the first few days, you won't be able to eat any food. Then you'll be on a clear liquid diet. This gives your digestive tract a chance to heal. Instead, you'll be fed through an IV in your vein or a catheter (tube) that goes into your belly. After about a week, you should be ready to start a light diet again.
	
	• Because your stomach is smaller now, be prepared to make some changes to how you eat:
	    ○ Small meals throughout the day. Six small meals will be easier for you to digest than three large ones.
	    ○ Drink and eat at different times. Have fluids 1 hour before or after meals instead of during them.
	    ○ Watch your fiber intake. High-fiber foods like beans, lentils, and whole grains can fill you up too fast. Add them back slowly.
	    ○ Go easy on dairy. After this surgery, many people can't digest lactose, the sugar in milk. If you're one of them, you'll have gas, bloating, and diarrhea after you have dairy foods.
	
	• Take a supplement. Some nutrients like iron, calcium, and vitamins B12 and D are harder for your body to absorb from food after a gastrectomy. Your doctor may do blood tests to check these levels. If they're low, you may need to start taking a supplement.
	
	Side Effects – Dumping Syndrome
	• You could get what's called dumping syndrome. When your small intestine has to digest a large amount of food at once, you may throw up or have nausea, cramps, or diarrhea.
	    ○ Many people notice these symptoms within an hour of eating.
	• If you feel sick a few hours later, your blood sugar may be rising and falling too fast.
	    ○ It's common to sweat, have a fast heart rate, or feel tired or confused.
	• Changing what you eat can help you manage these symptoms. Remember, too, to be patient.
	
	After your gastrectomy, it may take 3 to 6 months to adjust.
	
	(Web MD – What is a gastrectomy?)

References	CETI- Cancer Exercise Training Institute: *https://www.thecancerspecialist.com/* National Cancer Institute *(NCI)* - Gastric Cancer Treatment: *https://www.cancer.gov/types/stomach/patient/stomach-treatment-pdq* Web MD – What is a gastrectomy? *https://www.webmd.com/cancer/what-is-gastrectomy*

Recovery after Surgery
 	
*Information from **CETI-***
Cancer Exercise Training Institute
 	
Please follow MD/surgeon protocol, as every situation is unique.
	Partial Gastrectomy
	  ➤ **Hospital Stay:** 3-5 days
	  ➤ **Full Recovery:** 3-6 months
	  ➤ **Restrictions:** No heavy lifting per MD order
	  ➤ **Exercise:** Walking and slow stair climbing
	
	Total Gastrectomy:
	  ➤ **Hospital Stay:** 5-8 days
	  ➤ **Full Recovery: 3**-6 months
	  ➤ **Restrictions:** No heavy lifting per MD order
	  ➤ **Exercise:** Walking and slow stair climbing
	
	Possible Side Effects: Increased Heartburn, Weight Loss, Abdominal Pain and Cramping, Ulcers, Nausea, Vomiting, Diarrhea, Vitamin Deficiency (poor nutrient absorption), Dumping Syndrome *(see above under side effects)*
	  • Splenectomy - Risk of Infection
	  • Lymphedema if lymph nodes are removed *(see Lymphedema)*
	
	Gastric Feeding Tube (G or J Tube) – *also see side effects above under WebMD*:
	Caution – discuss the following with MD:
	  ➤ Yoga, Pilates or other core exercises
	  ➤ Swimming
	  ➤ Contact sports – can dislodge tube

THYROID

Information and pictures from *National Cancer Institute* unless otherwise specified

| **Description** | Thyroid cancer is a disease in which malignant (cancer) cells form in the tissues of the thyroid gland.

Thyroid hormones do the following:
- Control heart rate, body temperature, and how quickly food is changed into energy (metabolism).
- Control the amount of calcium in the blood.

Anatomy of the Thyroid and Parathyroid Glands

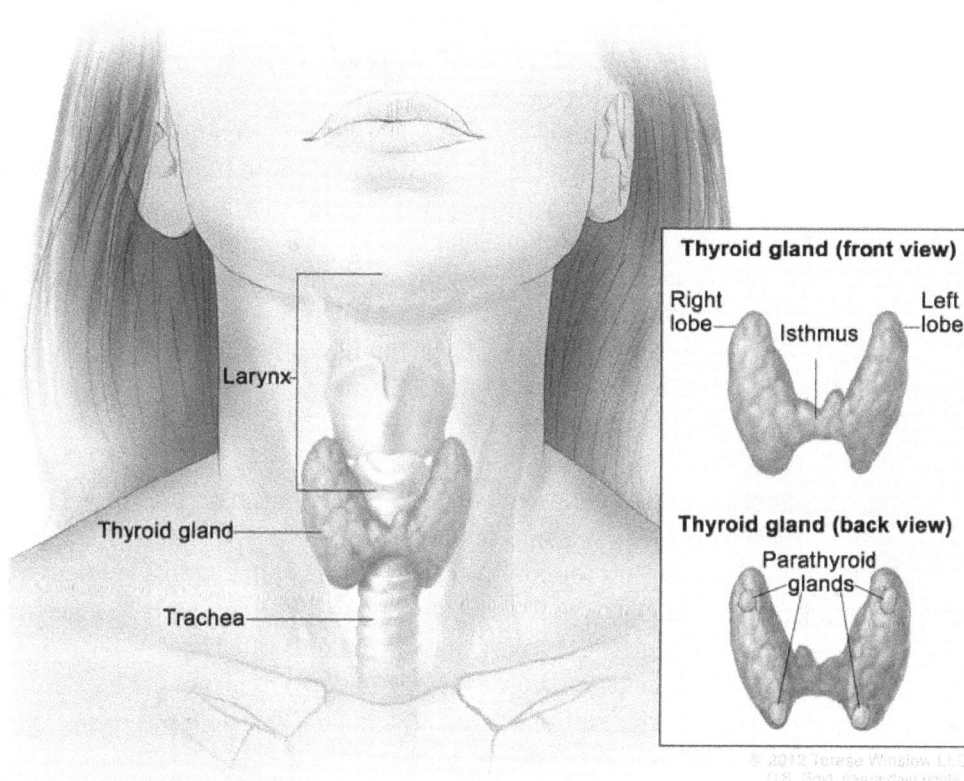

The thyroid is a gland at the base of the throat near the trachea (windpipe). It is shaped like a butterfly, with a right lobe and a left lobe.
- *The isthmus, a thin piece of tissue, connects the two lobes. A healthy thyroid is a little larger than a quarter. It usually cannot be felt through the skin.*
- *The thyroid uses iodine, a mineral found in some foods and in iodized salt, to help make several hormones.*
- *The parathyroid glands are four pea-sized organs found in the neck near the thyroid.*
- *The thyroid and parathyroid glands make hormones.* |

Description and Stages
 	
Continued
	There are four main types of thyroid cancer:
	• **Papillary thyroid cancer:** The most common type of thyroid cancer.
	    o Well-differentiated tumors (papillary thyroid cancer and follicular thyroid cancer) can be treated and can usually be cured.
	• **Follicular thyroid cancer.**
	    o Well-differentiated tumors (papillary thyroid cancer and follicular thyroid cancer) can be treated and can usually be cured.
	• **Medullary thyroid cancer.**
	    o Cancer that develops in C cells of the thyroid. The C cells make a hormone (calcitonin) that helps maintain a healthy level of calcium in the blood.
	    o Medullary thyroid cancer is a neuroendocrine tumor that forms from cells that release hormones into the blood in response to a signal from the nervous system. Neuroendocrine tumors may make higher-than-normal amounts of hormones, which can cause many different symptoms. These tumors may be benign (not cancer) or malignant (cancer).
	• **Anaplastic thyroid cancer.**
	    o Poorly differentiated and undifferentiated tumors (anaplastic thyroid cancer) are less common. These tumors grow and spread quickly and have a poorer chance of recovery. Patients with anaplastic thyroid cancer should have molecular testing for a mutation in the BRAF gene.
	• Papillary and follicular thyroid cancer are sometimes called differentiated thyroid cancer.
	• Medullary and anaplastic thyroid cancer are sometimes called poorly differentiated or undifferentiated thyroid cancer.
	
	Stages:
	Stages are used to describe thyroid cancer based on the type of thyroid cancer and the age of the patient:
	• Papillary and follicular thyroid cancer in patients younger than 55 years
	• Papillary and follicular thyroid cancer in patients 55 years and older
	• Anaplastic thyroid cancer in patients of all ages
	• Medullary thyroid cancer in patients of all ages
	• Thyroid cancer can recur (come back) after it has been treated.

Risk Factors	**Risk Factors for Thyroid Cancer:** • Being between 25 and 65 years old. • Being female. • Being exposed to radiation to the head and neck as an infant or child or being exposed to radioactive fallout. The cancer may occur as soon as 5 years after exposure. • Having a history of goiter (enlarged thyroid). • Having a family history of thyroid disease or thyroid cancer. • Having certain genetic conditions such as familial medullary thyroid cancer (FMTC), multiple endocrine neoplasia type 2A syndrome (MEN2A), or multiple endocrine neoplasia type 2B syndrome (MEN2B). • Being Asian.

Treatment	Chemotherapy Targeted therapy Watchful waiting **Surgery** Surgery is the most common treatment for thyroid cancer. One of the following procedures may be used: • **Lobectomy:** Removal of the lobe in which thyroid cancer is found. Lymph nodes near the cancer may also be removed and checked under a microscope for signs of cancer. • **Near-total thyroidectomy**: Removal of all but a very small part of the thyroid. Lymph nodes near the cancer may also be removed and checked under a microscope for signs of cancer. • **Total thyroidectomy**: Removal of the whole thyroid. Lymph nodes near the cancer may also be removed and checked under a microscope for signs of cancer. • **Tracheostomy:** Surgery to create an opening (stoma) into the windpipe to help you breathe. The opening itself may also be called a tracheostomy. **Radiation therapy**, including radioactive iodine therapy. • Radiation therapy may be given after surgery to kill any thyroid cancer cells that were not removed. **Radioactive iodine (RAI) therapy** • Follicular and papillary thyroid cancers are sometimes treated with radioactive iodine (RAI) therapy. RAI is taken by mouth and collects in any remaining thyroid tissue, including thyroid cancer cells that have spread to other places in the body. ○ Since only thyroid tissue takes up iodine, the RAI destroys thyroid tissue and thyroid cancer cells without harming other tissue. • Before a full treatment dose of RAI is given, a small test-dose is given to see if the tumor takes up the iodine. **Thyroid hormone therapy** • In the treatment of thyroid cancer, drugs may be given to prevent the body from making thyroid- stimulating hormone (TSH), a hormone that can increase the chance that thyroid cancer will grow or recur. • Also, because thyroid cancer treatment kills thyroid cells, the thyroid is not able to make enough thyroid hormone. • Patients are given thyroid hormone replacement pills.

Possible Side Effects	Surgery
	
	• **Total Thyroidectomy:**
	    o Pain and aches in neck and shoulders
	    o Will need to be on replacement medication
	    o Hoarseness
	    o Sore throat
	    o Difficulty swallowing
	    o Transient (temporary) hypoparathyroidism can happen after thyroid surgery. Hypoparathyroidism is when you have too little parathyroid hormone, which can lead to low calcium levels.
	• **Tracheotomy:**
	    o Bleeding
	    o Air trapped around the lungs (pneumothorax)
	    o Air trapped in the deeper layers of the chest(pneumomediastinum)
	    o Air trapped underneath the skin around the tracheostomy (subcutaneous emphysema)
	    o Damage to the swallowing tube (esophagus)
	    o Injury to the nerve that moves the vocal cords (recurrent laryngeal nerve)
	    o Tracheostomy tube can be blocked by blood clots, mucus or pressure of the airway walls. Blockages can be prevented by suctioning, humidifying the air, and selecting the appropriate tracheostomy tube. *(John Hopkins - Complications and Risks of Tracheostomy)*
	
	Radioactive Iodine Treatment
	• Dry eyes
	• Dry mouth
	• Salivary gland swelling or pain
	• Neck swelling and pain
	
	Radiation to the neck
	• Dry, sore mouth and throat
	• Hoarseness
	• Difficulty swallowing
	• Fatigue

References	CETI - Cancer Exercise Training Institute: *https://www.thecancerspecialist.com/* John Hopkins - Complications and Risks of Tracheostomy *https://www.hopkinsmedicine.org/tracheostomy/about/complications.html)* National Cancer Institute (NCI) - Thyroid Cancer Treatment (Adult) (PDQ®): *https://www.cancer.gov/types/thyroid/patient/thyroid-treatment-pdq* National Cancer Institute (NCI) Thyroid Cancer: *https://www.cancer.gov/types/thyroid*

Recovery after Surgery
 	
Information from **CETI-** *Cancer Exercise Training Institute*
 	
Please follow MD/surgeon protocol, as every situation is unique.
	Thyroidectomy - Total
	Hospital Stay: 1 day
	➢ **Full Recovery:** 3-4 weeks
	➢ **Restrictions:** No heavy lifting, bending or strenuous activity for 3-4 weeks. No lifting over 10 lbs. for 2 or more weeks.
	➢ **Exercise:** Walking. Gentle shoulder rolls and moving head from side to side to prevent stiffness.
	➢ **Possible Side Effects:** Excessive Bleeding / Hematoma in the Neck, Wound Infection, Hoarseness, Trouble Speaking or Breathing, Weight Gain, Lethargy, Decreased Metabolism
	    o **Parathyroid Gland Damage –** Regulates calcium level.
	        ▪ Hypocalcemia
	    o **Higher Risk of Osteoporosis**
	    o **Lymphedema** – Cervical if lymph nodes are removed *(see Lymphedema)*.
	    o **Hormonal Replacement Dependence**
	
	Tracheotomy:
	➢ **Hospital Stay:** 3-5 days
	➢ **Full Recovery:** 6-8 weeks
	➢ **Restrictions:** No heavy lifting, bending or strenuous activity for 3-4 weeks. No lifting over 5 lbs. for at least weeks.
	➢ **Exercise:** Walking
	➢ **Possible Side Effects:** Bleeding, Subcutaneous Emphysema, Pneumothorax, Damage to the Esophagus, Injury to the Nerve that Moves the Vocal Cords, Hematoma, Infection
	    o **Lymphedema** if lymph nodes are removed *(see Lymphedema)*.

Exercise, Special Considerations & Precautions – Short and Long Term
 	
Please follow MD/surgeon protocol, as every situation is unique.
	• Start exercises or stretches after clearance from MD
	• You may have some minor muscle spasms in the upper back and neck.
	   ○ It will be important for you to keep these muscles relaxed, and to maintain normal posture as much as possible to reduce these spasms.
	• Your voice may sound different for a few days to weeks after the surgery.
	   ○ Some patients are hoarse and some have "voice fatigue," meaning their voice is "tired" at the end of the day.
	   ○ There are a small percentage of patients that will need special voice therapy if your voice does not return in 6-8 weeks.
	• **Higher Risk of Osteoporosis –** Need for weight bearing exercises
	• **Lymphedema** (Cervical) if lymph nodes are removed *(see Lymphedema).*

Exercise or Stretches after Thyroid Surgery per MD protocol

Sections from HEP portion of book

Flex = Flexibility   *Strength* – UE = Upper Extremity

Exercise	Section	Number
Head turns – Neck rotation	Flex	47
Head tilt – Side bend	Flex	47
Neck flexion and extension – look up and down	Flex	48
Shoulder shrugs	UE	87
Shoulder roll	UE	89
Scapular squeezes / retractions	UE	91
Shoulder flexion – no weight	UE	44
Shoulder abduction – no weight	UE	77

Cancer Therapies
Information and pictures from *National Cancer Institute* unless otherwise specified

Quick Summary this Section

Chemotherapy:
- Chemotherapy works by stopping or slowing the growth of cancer cells, which grow and divide quickly.

Radiation:
- Radiation therapy (also called radiotherapy) is a cancer treatment that uses high doses of radiation to kill cancer cells and shrink tumors.

Hormone Therapy:
- Hormone therapy is a cancer treatment that removes hormones or blocks their action and stops cancer cells from growing. Hormones are substances made by glands in the body and circulated in the bloodstream.

Targeted Therapy:
- Targeted therapy is a type of treatment that uses drugs or other substances to identify and attack specific cancer cells without harming normal cells

Immunotherapy:
- Immunotherapy is a type of cancer treatment that helps your immune system fight cancer. The immune system helps your body fight infections and other diseases.
- It is made up of white blood cells and organs and tissues of the lymph system.

Stem Cell Therapy / Transplant:
- Stem cell transplants are procedures that restore blood-forming stem cells in people who have had theirs destroyed by the high doses of chemotherapy or radiation therapy that are used to treat certain cancers.

Other Therapies / Treatments:
- Ablation, Active surveillance, Biological, Bisphosphonate therapy, Chemoprevention, Chimeric antigen receptor, Electrocautery, Embolization therapy, Endoscopic stent placement, High-intensity–focused ultrasound therapy and more.

Side Effects and Late Side Effects:
- Side Effects and Late Side Effects of therapies and surgeries

Eating Hints: Before, during, and after Cancer Treatment:
- Clear Liquids, Full Liquid Diet, Foods and Drinks that Are Easy on the Stomach
- Low Fiber, High Fiber, High Protein, Foods and Drinks that Are Easy to Chew and Swallow

CHEMOTHERAPY
Information and pictures from *National Cancer Institute* unless otherwise specified

Quick Summary of Section

How Chemotherapy Works against Cancer and Who Receives It:
- Chemotherapy works by stopping or slowing the growth of cancer cells, which grow and divide quickly.

How Your Doctor Decides Which Chemotherapy Drugs to Give You:
- There are many different chemotherapy drugs.

How Chemotherapy Is Used with Other Cancer Treatments:
- When used with other treatments

How Often You Receive Chemotherapy
- Treatment schedules for chemotherapy vary widely. You may receive chemotherapy in cycles.
- A cycle is a period of chemotherapy treatment followed by a period of rest.

Ways Chemotherapy May be Given:
- Oral, intravenous, intrathecal, intraperitoneal, intra-arterial, topical, catheter, port, pump

The Most Common Chemotherapy Drugs/ Examples AND for Each Cancer Type *(Medical News Today)*

Side Effects and Exercise Precautions:
- Chemotherapy not only kills fast-growing cancer cells but also kills or slows the growth of healthy cells that grow and divide quickly.

How Chemotherapy Works against Cancer and Who Receives it	Chemotherapy is used to treat many types of cancer. For some people, chemotherapy may be the only treatment you receive. But most often, you will have chemotherapy and other cancer treatments. • The types of treatment that you need depends on the type of cancer you have, if it has spread and where, and if you have other health problems. *NIH NCI (14)* Chemotherapy is used to: • Treat cancer: Chemotherapy can be used to cure cancer, lessen the chance it will return, or stop or slow its growth. • Ease cancer symptoms: Chemotherapy can be used to shrink tumors that are causing pain and other problems. *NIH NCI (14)* Chemotherapy is a drug treatment that works by stopping or slowing the growth of cancer cells, which grow and divide quickly. But it can also harm healthy cells that divide quickly, such as those that line your mouth and intestines or cause your hair to grow. • Damage to healthy cells may cause side effects. Often, side effects get better or go away after chemotherapy is over. *Cancer.gov publication – Chemotherapy and You*

How Your Doctor Decides Which Chemotherapy Drugs to Give You	There are many different chemotherapy drugs. Which ones are included in your treatment plan depends mostly on: • The type of cancer you have and how advanced it is • Whether you have had chemotherapy before • Whether you have other health problems, such as diabetes or heart disease *NIH NCI (14)*
How Chemotherapy Is Used with Other Cancer Treatments	When used with other treatments, chemotherapy can: • Make a tumor smaller before surgery or radiation therapy. This is called neoadjuvant chemotherapy. • Destroy cancer cells that may remain after treatment with surgery or radiation therapy. This is called adjuvant chemotherapy. • Help other treatments work better. • Kill cancer cells that have returned or spread to other parts of your body. *NIH NCI (14)*

How Often You Receive Chemotherapy	Treatment schedules for chemotherapy vary widely. How often and how long you get chemotherapy depends on:
	• Your type of cancer and how advanced it is
	• Whether chemotherapy is used to:
	    ○ Cure your cancer
	    ○ Control its growth
	    ○ Ease symptoms
	• The type of chemotherapy you are getting
	• How your body responds to chemotherapy
	
	You may receive chemotherapy in cycles. A cycle is a period of chemotherapy treatment followed by a period of rest.
	• For instance, you might receive chemotherapy every day for 1 week followed by 3 weeks with no chemotherapy. These 4 weeks make up one cycle.
	• The rest period gives your body a chance to recover and build new healthy cells.
	NIH NCI (14)

Ways Chemotherapy May be Given	**Oral** The chemotherapy comes in pills, capsules, or liquids that you swallow **Intravenous (IV)** The chemotherapy goes directly into a vein **Injection** Chemotherapy is given by a shot in a muscle in your arm, thigh, or hip, or right under the skin in the fatty part of your arm, leg, or belly **Intrathecal** Chemotherapy is injected into the space between the layers of tissue that cover the brain and spinal cord **Intraperitoneal (IP)** Chemotherapy goes directly into the peritoneal cavity, which is the area in your body that contains organs such as your intestines, stomach, and liver **Intra-arterial (IA)** Chemotherapy is injected directly into the artery that leads to the cancer **Topical** The chemotherapy comes in a cream that you rub onto your skin Chemotherapy is often given through a thin needle that is placed in a vein on your hand or lower arm. Your nurse will put the needle in at the start of each treatment and remove it when the treatment is over. IV chemotherapy may also be given through catheters or ports, sometimes with the help of a pump. **Catheter** • A catheter is a thin, soft tube. A doctor or nurse places one end of the catheter in a large vein, often in your chest area. The other end of the catheter stays outside your body. • Most catheters stay in place until you have finished your chemotherapy treatments. • Catheters can also be used to give you other drugs and to draw blood. Be sure to watch for signs of infection around your catheter. **Port** • A port is a small, round disc that is placed under your skin during minor surgery. A surgeon puts it in place before you begin your course of treatment, and it remains there until you have finished. A catheter connects the port to a large vein, most often in your chest. • Your nurse can insert a needle into your port to give you chemotherapy or draw blood. • This needle can be left in place for chemotherapy treatments that are given for longer than one day. • Be sure to watch for signs of infection around your port. **Pump** • Pumps are often attached to catheters or ports. They control how much and how fast chemotherapy goes into a catheter or port, allowing you to receive your chemotherapy outside of the hospital. • Pumps can be internal or external. External pumps remain outside your body. • Internal pumps are placed under your skin during surgery. *NIH NCI (14)*

Types of Chemotherapy Drugs and Examples *Medical News Today* **See also References** *National Cancer Institute* **List of Cancer Drugs and Side Effects A-Z**	There are several main types of chemotherapy drugs that doctors use to target different types of cancer. The sections below look at these in more detail. **Alkylating agents** These were some of the earliest cancer treatments, and they are still common. They work by disrupting the DNA inside cells, which prevents them from dividing. They can help treat many types of cancer, but they are most effective against slow-growing cancers. Some *examples* of alkylating agents include: <ul><li>altretamine</li><li>busulfan</li><li>carboplatin</li><li>carmustine</li><li>cisplatin</li><li>cyclophosphamide</li><li>dacarbazine</li><li>ifosfamide</li><li>lomustine</li><li>melphalan</li><li>temozolomide</li><li>trabectedin</li></ul> **Antimetabolites** These drugs work by pretending to be nutrients that cells need to grow. The cell eventually starves to death after consuming them. These medications only work at specific stages in a cell's growth cycle. Some *examples* of antimetabolites include: <ul><li>5-fluorouracil</li><li>6-mercaptopurine</li><li>azacitidine</li><li>capecitabine</li><li>clofarabine</li><li>cytarabine</li><li>floxuridine</li><li>fludarabine</li><li>gemcitabine</li><li>methotrexate</li><li>pemetrexed</li><li>pentostatin</li><li>pralatrexate</li><li>trifluridine and tipiracil, which is a combination drug that comes in the form of a pill</li></ul>

Types of Chemotherapy Drugs and Examples *and* **The Most Common Chemotherapies for Each Cancer Type** *Continued* *Medical News Today*	**Plant alkaloids** Plant alkaloids are plant-based substances that prevent cancerous cells from dividing and growing into more cells. They can work throughout a cell's growth cycle, but they are most effective during certain phases. Some *examples* of plant alkaloids include: • vincristine • vinblastine • vinorelbine • paclitaxel • docetaxel • etoposide • teniposide • irinotecan • topotecan **Anti-tumor antibiotics** These drugs differ from antibiotics for treating infections. They work by causing DNA strands to unravel, which prevents the cell from dividing. Some *examples* of anti-tumor antibiotics include: • daunorubicin • doxorubicin • doxorubicin liposomal • epirubicin • idarubicin • valrubicin <p align="center">**The Most Common Chemotherapies for Each Cancer Type**</p>Doctors administer chemotherapy in cycles of treatment and recovery. These cycles are generally 2–3 weeks long and may repeat for 3–6 months. Most people receive chemotherapy drugs through an injection or infusion. The following sections look at some common chemotherapy medications for each common type of cancer. **Breast cancer** For breast cancer, a variety of chemotherapy drugs may be necessary, including: • anthracyclines, such as doxorubicin • cyclophosphamide • epirubicin • fluorouracil • methotrexate • taxanes, such as paclitaxel • docetaxel

The Most Common Chemotherapies for Each Cancer Type *Continued* *Medical News Today*	**Lung cancer** Chemotherapy drugs for non-small cell lung cancer include: • cisplatin • carboplatin • paclitaxel • albumin-bound paclitaxel • docetaxel • gemcitabine • vinorelbine • etoposide • pemetrexed **Prostate cancer** Doctors only use chemotherapy for prostate cancer if it spreads outside of the prostate and if hormone therapy is unsuccessful. Some chemotherapy drugs for prostate cancer include: • docetaxel • cabazitaxel • mitoxantrone • estramustine Doctors may start with a combination of docetaxel and prednisone, which is a steroid-based treatment. They may try cabazitaxel if the first combination does not treat the cancer. **Colorectal cancer** Chemotherapy drugs for colorectal cancer might include: • 5-fluorouracil • capecitabine • irinotecan • oxaliplatin • trifluridine and tipiracil Doctors may use combinations of two or three drugs at a time for treating colorectal cancer. **Melanoma** The two most common chemotherapy drugs for treating melanoma are • dacarbazine and temozolomide. Doctors may use these drugs on their own or combined with other medications.

The Most Common Chemotherapies for Each Cancer Type ***Continued*** *Medical News Today*	**Bladder cancer** Doctors may administer chemotherapy for bladder cancer indirectly through a vein or muscle or directly into the bladder. They typically opt for direct administration when the cancer is only present in the bladder's lining. People with bladder cancer might receive a combination of radiation therapy and chemotherapy drugs that include: • cisplatin • cisplatin plus fluorouracil • mitomycin plus fluorouracil When using chemotherapy without radiation therapy, the options include: • gemcitabine and cisplatin • dose-dense methotrexate, vinblastine, doxorubicin, and cisplatin • cisplatin, methotrexate, and vinblastine • gemcitabine and paclitaxel Doctors may suggest receiving chemotherapy drugs individually if treatment combinations affect the body too strongly. **Non-Hodgkin lymphoma** Chemotherapy is the main course of treatment for non-Hodgkin lymphoma. Doctors typically combine several drugs, including: • cyclophosphamide • chlorambucil • bendamustine • ifosfamide • prednisone • dexamethasone • cisplatin • carboplatin • oxaliplatin • fludarabine • pentostatin • cladribine (2-CdA) • cytarabine (ara-C) • gemcitabine • methotrexate • pralatrexate • doxorubicin • liposomal doxorubicin • vincristine • mitoxantrone • etoposide • bleomycin Doctors may use a combination of drugs called **CHOP**. This stands for cyclophosphamide, hydroxydaunorubicin, Oncovin (vincristine), and prednisone.

Side Effects (See *Side Effects* and *Late Effects* for more information)	**Possible Side Effects:** • Chemotherapy not only kills fast-growing cancer cells but also kills or slows the growth of healthy cells that grow and divide quickly. • Examples are cells that line your mouth and intestines and those that cause your hair to grow. • Damage to healthy cells may cause side effects, such as mouth sores, nausea, and hair loss. Side effects often get better or go away after you have finished chemotherapy. Cancer treatments can cause side effects—problems that occur when treatment affects healthy tissues or organs. Ask your health care team what side-effects you are likely to have. • Anemia • Appetite Loss • Bleeding and Bruising (Thrombocytopenia) • Constipation • Delirium • Diarrhea • Edema (Swelling) • Fatigue • Fertility Issues in Boys and Men • Fertility Issues in Girls and Women • Hair Loss (Alopecia) • Infection and Neutropenia • Lymphedema • Memory or Concentration Problems • Mouth and Throat Problems • Nausea and Vomiting • Nerve Problems (Peripheral Neuropathy) • Pain • Sexual Health Issues in Men • Sexual Health Issues in Women • Skin and Nail Changes • Sleep Problems • Urinary and Bladder Problems The most common side effect is fatigue, which is feeling exhausted and worn out. You can prepare for fatigue by: • Asking someone to drive you to and from chemotherapy • Planning time to rest on the day of and day after chemotherapy • Asking for help with meals and childcare on the day of and at least one day after chemotherapy *NIH NCI (14)*

Exercise Precautions or per MD Recommendations **CETI**	**CETI – Exercise Precautions:** • **IV Chemotherapy** – No exercise for 24 hours • **Hematocrit** less than 25% - No Exercise • **Hemoglobin** less than 24% 8g/dl due to anemia – No Exercise • **White blood** cell counts *less than 300 mm3* – No Exercise • **White blood** cell counts – Avoid public gyms unless blood cell count is *above 500 mm3* • **Platelet count** *less than 5000 mm3* – No resistance training – risk of internal bleeding/hemorrhage • **Platelet count** *less than 30,000 mm3* – Gentle Active Range of Motion • **Adriamycin use (doxorubicin)** – No exercise on the day of chemotherapy. May cause heart to bear irregularly for 24 hours, so only low impact exercise for 24- 48 post treatment – no more than 15-20 beats over resting heart rate.
References	Cancer.gov publication – Chemotherapy and *You* *https://www.cancer.gov/publications/patient-education/chemotherapy-and-you.pdf* CETI: Cancer Exercise Training Institute https*: //www.thecancerspecialist.com/* Medical News Today – Types of Chemotherapy Drugs: *https://www.medicalnewstoday.com/articles/most-common-chemo-drugs#types-of-chemotherapy-drugs* NIH NCI (14) *Chemotherapy https://www.cancer.gov/about-cancer/treatment/types/chemotherapy* **List of Cancer Drugs and Side Effects A-Z** National Cancer Institute - *https://www.cancer.gov/about-cancer/treatment/drugs*

RADIATION
Information and pictures from *National Cancer Institute* unless otherwise specified

Quick Summary of Section

What is Radiation?
- Radiation therapy (also called radiotherapy) is a cancer treatment that uses high doses of radiation to kill cancer cells and shrink tumors.

How Radiation Works against Cancer:
- At high doses, radiation therapy kills cancer cells or slows their growth by damaging their DNA.

Types of Radiation Therapy:
- There are two main types of radiation therapy, external beam and internal.

How Often will I have External Beam Radiation Therapy?
- Most people have external beam radiation therapy once a day, five days a week, Monday through Friday.
- Treatment lasts anywhere from 2 to 10 weeks, depending on the type of cancer you have and the goal of your treatment.

Positioning for Breast Cancer:
- Must have adequate shoulder range of motion lying on your back
- Pillows and supports are used to keep your arm out of the treatment field.

Side Effects *(also see Side Effects)*:
- Fatigue
- Hair loss in the radiation field
- Swelling / Edema *(also see lymphedema)*
- Tenderness
- Skin changes

Late Effects:
- Late Effects are not common, but may include Inflammation in the lung or lymphedema
- In breast cancer, possibility of cancer in the opposite breast.

Treatment Areas And Possible Side Effects
- Other radiation therapy side effects you may have depend on the part of the body that is treated.

What is Radiation	Radiation therapy (also called radiotherapy) is a cancer treatment that uses high doses of radiation to kill cancer cells and shrink tumors. • At low doses, radiation is used in x-rays to see inside your body, as with x-rays of your teeth or broken bones. *NIH NCI (15)*

How Radiation Works against Cancer	• At high doses, radiation therapy kills cancer cells or slows their growth by damaging their DNA. • Cancer cells whose DNA is damaged beyond repair stop dividing or die. When the damaged cells die, they are broken down and removed by the body. • Radiation therapy does not kill cancer cells right away. It takes days or weeks of treatment before DNA is damaged enough for cancer cells to die. Then, cancer cells keep dying for weeks or months after radiation therapy ends. *NIH NCI (15)*
Types of Radiation Therapy	There are two main types of radiation therapy, external beam and internal. **External Beam Radiation Therapy** • External beam radiation therapy comes from a machine that aims radiation at your cancer. The machine is large and may be noisy. It does not touch you, but can move around you, sending radiation to a part of your body from many directions. • External beam radiation therapy is a local treatment, which means it treats a specific part of your body. For example, if you have cancer in your breast, you will have radiation only to your chest/breast, not to your whole body. **Internal Radiation Therapy** • Internal radiation therapy is a treatment in which a source of radiation is put inside your body. The radiation source can be solid or liquid. • Internal radiation therapy with a solid source is called **brachytherapy**. • In this type of treatment, *seeds, ribbons,* or *capsules* that contain a radiation source are placed in your body, in or near the tumor. • Like external beam radiation therapy, brachytherapy is a local treatment and treats only a specific part of your body. • With brachytherapy, the radiation source in your body will give off radiation for a while. *NIH NCI (15)*
How Often Will I Have External Beam Radiation Therapy?	• Most people have external beam radiation therapy once a day, five days a week, Monday through Friday. • Treatment lasts anywhere from 2 to 10 weeks, depending on the type of cancer you have and the goal of your treatment. • This span of time is called a course of treatment. Radiation therapy may also be given on other schedules. These schedules include: • Accelerated fractionation, which is treatment given in larger daily or weekly doses to reduce the number of weeks of treatment • Hyperfractionation, which is smaller doses of radiation given more than once a day • Hypofractionation, which is larger doses given once a day (or less often) to reduce the number of treatments Your doctor may prescribe one of these treatment schedules if he or she feels that it will work better for you. *NIH NCI (16)*

Positioning *(Breast Cancer)*	• Must have adequate shoulder range of motion lying on your back • Pillows and supports are used to keep your arm out of the treatment field.
	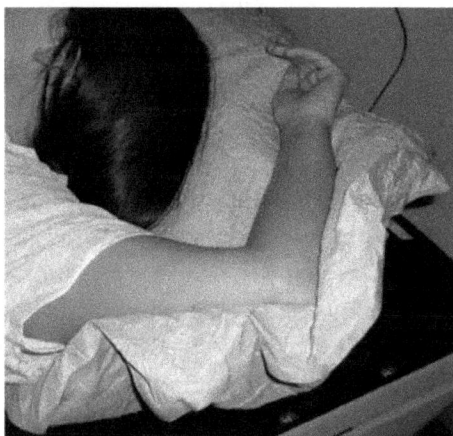
Skin Changes	Radiation therapy can cause skin changes in your treatment area. Here are some common skin changes: • Redness. Your skin in the treatment area may look as if you have a mild to severe sunburn or tan. • Severe itching. The skin in your treatment area may itch very badly. It is important to avoid scratching, which can cause skin breakdown and infection. Skin breakdown is a problem that happens when the skin in the treatment area peels off faster than it can grow back. • Dry and peeling skin. The skin in your treatment area can get very dry. It may get so dry that it starts to peel, as if you have had a bad sunburn. If it peels off faster than it can grow back, you may develop sores or ulcers. • Moist reaction. The skin in your treatment area can become wet, sore, and infected. This problem is more common where you have skin folds, such as your buttocks, behind your ears, and under your breasts. It may also occur where your skin is very thin, such as your neck. • Swollen skin. The skin in your treatment area may be swollen and puffy. **Why they occur:** Radiation kills healthy skin cells in the treatment area. When people get radiation therapy almost every day, their skin cells do not have enough time to grow back between treatments. Skin changes can happen anywhere on the body that gets radiation. **How long they last:** • Skin changes may start a few weeks after you begin radiation therapy. Many of these changes go away a few weeks after treatment is over. But even after radiation therapy ends, some skin changes may remain. • Skin in the treatment area may always look darker and blotchy. • It may feel very dry or thicker than before. • You will always burn quickly and be sensitive to the sun.

Skin Changes
 	
Continued
	Ways to manage
	• Skin care. Take extra good care of your skin during radiation therapy. Be gentle and do not rub, scrub, or scratch in the treatment area. Use creams that your doctor or nurse suggests.
	• Do not put anything on your skin that is very hot or cold. Do not use heating pads, ice packs, or other hot or cold items on the treatment area.
	• Be gentle when you shower or take a bath. You can take a lukewarm shower every day. If you prefer to take a lukewarm bath, do so only every other day and don't soak for too long. Whether you take a shower or bath, make sure to use a mild soap. Dry yourself with a soft towel by patting, not rubbing, your skin. Be careful not to wash off the ink markings that you need for radiation therapy.
	• Use only those lotions and skin products that your doctor or nurse suggests. If you are using a prescribed cream for a skin problem or acne, tell your doctor or nurse before you begin radiation treatment.
	• Check with your doctor or nurse before using any of the following skin products: *Bubble bath * Cornstarch * Cream * Deodorant * Hair removers * Makeup * Oil *
	Ointment * Perfume * Powder * Soap * Sunscreen
	• Cool, humid places. Your skin may feel much better when you are in cool, humid places. You can make rooms more humid by putting a bowl of water on the radiator or using a humidifier. If you use a humidifier, be sure to follow the directions about cleaning it to prevent bacteria.
	• Soft fabrics. Wear clothes and use bed sheets that are made of very soft fabrics.
	• Do not wear clothes in your treatment area that are tight and do not breathe, such as girdles, body shapers, and pantyhose.
	• Protect your skin from the sun every day. The sun can burn you even on cloudy days or when you are outside for just a few minutes.
	    o Do not go to the beach or sunbathe.
	    o Wear a broad-brimmed hat, long-sleeved shirt, and long pants when you are outside.
	    o Talk with your doctor or nurse about sunscreen lotions. He or she may suggest that you use a sunscreen with an SPF of 30 or higher. You will need to protect your skin from the sun even after radiation therapy is over. Do not use tanning beds. Tanning beds expose you to the same harmful effects as the sun.
	• Adhesive tape. Do not put adhesive bandages or other types of sticky tape on your skin in the treatment area. Talk with your doctor or nurse about ways to bandage without tape.
	• Shaving. Ask your doctor or nurse if you can shave the treatment area. If you can shave use an electric razor, but do not use a pre-shave liquid.
	• Talk with your doctor or nurse. Some skin changes can be very serious. Your treatment team will check for skin changes each time you have radiation therapy. Make sure to report any skin changes that you notice.
	• Medicine. Medicines can help with some skin changes. These include lotions for dry or itchy skin, antibiotics to treat infection, and drugs to reduce swelling or itching.
	NIH NCI (16)

Side Effects (Also see *Side Effects* and *Late Side Effects*)	• Fatigue • Hair loss in the radiation field • Swelling / Edema (also see lymphedema) • Tenderness • Skin changes *(see below)*

Late Effects (Also see *Side Effects* and *Late Side Effects*)	Late Effects are not common, but may include: • Inflammation of the lung after radiation therapy to the breast, especially when chemotherapy is given at the same time. • Arm lymphedema, especially when radiation therapy is given after lymph node dissection. • In women younger than 45 years who receive radiation therapy to the chest wall after mastectomy, there may be a higher risk of developing breast cancer in the other breast. *NIH NCI (15)*
Treatment Areas and Possible Side Effects	Other radiation therapy side effects you may have depend on the part of the body that is treated. See more information in the *Side Effects* section. Treatment areas and possible side effects: **Brain** • Fatigue • Hair loss • Memory or concentration problems • Nausea and vomiting • Skin changes • Headache • Blurry vision **Breast** • Fatigue • Hair loss • Skin changes • Swelling (edema) • Tenderness **Chest** • Fatigue • Hair loss • Skin changes • Throat problems, such as trouble swallowing • Cough • Shortness of breath **Head and Neck** • Fatigue • Hair loss • Mouth problems • Skin changes • Taste changes • Throat problems, such as trouble swallowing • Less active thyroid gland

Treatment areas and Possible Side Effects *Continued*	**Pelvis** • Diarrhea • Fatigue • Hair loss • Nausea and vomiting • Sexual problems (men) • Fertility problems (men) • Sexual problems (women) • Fertility problems (women) • Skin changes • Urinary and bladder problems **Rectum** • Diarrhea • Fatigue • Hair loss • Sexual problems (men) • Fertility problems (men) • Sexual problems (women) • Fertility problems (women) • Skin changes • Urinary and bladder problems **Stomach and Abdomen** • Diarrhea • Fatigue • Hair loss • Nausea and vomiting • Skin changes • Urinary and bladder problems
References	NCI – National Cancer Institute – Radiation Therapy Side Effects: *https://www.cancer.gov/about-cancer/treatment/types/radiation-therapy/side-effects* NIH NCI (15) Radiation *https://www.cancer.gov/about-cancer/treatment/types/radiation-therapy* *NIH NCI (16)* Radiation Therapy and You. *https://www.cancer.gov/publications/patient- education/radiationttherapy.pdf*

HORMONE THERAPY

Information and pictures from *National Cancer Institute* unless otherwise specified

Quick Summary of Section

Hormone Therapy:

Hormone therapy is a cancer treatment that removes hormones or blocks their action and stops cancer cells from growing. Hormones are substances made by glands in the body and circulated in the bloodstream.

Breast Cancer & Drugs Used *(Pink Ribbon Program®)*

- Tamoxifen
- Arimidex
- Herceptin

Prostate Cancer:

- What are male sex hormones?
- How does hormone therapy work against prostate cancer?
- What types of hormone therapy are used for prostate cancer?

Hormone Therapy	Hormone therapy is a cancer treatment that removes hormones or blocks their action and stops cancer cells from growing. Hormones are substances made by glands in the body and circulated in the bloodstream. • Some hormones can cause certain cancers to grow. If tests show that the cancer cells have places where hormones can attach (receptors), drugs, surgery, or radiation therapy is used to reduce the production of hormones or block them from working. *Hormone therapy is used to* • Treat cancer. Hormone therapy can lessen the chance that cancer will return or stop or slow its growth. • Ease cancer symptoms. Hormone therapy may be used to reduce or prevent symptoms in men with prostate cancer who are not able to have surgery or radiation therapy. *Types of hormone therapy* • Hormone therapy falls into two broad groups, those that block the body's ability to produce hormones and those that interfere with how hormones behave in the body. *Who receives hormone therapy?* • Hormone therapy is used to treat prostate and breast cancers that use hormones to grow. Hormone therapy is most often used along with other cancer treatments. • The types of treatment that you need depend on the type of cancer, if it has spread and how far, if it uses hormones to grow, and if you have other health problems. *How hormone therapy is used with other cancer treatments* • Range of scores for the Decipher test showing low, intermediate, and high risk of prostate cancer metastasis • Genetic Test May Help Predict Whether Prostate Cancer Will Spread • The test may help determine whether to treat with hormone therapy.

Hormone Therapy *Continued*	**When used with other treatments, hormone therapy can** • Make a tumor smaller before surgery or radiation therapy. This is called neoadjuvant therapy. • Lower the risk that cancer will come back after the main treatment. This is called adjuvant therapy. • Destroy cancer cells that have returned or spread to other parts of your body. *(Hormone Therapy to Treat Cancer – NCI)*
Hormone Therapy **Breast Cancer** **See also References** *National Cancer Institute* **List of Cancer Drugs and Side Effects A-Z**	• The hormone estrogen, which makes some breast cancers grow, is made mainly by the ovaries. Treatment to stop the ovaries from making estrogen is called ovarian ablation. • Hormone therapy with tamoxifen is often given to patients with early localized breast cancer that can be removed by surgery and those with metastatic breast cancer (cancer that has spread to other parts of the body). Hormone therapy with tamoxifen or estrogens can act on cells all over the body and may increase the chance of developing endometrial cancer. Women taking tamoxifen should have a pelvic exam every year to look for any signs of cancer. Any vaginal bleeding, other than menstrual bleeding, should be reported to a doctor as soon as possible. • Hormone therapy with a luteinizing hormone-releasing hormone (LHRH) agonist is given to some premenopausal women who have just been diagnosed with hormone receptor positive breast cancer. LHRH agonists decrease the body's estrogen and progesterone. • Hormone therapy with an aromatase inhibitor is given to some postmenopausal women who have hormone receptor positive breast cancer. Aromatase inhibitors decrease the body's estrogen by blocking an enzyme called aromatase from turning androgen into estrogen. Anastrozole, letrozole, and exemestane are types of aromatase inhibitors. • For the treatment of early localized breast cancer that can be removed by surgery, certain aromatase inhibitors may be used as adjuvant therapy instead of tamoxifen or after 2 to 3 years of tamoxifen use. For the treatment of metastatic breast cancer, aromatase inhibitors are being tested in clinical trials to compare them to hormone therapy with tamoxifen. • In women with hormone receptor positive breast cancer, at least 5 years of adjuvant hormone therapy reduces the risk that the cancer will recur (come back). • Other types of hormone therapy include megestrol acetate or anti-estrogen therapy such as fulvestrant. *NIH NCI (17)*

Tamoxifen **Arimidex** **Herceptin** *Pink Ribbon* *Program®*	**Tamoxifen** was approved for treating breast cancer more than two decades ago. The standard treatment used to last 5 years, but researchers have found that taking tamoxifen for 10 years produced more reductions in breast cancer recurrence and death than taking tamoxifen for 5 years. • Tamoxifen: slows cancer growth by blocking estrogen-positive receptor sites. Some breast cancers are spread through estrogen. These are classified as estrogen-positive cancers. • By blocking the estrogen receptors, the drug slows or stops the growth of cancer cells that are already present in the body. Needs to be taken for 5 years after surgery/treatment. **Side effects:** • Menopause • Fatigue • Weight Gain • Hot Flashes • Depression • Osteoporosis due to menopause • Endometrial Cancer (cancer of the lining of the uterus) • Uterine sarcoma (cancer of the connective tissue of the uterus • Pulmonary embolism (blood clot in the lung) • Deep vein thrombosis (blood clot in a major vein) **Arimidex** is an aromatase inhibitor, which reduces the body's production of estrogen. An aromatase inhibitor is a drug that blocks aromatase, an enzyme needed to make estrogen. • Prescribed for post-menopausal women only • Prescribed after Tamoxifen • Has fewer side effects • Joint pain is a significant side effect **Herceptin:** Some breast cancers make excessive amounts of a protein called human growth factor receptor 2 (HER2), which helps breast cancer cells grow and survive. • Trastuzumab is a biological class of drugs known as monoclonal antibodies. It blocks HER2 and cause the cancer cells to die. • For women with HER2-positive breast cancers, the drug Herceptin has been shown to dramatically reduce the risk of recurrence. • It has now become standard treatment to give Herceptin along with adjuvant (after-surgery) chemotherapy in those with metastatic breast cancer. • Herceptin has far fewer immediate side effects than chemotherapy -- for example, there is usually no nausea or hair loss. • However, it causes muscle weakness and there is a small but real risk of heart damage (cardiac dysfunction) and possible lung damage. • Some other adverse effects have been reported as anaphylaxis and severe dyspnea, allergic or hypersensitivity reactions, hematological toxicity hepatic and renal toxicity, diarrhea and an increased risk of infections. *Pink Ribbon Program®*

Hormone Therapy
 	
Prostate Cancer
 	
See also References
National Cancer Institute
List of Cancer Drugs and Side Effects A-Z
	What are male sex hormones?
	
	• Hormones are substances that are made by glands in the body. Hormones circulate in the bloodstream and control the actions of certain cells or organs.
	• Androgens (male sex hormones) are a class of hormones that control the development and maintenance of male characteristics. The most abundant androgens in men are testosterone and dihydrotestosterone (DHT).
	• Androgens are required for normal growth and function of the prostate, a gland in the male reproductive system that helps make semen. Androgens are also necessary for prostate cancers to grow. Androgens promote the growth of both normal and cancerous prostate cells by binding to and activating the androgen receptor, a protein that is expressed in prostate cells. Once activated, the androgen receptor stimulates the expression of specific genes that cause prostate cells to grow.
	• Almost all testosterone is produced in the testicles; a small amount is produced by the adrenal glands. Although prostate cells do not normally make testosterone, some prostate cancer cells acquire the ability to do so.
	
	How does hormone therapy work against prostate cancer?
	
	• Early in their development, prostate cancers need androgens to grow. Hormone therapies, which are treatments that decrease androgen levels or block androgen action, can inhibit the growth of such prostate cancers, which are therefore called castration sensitive, androgen dependent, or androgen sensitive.
	• Most prostate cancers eventually stop responding to hormone therapy and become castration (or castrate) resistant. That is, they continue to grow even when androgen levels in the body are extremely low or undetectable. In the past, these tumors were also called hormone resistant, androgen independent, or hormone refractory; however, these terms are rarely used now because the tumors are not truly independent of androgens for their growth. In fact, some newer hormone therapies have become available that can be used to treat tumors that have become castration resistant.
	
	What types of hormone therapy are used for prostate cancer?
	
	• Hormone therapy for prostate cancer can block the production or use of androgens (4). Currently available treatments can do so in several ways:
	    ○ reducing androgen production by the testicles
	    ○ blocking the action of androgens throughout the body
	    ○ block androgen production (synthesis) throughout the body
	    (Hormone Therapy for Prostate Cancer – NCI)

References	*NIH NCI (17) https://www.cancer.gov/types/breast/patient/breast-treatment-pdq#_185* National Cancer Institute – NCI - Hormone Therapy to Treat Cancer: *https://www.cancer.gov/about- cancer/treatment/types/hormone-therapy* National Cancer Institute – NCI - Hormone Therapy for Prostate Cancer: *https://www.cancer.gov/types/prostate/prostate-hormone-therapy-fact-sheet* Pink Ribbon Program® *https://www.pinkribbonprogram.com/* **List of Cancer Drugs and Side Effects A-Z** National Cancer Institute - *https://www.cancer.gov/about-cancer/treatment/drugs*

TARGETED THERAPY
Information and pictures from *National Cancer Institute* unless otherwise specified

Quick Summary of Section

Targeted Therapy:

- Targeted therapy is a type of treatment that uses drugs or other substances to identify and attack specific cancer cells without harming normal cells.

Drugs Used in Targeted Therapy *(Breast Cancer)*:

- Monoclonal antibody therapy
- Tyrosine kinase inhibitors are targeted therapy drugs that block signals needed for tumors to grow.
- Cyclin-dependent kinase inhibitors are targeted therapy drugs that block proteins called cyclin-dependent kinases, which cause the growth of cancer cells.

Targeted Therapy	**What is targeted therapy?** Targeted therapy is a type of cancer treatment that targets proteins that control how cancer cells grow, divide, and spread. It is the foundation of precision medicine. As researchers learn more about the DNA changes and proteins that drive cancer, they are better able to design treatments that target these proteins. Targeted therapy is a type of treatment that uses drugs or other substances to identify and attack specific cancer cells without harming normal cells. • Monoclonal antibodies, tyrosine kinase inhibitors, cyclin-dependent kinase inhibitors, mammalian target of rapamycin (mTOR) inhibitors, and PARP inhibitors are types of targeted therapies used in the treatment of breast cancer. • Monoclonal antibody therapy is a cancer treatment that uses antibodies made in the laboratory, from a single type of immune system cell. **What are the types of targeted therapy?** • Most targeted therapies are either small-molecule drugs or monoclonal antibodies. • Small-molecule drugs are small enough to enter cells easily, so they are used for targets that are inside cells. • Monoclonal antibodies, also known as therapeutic antibodies, are proteins produced in the lab. These proteins are designed to attach to specific targets found on cancer cells. Some monoclonal antibodies mark cancer cells so that they will be better seen and destroyed by the immune system. Other monoclonal antibodies directly stop cancer cells from growing or cause them to self-destruct. Still others carry toxins to cancer cells. **Who is treated with targeted therapy?** • For some types of cancer, most patients with that cancer will have a target for a certain drug, so they can be treated with that drug. Most of the time, the tumor will need to be tested to see if it contains targets for which we have drugs. • Testing your cancer for targets that could help you and your doctor choose your treatment is called biomarker testing. • You may need to have a biopsy for biomarker testing. A biopsy is a procedure in which your doctor removes a piece of the tumor for testing. There are some risks to having a biopsy. These risks vary depending on the size of the tumor and where it is located. Your doctor will explain the risks of having a biopsy for your type of tumor.

Targeted Therapy *Continued*	**How does targeted therapy work against cancer?** Most types of targeted therapy help treat cancer by interfering with specific proteins that help tumors grow and spread throughout the body. They treat cancer in many ways. They can: • Help the immune system destroy cancer cells. One reason that cancer cells thrive is because they can hide from your immune system. Certain targeted therapies can mark cancer cells, so it is easier for the immune system to find and destroy them. Other targeted therapies help boost your immune system to work better against cancer. • Stop cancer cells from growing. Healthy cells in your body usually divide to make new cells only when they receive strong signals to do so. These signals bind to proteins on the cell surface, telling the cells to divide. This process helps new cells form only as your body needs them. Some cancer cells have changes in the proteins on their surface that tell them to divide whether or not signals are present. Some targeted therapies interfere with these proteins, preventing them from telling the cells to divide. This process helps slow cancer's uncontrolled growth. • Stop signals that help form blood vessels. Tumors need to form new blood vessels to grow beyond a certain size. In a process called angiogenesis, these new blood vessels form in response to signals from the tumor. Some targeted therapies called angiogenesis inhibitors are designed to interfere with these signals to prevent a blood supply from forming. Without a blood supply, tumors stay small. Or, if a tumor already has a blood supply, these treatments can cause blood vessels to die, which causes the tumor to shrink. Learn more about Angiogenesis Inhibitors. • Deliver cell-killing substances to cancer cells. Some monoclonal antibodies are combined with toxins, chemotherapy drugs, and radiation. Once these monoclonal antibodies attach to targets on the surface of cancer cells, the cells take up the cell-killing substances, causing them to die. Cells that don't have the target will not be harmed. • Cause cancer cell death. Healthy cells die in an orderly manner when they become damaged or are no longer needed, but cancer cells have ways of avoiding this dying process. Some targeted therapies can cause cancer cells to go through this process of cell death. • Starve cancer of the hormones it needs to grow. Some breast and prostate cancers require certain hormones to grow. Hormone therapies are a type of targeted therapy that can work in two ways. Some hormone therapies prevent your body from making specific hormones. Others prevent the hormones from acting on your cells, including cancer cells. **Are there drawbacks to targeted therapy?** • Targeted therapy does have some drawbacks. These include: • Cancer cells can become resistant to targeted therapy. For this reason, they may work best when used with other types of targeted therapy or with other cancer treatments, such as chemotherapy and radiation. • Drugs for some targets are hard to develop. Reasons include the target's structure, the target's function in the cell, or both.

Targeted Therapy *Continued*	**What are the side effects of targeted therapy?** • Targeted therapy can cause side effects. The side effects you may have depend on the type of targeted therapy you receive and how your body reacts to the therapy. • The most common side effects of targeted therapy include diarrhea and liver problems. Other side effects might include problems with blood clotting and wound healing, high blood pressure, fatigue, mouth sores, nail changes, the loss of hair color, and skin problems. Skin problems might include rash or dry skin. Very rarely, a hole might form through the wall of the esophagus, stomach, small intestine, large bowel, rectum, or gallbladder. • There are medicines for many of these side effects. These medicines may prevent the side effects from happening or treat them once they occur. • Most side effects of targeted therapy go away after treatment ends. *(Targeted Therapy to Treat Cancer)*

Drugs used in Targeted Therapy For Breast Cancer
 	
See also References
National Cancer Institute
List of Cancer Drugs and Side Effects A-Z
	Types of monoclonal antibody therapy include the following:
	 • ***Trastuzumab*** is a monoclonal antibody that blocks the effects of the growth factor protein HER2, which sends growth signals to breast cancer cells. It may be used with other therapies to treat HER2 positive breast cancer.
	 • ***Pertuzumab*** is a monoclonal antibody that may be combined with trastuzumab and chemotherapy to treat breast cancer. It may be used to treat certain patients with HER2 positive breast cancer that has metastasized (spread to other parts of the body). It may also be used as neoadjuvant therapy in certain patients with early stage HER2 positive breast cancer.
	 • ***Ado-trastuzumab emtansine*** is a monoclonal antibody linked to an anticancer drug. This is called an antibody-drug conjugate. It is used to treat HER2 positive breast cancer that has spread to other parts of the body or recurred (come back).
	 • ***Sacituzumab govitecan*** is a monoclonal antibody that carries an anticancer drug to the tumor. This is called an antibody-drug conjugate. It is being studied to treat women with triple-negative breast cancer who have received at least two previous chemotherapy regimens.
	
	 Tyrosine kinase inhibitors are targeted therapy drugs that block signals needed for tumors to grow. Tyrosine kinase inhibitors may be used with other anticancer drugs as adjuvant therapy. Tyrosine kinase inhibitors include the following:
	 • **Lapatinib** is a tyrosine kinase inhibitor that blocks the effects of the HER2 protein and other proteins inside tumor cells. It may be used with other drugs to treat patients with HER2 positive breast cancer that has progressed after treatment with trastuzumab.
	 • **Neratinib** is a tyrosine kinase inhibitor that blocks the effects of the HER2 protein and other proteins inside tumor cells. It may be used to treat patients with early stage HER2 positive breast cancer after treatment with trastuzumab.
	
	 Cyclin-dependent kinase inhibitors are targeted therapy drugs that block proteins called cyclin- dependent kinases, which cause the growth of cancer cells. Cyclin-dependent kinase inhibitors include the following:
	 • **Palbociclib** is a cyclin-dependent kinase inhibitor used with the drug letrozole to treat breast cancer that is estrogen receptor positive and HER2 negative and has spread to other parts of the body.
	     o It is used in postmenopausal women whose cancer has not been treated with hormone therapy.
	     o Palbociclib may also be used with fulvestrant in women whose disease has gotten worse after treatment with hormone therapy.

Drugs used in Targeted Therapy For Breast Cancer
 	
Continued
	• ***Ribociclib*** *is a cyclin-dependent kinase inhibitor* used with letrozole to treat breast cancer that is hormone receptor positive and HER2 negative and has come back or spread to other parts of the body.
	    ○ It is used in postmenopausal women whose cancer has not been treated with hormone therapy.
	    ○ It is also used with fulvestrant in postmenopausal women with hormone receptor positive and HER2 negative breast cancer that has spread to other parts of the body or has recurred.
	    ○ It is also used in premenopausal women with hormone receptor positive and HER2 negative breast cancer that has spread to other parts of the body or has recurred..
	• ***Abemaciclib is*** *a cyclin-dependent kinase inhibitor* used to treat hormone receptor positive and HER2 negative breast cancer that is advanced or has spread to other parts of the body. It may be used alone or with other drugs to treat breast cancer that has gotten worse after other treatment.
	• ***Alpelisib*** *is a cyclin-dependent kinase inhibitor* used with the drug fulvestrant to treat hormone receptor positive and HER2 negative breast cancer that has a certain gene change and is advanced or has spread to other parts of the body.
	    ○ It is used in postmenopausal women whose breast cancer has gotten worse during or after treatment with hormone therapy.
	
	Mammalian target of rapamycin (mTOR) inhibitors block a protein called mTOR, which may keep cancer cells from growing and prevent the growth of new blood vessels that tumors need to grow. mTOR inhibitors include the following:
	• **Everolimus** is an mTOR inhibitor used in postmenopausal women with advanced hormone receptor positive breast cancer that is also HER2 negative and has not gotten better with other treatment.
	
	PARP inhibitors are a type of targeted therapy that block DNA repair and may cause cancer cells to die. PARP inhibitors include the following:
	• **Olaparib** is a PARP inhibitor used to treat patients with mutations in the BRCA1 or BRCA2 gene and HER2 negative breast cancer that has spread to other parts of the body. PARP inhibitor therapy is being studied for the treatment of patients with triple-negative breast cancer.
	• **Talazoparib** is a PARP inhibitor used to treat patients with mutations in the BRCA1 or BRCA2 genes and HER2 negative breast cancer that is locally advanced or has spread to other parts of the body.
	NIH NCI (17)

References	*NIH NCI (17) https://www.cancer.gov/types/breast/patient/breast-treatment-pdq#_185* National Cancer Institute – NCI - Targeted Therapy to Treat Cancer: *https://www.cancer.gov/about- cancer/treatment/types/targeted-therapies* **List of Cancer Drugs and Side Effects A-Z** National Cancer Institute - *https://www.cancer.gov/about-cancer/treatment/drugs*

Immunotherapy
Information and pictures from *National Cancer Institute* unless otherwise specified

Quick Summary of Section

Immunotherapy:

Immunotherapy is a type of treatment that helps your immune system fight against cancer.

- The immune system helps your body fight infections and other diseases. It is made up of white blood cells and organs and tissues of the lymph system.

Types:

Several types of immunotherapies are used to treat cancer.

- These treatments can either help the immune system attack the cancer directly or stimulate the immune system in a more general way.

Side Effects:

- The most common side effects are skin reactions at the needle site.
- You may also have flu-like symptoms.

Description	Immunotherapy is a type of cancer treatment that helps your immune system fight cancer. The immune system helps your body fight infections and other diseases. It is made up of white blood cells and organs and tissues of the lymph system. • Immunotherapy is a type of biological therapy. Biological therapy is a type of treatment that uses substances made from living organisms to treat cancer. • One reason that cancer cells thrive is because they are able to hide from your immune system. Certain immunotherapies can mark cancer cells so it is easier for the immune system to find and destroy them. • Other immunotherapies boost your immune system to work better against cancer. Different forms of immunotherapy may be given in different ways. These include: • **Intravenous (IV)** - The immunotherapy goes directly into a vein. • **Oral** - The immunotherapy comes in pills or capsules that you swallow. • **Topical** - The immunotherapy comes in a cream that you rub onto your skin. This type of immunotherapy can be used for very early skin cancer. • **Intravesical** - The immunotherapy goes directly into the bladder.
Types	Several types of immunotherapies are used to treat cancer. These treatments can either help the immune system attack the cancer directly or stimulate the immune system in a more general way. Types of immunotherapies that help the immune system act directly against the cancer include: • **Checkpoint inhibitors**, which are drugs that help the immune system respond more strongly to a tumor. These drugs work by releasing "brakes" that keep T cells (a type of white blood cell and part of the immune system) from killing cancer cells. These drugs do not target the tumor directly. Instead, they interfere with the ability of cancer cells to avoid immune system attack. • **Adoptive cell transfer**, which is a treatment that attempts to boost the natural ability of your T cells to fight cancer. In this treatment, T cells are taken from your tumor. Then those that are most active against your cancer are grown in large batches in the lab.

Types
 	
Continued
	• **Monoclonal antibodies,** also known as therapeutic antibodies, which are immune system proteins created in the lab. These antibodies are designed to attach to specific targets found on cancer cells.
	  ○ Some monoclonal antibodies mark cancer cells so that they will be better seen and destroyed by the immune system.
	  ○ Other monoclonal antibodies directly stop cancer cells from growing or cause them to self-destruct.
	  ○ Still others carry toxins to cancer cells.
	  ○ Because therapeutic monoclonal antibodies recognize specific proteins on cancer cells, they are also considered *targeted* therapies.
	• *Treatment vaccines,* which work against cancer by boosting your immune system's response to cancer cells. Treatment vaccines are different from the ones that help prevent disease.
	
	Types of immunotherapies that enhance the body's immune response to fight the cancer include:
	• **Cytokines,** which are proteins made by your body's cells. They play important roles in the body's normal immune responses and also in the immune system's ability to respond to cancer. The two main types of cytokines used to treat cancer are called interferons and interleukins.
	• **BCG**, which stands for Bacillus Calmette-Guérin, is an immunotherapy that is used to treat bladder cancer. It is a weakened form of the bacteria that causes tuberculosis. When inserted directly into the bladder with a catheter, BCG causes an immune response against cancer cells.

Side Effects	The most common side effects are skin reactions at the needle site. These side effects include: • Pain, Soreness • Swelling • Redness, Itchiness, Rash You may have flu-like symptoms, which include: • Fever, Chills • Weakness, Dizziness • Nausea or vomiting • Muscle or joint aches • Fatigue • Headache • Trouble breathing • Low or high blood pressure Other side effects might include: • Swelling and weight gain from retaining fluid • Heart palpitations • Sinus congestion • Diarrhea • Risk of infection • *White blood cell counts – Avoid public gyms unless blood cell count is above 500 mm3* (CETI: Cancer Exercise Training Institute *https: //www.thecancerspecialist.com/)* *Immunotherapy rarely causes severe or even fatal allergic reactions.*

Stem Cell Therapy / Transplant
Information and pictures from *National Cancer Institute* unless otherwise specified

Quick Summary of Section

Stem Cell Therapy / Transplant

- Stem cell transplants are procedures that restore blood-forming stem cells in people who have had theirs destroyed by the high doses of chemotherapy or radiation therapy that are used to treat certain cancers.

Types:

- The blood-forming stem cells that are used in transplants can come from the bone marrow, bloodstream, or umbilical cord.

How Stem Cell Transplants Work Against Cancer:

- Stem cell transplants do not usually work against cancer directly. Instead, they help you recover your body's ability to produce stem cells after treatment with very high doses of radiation therapy, chemotherapy, or both.

Side Effects:

- The high doses of cancer treatment that you have before a stem cell transplant can cause problems such as bleeding and an increased risk of infection.

Description	Stem cell transplants are procedures that restore blood-forming stem cells in people who have had theirs destroyed by the high doses of chemotherapy or radiation therapy that are used to treat certain cancers. Blood-forming stem cells are important because they grow into different types of blood cells. The main types of blood cells are: <ul><li>white blood cells, which are part of your immune system and help your body fight infection</li><li>red blood cells, which carry oxygen throughout your body</li><li>platelets, which help the blood clot<ul><li>You need all three types of blood cells to be healthy.</li></ul></li></ul>
Types	In a stem cell transplant, you receive healthy blood-forming stem cells through a needle in your vein. Once they enter your bloodstream, the stem cells travel to the bone marrow, where they take the place of the cells that were destroyed by treatment. The blood-forming stem cells that are used in transplants can come from the bone marrow, bloodstream, or umbilical cord. Transplants can be: <ul><li>**Autologous**, which means the stem cells come from you, the patient</li><li>**Allogeneic**, which means the stem cells come from someone else. The donor may be a blood relative but can also be someone who is not related.</li><li>**Syngeneic**, which means the stem cells come from your identical twin, if you have one</li></ul>To reduce possible side effects and improve the chances that an allogeneic transplant will work, the donor's blood-forming stem cells must match yours in certain ways.

How Stem Cell Transplants Work Against Cancer	Stem cell transplants do not usually work against cancer directly. Instead, they help you recover your body's ability to produce stem cells after treatment with very high doses of radiation therapy, chemotherapy, or both.. • However, in multiple myeloma and some types of leukemia, the stem cell transplant may work against cancer directly. This happens because of an effect called graft-versus-tumor that can occur after allogeneic transplants. • *Graft-versus-tumor* occurs when white blood cells from your donor (the graft) attack any cancer cells that remain in your body (the tumor) after high-dose treatments. This effect improves the success of the treatments. **Who receives stem cell transplants?** Stem cell transplants are most often used to help people with leukemia and lymphoma. • They may also be used for neuroblastoma and multiple myeloma.
Side Effects	The high doses of cancer treatment that you have before a stem cell transplant can cause problems such as bleeding and an increased risk of infection. Talk with your doctor or nurse about other side effects that you might have and how serious they might be. If you have an allogeneic transplant, you might develop a serious problem called graft-versus-host disease. • **Graft-versus-host disease** can occur when white blood cells from your donor (the graft) recognize cells in your body (the host) as foreign and attack them. • This problem can cause damage to your skin, liver, intestines, and many other organs. • It can occur a few weeks after the transplant or much later. • Graft-versus-host disease can be treated with steroids or other drugs that suppress your immune system. The closer your donor's blood-forming stem cells match yours, the less likely you are to have graft-versus-host disease. • Your doctor may also try to prevent it by giving you drugs to suppress your immune system.
References	National Cancer Institute - NCI - Stem Cell Transplants in Cancer Treatment: *https://www.cancer.gov/about-cancer/treatment/types/stem-cell-transplant*

Other Therapies / Treatment
Information and pictures from National Cancer Institute unless otherwise specified

Ablation therapy	Ablation therapy removes or destroys tissue. Different types of ablation therapy are used for liver cancer: **Radiofrequency ablation:** - The use of special needles that are inserted directly through the skin or through an incision in the abdomen to reach the tumor. High-energy radio waves heat the needles and tumor which kills cancer cells. **Microwave therapy:** - A type of treatment in which the tumor is exposed to high temperatures created by microwaves. This can damage and kill cancer cells or make them more sensitive to the effects of radiation and certain anticancer drugs. **Percutaneous ethanol injection:** - A cancer treatment in which a small needle is used to inject ethanol (pure alcohol) directly into a tumor to kill cancer cells. Several treatments may be needed. Usually local anesthesia is used, but if the patient has many tumors in the liver, general anesthesia may be used. **Cryoablation:** - A treatment that uses an instrument to freeze and destroy cancer cells. This type of treatment is also called cryotherapy and cryosurgery. The doctor may use ultrasound to guide the instrument. **Electroporation therapy:** - A treatment that sends electrical pulses through an electrode placed in a tumor to kill cancer cells. Electroporation therapy is being studied in clinical trials.
Active surveillance	Active surveillance is closely following a patient's condition without giving any treatment unless there are changes in test results. It is used to find early signs that the condition is getting worse. • In active surveillance, patients are given certain exams and tests, including digital rectal exam, PSA test, transrectal ultrasound, and transrectal needle biopsy, to check if the cancer is growing. • When the cancer begins to grow, treatment is given to cure the cancer.
Biologic therapy	Biologic therapy is a treatment that uses the patient's immune system to fight cancer. Substances made by the body or made in a laboratory are used to boost, direct, or restore the body's natural defenses against cancer. This type of cancer treatment is also called biotherapy or immunotherapy. The following types of biologic therapy are being used or studied in the treatment of renal cell cancer: • **Nivolumab:** Nivolumab is a monoclonal antibody that boosts the body's immune response against renal cell cancer cells. • **Interferon:** Interferon affects the division of cancer cells and can slow tumor growth. Interleukin-2 (IL-2): IL-2 boosts the growth and activity of many immune cells, especially lymphocytes (a type of white blood cell)
Bisphosphonate therapy	Bisphosphonate drugs, such as clodronate or zoledronate, reduce bone disease when cancer has spread to the bone. • Men who are treated with antiandrogen therapy or orchiectomy are at an increased risk of bone loss. In these men, bisphosphonate drugs lessen the risk of bone fracture (breaks). • The use of bisphosphonate drugs to prevent or slow the growth of bone metastases is being studied in clinical trials.
Chemoprevention	Chemoprevention is the use of drugs, vitamins, or other substances to reduce the risk of cancer or to reduce the risk cancer will recur (come back).

Chimeric antigen receptor (CAR) T-cell therapy	CAR T-cell therapy is a type of immunotherapy that changes the patient's T cells (a type of immune system cell) so they will attack certain proteins on the surface of cancer cells. T cells are taken from the patient and special receptors are added to their surface in the laboratory. The changed cells are called chimeric antigen receptor (CAR) T cells. • The CAR T cells are grown in the laboratory and given to the patient by infusion. The CAR T cells multiply in the patient's blood and attack cancer cells. CAR T-cell therapy is being studied in the treatment of adult ALL that has recurred (come back).
Electrocautery	Electrocautery is a treatment that uses a probe or needle heated by an electric current to destroy abnormal tissue. For tumors in the airways, electrocautery is done through an endoscope.
Embolization therapy **AKA** **Chemoembolization**	Embolization therapy is the use of substances to block or decrease the flow of blood through the hepatic artery to the tumor. When the tumor does not get the oxygen and nutrients it needs, it will not continue to grow. Embolization therapy is used for patients who cannot have surgery to remove the tumor or ablation therapy and whose tumor has not spread outside the liver. *The liver receives blood from the hepatic portal vein and the hepatic artery. Blood that comes into the liver from the hepatic portal vein usually goes to the healthy liver tissue. Blood that comes from the hepatic artery usually goes to the tumor. When the hepatic artery is blocked during embolization therapy, the healthy liver tissue continues to receive blood from the hepatic portal vein.* There are two main types of embolization therapy: • **Transarterial embolization (TAE):** A small incision (cut) is made in the inner thigh and a catheter (thin, flexible tube) is inserted and threaded up into the hepatic artery. Once the catheter is in place, a substance that blocks the hepatic artery and stops blood flow to the tumor is injected. • **Transarterial chemoembolization (TACE):** This procedure is like TAE except an anticancer drug is also given. The procedure can be done by attaching the anticancer drug to small beads that are injected into the hepatic artery or by injecting the anticancer drug through the catheter into the hepatic artery and then injecting the substance to block the hepatic artery. Most of the anticancer drug is trapped near the tumor and only a small amount of the drug reaches other parts of the body. This type of treatment is also called *chemoembolization.*
Endoscopic stent placement	An endoscope is a thin, tube-like instrument used to look at tissues inside the body. An endoscope has a light and a lens for viewing and may be used to place a stent in a body structure to keep the structure open. An endoscopic stent can be used to open an airway blocked by abnormal tissue.
High-intensity–focused ultrasound therapy	High-intensity–focused ultrasound therapy is a treatment that uses ultrasound (high-energy sound waves) to destroy cancer cells. To treat prostate cancer, an endorectal probe is used to make sound waves.
Monoclonal antibody therapy	Monoclonal antibody therapy is a cancer treatment that uses antibodies made in the laboratory, from a single type of immune system cell. These antibodies can identify substances on cancer cells or normal substances that may help cancer cells grow. • The antibodies attach to the substances and kill the cancer cells, block their growth, or keep them from spreading. Monoclonal antibodies are given by infusion. They may be used alone or to carry drugs, toxins, or radioactive material directly to cancer cells.

Proton beam radiation therapy	Proton beam radiation therapy is a type of high-energy, external radiation therapy that targets tumors with streams of protons (small, positively charged particles). • This type of radiation therapy is being studied in the treatment of prostate cancer.
Radioactive iodine	A radioactive form of iodine, often used for imaging tests or to treat an overactive thyroid, thyroid cancer, and certain other cancers. For imaging tests, the patient takes a small dose of radioactive iodine that collects in thyroid cells and certain kinds of tumors and can be detected by a scanner. • To treat thyroid cancer, the patient takes a large dose of radioactive iodine, which kills thyroid cells. • Radioactive iodine is also used in internal radiation therapy for prostate cancer, intraocular (eye) melanoma, and carcinoid tumors. • Radioactive iodine is given by mouth as a liquid or in capsules, by infusion, or sealed in seeds, which are placed in or near the tumor to kill cancer cells.
Radiofrequency ablation	Radiofrequency ablation is the use of a special probe with tiny electrodes that kill cancer cells. • Sometimes the probe is inserted directly through the skin and only local anesthesia is needed. • In other cases, the probe is inserted through an incision in the abdomen. • This is done in the hospital with general anesthesia.
Radiopharmaceutical therapy	Radiopharmaceutical therapy uses a radioactive substance to treat cancer. Radiopharmaceutical therapy includes the following: • Alpha emitter radiation therapy uses a radioactive substance to treat prostate cancer that has spread to the bone. • A radioactive substance called radium-223 is injected into a vein and travels through the bloodstream. The radium-223 collects in areas of bone with cancer and kills the cancer cells.
Radiosensitizers	Radiosensitizers are substances that make tumor cells easier to kill with radiation therapy. The combination of chemotherapy and radiation therapy given with a radiosensitizer is being studied in the treatment of non-small cell lung cancer.
Steroid therapy	Steroids are hormones made naturally in the body by the adrenal glands and by reproductive organs. Some types of steroids are made in a laboratory. • Certain steroid drugs have been found to help chemotherapy work better and help stop the growth of cancer cells. • Steroids can also help the lungs of the fetus develop faster than normal. This is important when delivery is induced early.
Vaccine therapy	Vaccine therapy uses a substance or group of substances meant to cause the immune system to respond to a tumor and kill it. Vaccine therapy is being studied in the treatment of stage III melanoma that can be removed by surgery.
Watchful waiting	Watchful waiting is closely monitoring a patient's condition without giving any treatment until signs or symptoms appear or change. This is also called observation. • During this time, problems caused by the disease, such as infection, are treated.

SIDE EFFECTS and LATE SIDE EFFECTS
Information and pictures from *National Cancer Institute* unless otherwise specified

Quick Summary
of Section

NIH (NCI)
https://www.cancer.gov/about-cancer/treatment/side-effects

SIDE EFFECTS

- Anemia
- Appetite Loss
- Bleeding & Bruising (Thrombocytopenia)
- Constipation
- Delirium
- Diarrhea
- Edema (Swelling)
- Fatigue
- Fertility Issues in Girls and Women
- Hair Loss (Alopecia)
- Infection and Neutropenia
- Memory or Concentration Issues
- Mouth and Throat Problems
- Nausea and Vomiting
- Nerve Problems (Peripheral Neuropathy)
- Pain
- Skin and Nail Changes
- Sleep Problems
- Urinary and Bladder Problems
- Bone Loss
- Brain Changes

LATE EFFECTS

- Eye Problems
- Hearing Loss
- Heart Problems
- Hot Flashes and Night Sweats
- Joint Changes
- Lung Problems
- Mouth Changes
- Joint Changes

SIDE EFFECT AND POSSIBLE CAUSE	DESCRIPTION	WAYS TO MANAGE
Anemia *Chemotherapy *Radiation therapy	• Anemia is a condition that can make you feel very tired, short of breath, and lightheaded. • Other signs of anemia may include feeling dizzy or faint, headaches, a fast heartbeat, and/or pale skin. • Cancer treatments, such as chemotherapy and radiation therapy can cause anemia. • When you are anemic, your body does not have enough red blood cells. Red blood cells are the cells that that carry oxygen from the lungs throughout your body to help it work properly. • You will have blood tests to check for anemia. Treatment for anemia is also based on your symptoms and on what is causing the anemia.	**Save your energy and ask for help**. Choose the most important things to do each day. When people offer to help, let them do so. They can take you to the doctor, make meals, or do other things you are too tired to do. **Balance rest with activity.** Take short naps during the day, but keep in mind that too much bed rest can make you feel weak. You may feel better if you take short walks or exercise a little every day. **Eat and drink well. Talk** with your doctor, nurse, or a registered dietitian to learn what foods and drinks are best for you. You may need to eat foods that are high in protein or iron.
Appetite Loss *Chemotherapy *Radiation therapy	• Cancer treatments may lower your appetite or change the way food tastes or smells. • Side effects such as mouth and throat problems, or nausea and vomiting can also make eating difficult. • Cancer-related fatigue can also lower your appetite. • Talk with your health care team if you are not hungry or if your find it difficult to eat. Don't wait until you feel weak, have lost too much weight, or are dehydrated, to talk with your doctor or nurse. It's important to eat well, especially during treatment for cancer.	**Drink plenty of liquids.** Drinking plenty of liquids is important, especially if you have less of an appetite. Losing fluid can lead to dehydration, a dangerous condition. You may become weak or dizzy and have dark yellow urine if you are not drinking enough liquids. **Choose healthy and high-nutrient foods**. Eat a little, even if you are not hungry. It may help to have five or six small meals throughout the day instead of three large meals. Most people need to eat a variety of nutrient-dense foods that are high in protein and calories. **Be active.** Being active can actually increase your appetite. Your appetite may increase when you take a short walk each day.

SIDE EFFECT AND POSSIBLE CAUSE	DESCRIPTION	WAYS TO MANAGE

Bleeding & Bruising (Thrombocytopenia)
 	
*Chemotherapy
*Targeted therapy
	• Some cancer treatments, such as chemotherapy and targeted therapy, can increase your risk of bleeding and bruising.
	• These treatments can lower the number of platelets in the blood. Platelets are the cells that help your blood to clot and stop bleeding. When your platelet count is low, you may bruise or bleed a lot or very easily and have tiny purple or red spots on your skin. This condition is called thrombocytopenia.
	• It is important to tell your doctor or nurse if you notice any of these changes.
	• Call your doctor or nurse if you have more serious problems, such as:
	   o Bleeding that doesn't stop after a few minutes; bleeding from your mouth, nose, or when you vomit; bleeding from your vagina when you are not having your period (menstruation); urine that is red or pink; stools that are black or bloody; or bleeding during your period that is heavier or lasts longer than normal.
	   o Head or vision changes such as bad headaches or changes in how well you see, or if you feel confused or very sleepy.
		Avoid certain medicines. Many over-the-counter medicines contain aspirin or ibuprofen, which can increase your risk of bleeding. When in doubt, be sure to check the label. Get a list of medicines and products from your health care team that you should avoid taking. You may also be advised to limit or avoid alcohol if your platelet count is low.
		
		Take extra care to prevent bleeding. Brush your teeth gently, with a very soft toothbrush. Wear shoes, even when you are inside. Be extra careful when using sharp objects. Use an electric shaver, not a razor. Use lotion and a lip balm to prevent dry, chapped skin and lips. Tell your doctor or nurse if you are constipated or notice bleeding from your rectum.
		
		Care for bleeding or bruising. If you start to bleed, press down firmly on the area with a clean cloth. Keep pressing until the bleeding stops. If you bruise, put ice on the area.

SIDE EFFECT AND POSSIBLE CAUSE	DESCRIPTION	WAYS TO MANAGE
Constipation *Chemotherapy *Pain medications	• Constipation is when you have infrequent bowel movements and stool that may be hard, dry, and difficult to pass. • You may also have stomach cramps, bloating, and nausea when you are constipated. • Cancer treatments such as chemotherapy can cause constipation. • Certain medicines (such as pain medicines), changes in diet, not drinking enough fluids, and being less active may also cause constipation. • It is easier to prevent constipation than to treat its complications which may include fecal impaction or bowel obstruction.	**Eat high-fiber foods.** Adding bran to foods such as cereals or smoothies is an easy way to get more fiber in your diet. Ask your health care team how many grams of fiber you should have each day. If you have had an intestinal obstruction or intestinal surgery, you should not eat a high-fiber diet. **Drink plenty of liquids.** Most people need to drink at least 8 cups of liquid each day. You may need more based on your treatment, medications you are taking, or other health factors. Drinking warm or hot liquids may also help. **Try to be active every day.** Ask your health care team about exercises that you can do. Most people can do light exercise, even in a bed or chair. Other people choose to walk or ride an exercise bike for 15 to 30 minutes each day. **Learn about medicine.** Use only medicines and treatments for constipation that are prescribed by your doctor, since some may lead to bleeding, infection, or other harmful side effects in people being treated for cancer. Keep a record of your bowel movements to share with your doctor or nurse.

SIDE EFFECT AND POSSIBLE CAUSE	DESCRIPTION	WAYS TO MANAGE
Delirium Causes may include: *Advanced cancer *Older age *Dehydration *Infection *Taking certain medicines, such as high doses of opioids *Withdrawal from or stopping certain medicines *Early monitoring of someone with these risk factors for delirium may prevent it or allow it to be treated more quickly.*	• Delirium is a confused mental state that includes changes in awareness, thinking, judgment, sleeping patterns, as well as behavior. • Although delirium can happen at the end of life, many episodes of delirium are caused by medicine or dehydration and are reversible. • The symptoms of delirium usually occur suddenly (within hours or days) over a short period of time and may come and go. • Although delirium may be mistaken for depression or dementia, these conditions are different and have different treatments. Types of Delirium: • *Hypoactive delirium:* The patient seems sleepy, tired, or depressed • *Hyperactive delirium:* The patient is restless, anxious, or suddenly agitated and uncooperative • *Mixed delirium:* The patient changes back and forth between hypoactive delirium and hyperactive delirium Changes caused by delirium can be upsetting for family members and dangerous to the person with cancer, especially if judgment is affected. People with delirium may be more likely to fall, unable to control their bladder and/or bowels, and more likely to become dehydrated. Their confused state may make it difficult to talk with others about their needs and make decisions about care.	**Treat the causes of delirium**: If medicines are causing delirium, then reducing the dose or stopping them may treat delirium. If conditions such as dehydration, poor nutrition, and infections are causing the delirium, then treating these may help. **Control surroundings:** If the symptoms of delirium are mild, it may help to keep the room quiet and well lit, with a clock or calendar and familiar possessions. Having family members around and keeping the same caregivers, as much as possible, may also help. **Consider medicines:** Medicines are sometimes given to treat the symptoms of delirium. However, these medicines have serious side effects and patients receiving them require careful observation by a doctor. **Sometimes sedation may help**: After discussion with family members, sedation is sometimes used for delirium at the end of life, if it does not get better with other treatments. The doctor will discuss the decisions involved in using sedation to treat delirium with the family.

SIDE EFFECT AND POSSIBLE CAUSE	DESCRIPTION	WAYS TO MANAGE
Diarrhea *Treatments for cancer *Medications *Infections *Stress *Certain Cancers	• Diarrhea means having bowel movements that are soft, loose, or watery more often than normal. • If diarrhea is severe or lasts a long time, the body does not absorb enough water and nutrients. This can cause you to become dehydrated or malnourished. • Cancer treatments, or the cancer itself, may cause diarrhea or make it worse. • Some medicines, infections, and stress can also cause diarrhea. • Tell your health care team if you have diarrhea. • Diarrhea that leads to dehydration (the loss of too much fluid from the body) and low levels of salt and potassium (important minerals needed by the body) can be life threatening. • Call your health care team if you feel dizzy or light headed, have dark yellow urine or are not urinating, or have a fever of 100.5 °F (38 °C) or higher.	**Drink plenty of fluid each day.** Most people need to drink 8 to 12 cups of fluid each day. Ask your doctor or nurse how much fluid you should drink each day. For severe diarrhea, only clear liquids or IV (intravenous) fluids may be advised for a short period. **Eat small meals that are easy on your stomach.** Eat six to eight small meals throughout the day, instead of three large meals. Foods high in potassium and sodium (minerals you lose when you have diarrhea) are good food choices, for most people. Limit or avoid foods and drinks that can make your diarrhea worse. **Check before taking medicine.** Check with your doctor or nurse before taking medicine for diarrhea. Your doctor will prescribe the correct medicine for you. **Keep your anal area clean and dry.** Try using warm water and wipes to stay clean. It may help to take warm, shallow baths. These are called sitz baths.
Edema (Swelling) *Chemotherapy *Radiation *Certain Cancers *Unrelated conditions	Edema, a condition in which fluid builds up in your body's tissues, may be caused by some types of chemotherapy, certain cancers, and conditions not related to cancer. Signs of edema may include: • Swelling in your feet, ankles, and legs • Swelling in your hands and arms • Swelling in your face or abdomen • Skin that is puffy, shiny, or looks slightly dented after being pressed • Shortness of breath, a cough, or irregular heartbeat Tell your health care team if you notice swelling. Your doctor or nurse will determine what is causing your symptoms, advise you on steps to take, and may prescribe medicine. Some problems related to edema are serious. Call your doctor or nurse if you feel short of breath, have a heartbeat that seems different or is not regular, have sudden swelling or swelling that is getting worse or is moving up your arms or legs, you gain weight quickly, or you don't urinate at all or urinate only a little.	**Get comfortable**. Wear loose clothing and shoes that are not too tight. When you sit or lie down, raise your feet with a stool or pillows. Avoid crossing your legs when you sit. Talk with your health care team about wearing special stockings, sleeves, or gloves that help with circulation if your swelling is severe. **Exercise.** Moving the part of your body with edema can help. Your doctor may give you specific exercises, including walking, to improve circulation. However, you may be advised not to stand or walk too much at one time. **Limit salt (sodium) in your diet.** Avoid foods such as chips, bacon, ham, and canned soup. Check food labels for the sodium content. Don't add salt or soy sauce to your food. **Take your medicine.** If your doctor prescribes a medicine called a diuretic, take it exactly as instructed. The medicine will help move the extra fluid and salt out of your body.

SIDE EFFECT AND POSSIBLE CAUSE	DESCRIPTION	WAYS TO MANAGE
Fatigue *Chemotherapy *Immunotherapy *Radiation therapy *Bone marrow transplant *Surgery *Anemia *Pain *Medications *Emotions	• Fatigue is a common side effect of many cancer treatments, including chemotherapy, immunotherapy, radiation therapy, bone marrow transplants, and surgery. • Conditions such as anemia, as well as pain, medications, and emotions, can also cause or worsen fatigue. • People often describe cancer-related fatigue as feeling extremely tired, weak, heavy, run down, and having no energy. • Resting does not always help with cancer-related fatigue. Cancer-related fatigue is one of the most difficult side effects for many people to cope with. • Tell your health care team if you feel extremely tired and are not able to do your normal activities or are very tired even after resting or sleeping. • There are many causes of fatigue. Keeping track of your levels of energy throughout the day will help your doctor to assess your fatigue. Write down how fatigue affects your daily activities and what makes the fatigue better or worse.	**Make a plan that balances rest and activity.** Choose activities that are relaxing for you. Many people choose to listen to music, read, meditate, practice guided imagery, or spend time with people they enjoy. Relaxing can help you save your energy and lower stress. Light exercise may also be advised by your doctor to give you more energy and help you feel better. **Plan time to rest.** If you are tired, take short naps of less than 1 hour during the day. However, too much sleep during the day can make it difficult to sleep at night. Choose the activities that are most important to you and do them when you have the most energy. Ask for help with important tasks such as making meals or driving. **Eat and drink well.** Meet with a registered dietitian to learn about foods and drinks that can increase your level of energy. Foods high in protein and calories will help you keep up your strength. Some people find it easier to eat many small meals throughout the day instead of three big meals. Stay well hydrated. Limit your intake of caffeine and alcohol. **Meet with a specialist.** It may help to meet with a counselor, psychologist, or psychiatrist. These experts help people to cope with difficult thoughts and feelings. Lowering stress may give you more energy. Since pain that is not controlled can also be major source of fatigue, it may help to meet with a pain or palliative care specialist.

SIDE EFFECT AND POSSIBLE CAUSE	DESCRIPTION	CANCER TREATMENTS MAY AFFECT YOURFERTILITY
Fertility Issues in Boys and Men **Possible Cause:** See 2nd column *Cancer Treatments May Affect Your Fertility*	Many cancer treatments can affect a boy's or a man's fertility. Most likely, your doctor will talk with you about whether or not cancer treatment may lower fertility or cause infertility. However, not all doctors bring up this topic. Sometimes you, a family member, or parents of a child being treated for cancer may need to initiate this conversation. Whether or not your fertility is affected depends on factors such as: • Your baseline fertility • Your age at the time of treatment • The type of cancer and treatment(s) • The amount (dose) of treatment • he length (duration) of treatment • The amount of time that has passed since treatment • Other personal health factors ***Emotional Considerations and Support for Fertility Issues*** For some men, infertility can be one of the most difficult and upsetting long-term effects of cancer treatment. Although it might feel overwhelming to think about your fertility right now, most people benefit from having talked with their doctor (or their child's doctor, when a child is being treated for cancer) about how treatment may affect their fertility and learning about options to preserve their fertility. Although most people want to have children at some point in their life, families can come together in many ways. For extra support during this time, reach out to your health care team with questions or concerns, as well as to professionally led support groups.	Cancer treatments are important for your future health, but they may harm reproductive organs and glands that control fertility. Changes to your fertility may be temporary or permanent. Talk with your healthcare team to learn what to expect based on your treatment(s): **Chemotherapy** (especially alkylating drugs) can damage sperm in men and sperm-forming cells (germ cells) in young boys. **Hormone therapy** (also called endocrine therapy) can decrease the production of sperm. **Radiation therapy** to the reproductive organs aswell as radiation near the abdomen, pelvis, or spine may lower sperm counts and testosterone levels, causing infertility. • Radiation may also destroy sperm cells and the stem cells that make sperm. Radiation therapy to the brain can damage the pituitary gland and decrease the production of testosterone and sperm. • For some types of cancers, the testicles can be protected from radiation through a procedure called testicular shielding. **Surgery** for cancers of the reproductive organs and for pelvic cancers (such as bladder, colon, prostate, and rectal cancer) can damage these organs and/or nearby nerves or lymph nodes in the pelvis, leading to infertility. **Stem cell transplants** such as bone marrow transplants and peripheral blood stem cell transplants, involve receiving high doses of chemotherapy and/or radiation. These treatments can damage sperm and sperm-forming cells. **Other treatments:** Talk with your doctor to learn whether other types of treatment, such as immunotherapy and targeted cancer therapy, may affect your fertility.

SIDE EFFECT AND POSSIBLE CAUSE	DESCRIPTION	CANCER TREATMENTS MAY AFFECT YOUR FERTILITY
Fertility Issues in Girls and Women **Possible Cause:** See 2nd column *Cancer Treatments May Affect Your Fertility*	Many cancer treatments can affect a girl's or woman's fertility. Most likely, your doctor will talk with you about whether or not cancer treatment may increase the risk of, or cause, infertility. However, not all doctors bring up this topic. Sometimes you, a family member, or parents of a child being treated for cancer may need to initiate this conversation. Whether or not your fertility is affected depends on factors such as: • Your baseline fertility • Your age at the time of treatment • The type of cancer and treatment(s) • The amount (dose) of treatment • The length (duration) of treatment • The amount of time that has passed since treatment • Other personal health factors ***Emotional Considerations and Support for Fertility Issues*** For some women, infertility can be one of the most difficult and upsetting long-term effects of cancer treatment. While it might feel overwhelming to think about your fertility right now, most people benefit from having talked with their doctor (or their child's doctor, when a child is being treated for cancer) about how treatment may affect their fertility and about options to preserve fertility.	Cancer treatments are important for your future health, but they may harm reproductive organs and glands that control fertility. Changes to your fertility may be temporary or permanent. Talk with your health care team to learn what to expect, based on your treatment(s): **Chemotherapy** (especially alkylating agents) can affect the ovaries, causing them to stop releasing eggs and estrogen. This is called primary ovarian insufficiency (POI). • Sometimes POI is temporary, and your menstrual periods and fertility return after treatment. Other times, damage to your ovaries is permanent and fertility doesn't return. • You may have hot flashes, night sweats, irritability, vaginal dryness, and irregular or no menstrual periods. • Chemotherapy can also lower the number of healthy eggs in the ovaries. • Women who are closer to the age of natural menopause may have a greater risk of infertility. • The National Institute for Child Health and Human Development (NICHD) has more information about primary ovarian insufficiency. **Hormone therapy** (also called endocrine therapy) used to treat cancer can disrupt the menstrual cycle, which may affect your fertility. Side effects depend on the specific hormones used and may include hot flashes, night sweats, and vaginal dryness. **Bone marrow transplants, peripheral blood stem cell transplants**, and other stem cell transplants involve receiving high doses of chemotherapy and/or radiation. These treatments can damage the ovaries and may cause infertility. **Other treatments:** Talk with your doctor to learn whether or not other types of treatment such as immunotherapy and targeted cancer therapy may affect your fertility.

SIDE EFFECT AND POSSIBLE CAUSE	DESCRIPTION	WAYS TO MANAGE
Hair Loss (Alopecia) *Chemotherapy *Radiation (Localized)	• Some types of chemotherapy cause the hair on your head and other parts of your body to fall out. • Radiation therapy can also cause hair loss on the part of the body that is being treated. • Hair loss is called alopecia. ***Ways to Care for Your Hair When It Grows Back*** **Be gentle.** When your hair starts to grow back, you will want to be gentle with it. Avoid too much brushing, curling, and blow-drying. You may not want to wash your hair as frequently. **After chemotherapy.** Hair often grows back in 2 to 3 months after treatment has ended. Your hair will be very fine when it starts to grow back. Sometimes your new hair can be curlier or straighter—or even a different color. In time, it may go back to how it was before treatment. **After radiation therapy.** Hair often grows back in 3 to 6 months after treatment has ended. If you received a very high dose of radiation your hair may grow back thinner or not at all on the part of your body that received radiation.	***Ways to Manage Hair Loss*** Talk with your health care team about ways to manage before and after hair loss: **Treat your hair gently.** You may want to use a hairbrush with soft bristles or a wide-tooth comb. Do not use hair dryers, irons, or products such as gels or clips that may hurt your scalp. Wash your hair with a mild shampoo. Wash it less often and be very gentle. Pat it dry with a soft towel. **You have choices.** Some people choose to cut their hair short to make it easier to deal with when it starts to fall out. Others choose to shave their head. If you choose to shave your head, use an electric shaver so you won't cut yourself. If you plan to buy a wig, get one while you still have hair so you can match it to the color of your hair. If you find wigs to be itchy and hot, try wearing a comfortable scarf or turban. **Protect and care for your scalp.** Use sunscreen or wear a hat when you are outside. Choose a comfortable scarf or hat that you enjoy and that keeps your head warm. If your scalp itches or feels tender, using lotions and conditioners can help it feel better. **Talk about your feelings.** Many people feel angry, depressed, or embarrassed about hair loss. It can help to share these feelings with someone who understands. Some people find it helpful to talk with other people who have lost their hair during cancer treatment. Talking openly and honestly with your children and close family members can also help you all. Tell them that you expect to lose your hair during treatment.

SIDE EFFECT AND POSSIBLE CAUSE	DESCRIPTION	WAYS TO MANAGE
Infection and Neutropenia *Surgery *Chemotherapy	<ul><li>An infection is the invasion and growth of germs in the body, such as bacteria, viruses, yeast, or other fungi.</li><li>An infection can begin anywhere in the body, may spread throughout the body, and can cause one or more of these signs:<ul><li>Fever of 100.5 °F (38 °C) or higher or chills</li><li>Cough or sore throat</li><li>Diarrhea</li><li>Ear pain, headache or sinus pain, or a stiff or sore neck</li><li>skin rash</li><li>Sores or white coating in your mouth or on your tongue</li><li>Swelling or redness, especially where a catheter enters your body</li><li>Urine that is bloody or cloudy, or pain when you urinate</li></ul></li><li>Call your health care team if you have signs of an infection.</li><li>Infections during cancer treatment can be life threatening and require urgent medical attention.</li><li>Be sure to talk with your doctor or nurse before taking medicine—even aspirin, acetaminophen (such as Tylenol®), or ibuprofen (such as Advil®) for a fever. These medicines can lower a fever but may also mask or hide signs of a more serious problem.</li><li>Some types of cancer and treatments such as chemotherapy may increase your risk of infection. This is because they lower the number of white blood cells, the cells that help your body to fight infection. During chemotherapy, there will be times in your treatment cycle when the number of white blood cells (called neutrophils) is particularly low, and you are at increased risk of infection.</li><li>Stress, poor nutrition, and not enough sleep can also weaken the immune system, making infection more likely.</li></ul>	*Ways to Prevent Infection* Your health care team will talk with you about these and other ways to prevent infection: **Wash your hands often and well**. Use soap and warm water to wash your hands well, especially before eating. Have people around you wash their hands well too. **Stay extra clean**. If you have a catheter, keep the area around it clean and dry. Clean your teeth well and check your mouth for sores or other signs of an infection each day. If you get a scrape or cut, clean it well. Let your doctor or nurse know if your bottom is sore or bleeds, as this could increase your risk of infection. **Avoid germs.** Stay away from people who are sick or have a cold. Avoid crowds and people who have just had a live vaccine, such as one for chicken pox, polio, or measles. Follow food safety guidelines; make sure the meat, fish, and eggs you eat are well cooked. Keep hot foods hot and cold foods cold. You may be advised to eat only fruits and vegetables that can be peeled, or to wash all raw fruits and vegetables very well.

SIDE EFFECT AND POSSIBLE CAUSE	DESCRIPTION	WAYS TO MANAGE
Memory or Concentration Issues *Chemotherapy *Immunotherapy *Radiation therapy (brain)	• Whether you have memory or concentration problems (sometimes described as a mental fog or chemo brain) depends on the type of treatment you receive, your age, and other health-related factors. • Cancer treatments such as chemotherapy may cause difficulty with thinking, concentrating, or remembering things. • So can some types of radiation therapy to the brain and immunotherapy. • These cognitive problems may start during or after cancer treatment. Some people notice very small changes, such as a bit more difficulty remembering things, whereas others have much greater memory or concentration problems. • Your doctor will assess your symptoms and advise you about ways to manage or treat these problems. Treating conditions such as poor nutrition, anxiety, depression, fatigue, and insomnia may also help.	It's important for you or a family member to tell your health care team if you have difficulty remembering things, thinking, or concentrating. Here are some steps you can take to manage minor memory or concentration problems: **Plan your day.** Do things that need the most concentration at the time of day when you feel best. Get extra rest and plenty of sleep at night. If you need to rest during the day, short naps of less than 1 hour are best. Long naps can make it more difficult to sleep at night. Keep a daily routine. **Exercise your body and mind.** Exercise can help to decrease stress and help you to feel more alert. Exercise releases endorphins, also known as "feel-good chemicals, "which give people a feeling of well-being. Ask what light physical exercises may be helpful for you. Mind–body practices such as meditation or mental exercises such as puzzles or games also help some people. **Get help to remember things.** Write down and keep a list handy of important information. Use a daily planner, recorder, or other electronic device to help you remember important activities. Make a list of important names and phone numbers. Keep it in one place so it's easy to find

SIDE EFFECT AND POSSIBLE CAUSE	DESCRIPTION	WAYS TO MANAGE

Mouth and Throat Problems
 	
*Chemotherapy
*Immunotherapy
*Radiation therapy (head & neck)
*Medications
 	
See Eating Hints
	• Cancer treatments may cause dental, mouth, and throat problems.
	• Radiation therapy to the head and neck may harm the salivary glands and tissues in your mouth and/or make it hard to chew and swallow safely.
	• Some types of chemotherapy and immunotherapy can also harm cells in your mouth, throat, and lips.
	• Drugs used to treat cancer and certain bone problems may also cause oral complications.
	Mouth and throat problems may include:
	  o Changes in taste or smell
	  o Dry mouth (xerostomia)
	  o Infections and mouth sores
	  o Pain or swelling in your mouth (oral mucositis)
	  o Sensitivity to hot or cold foods
	  o Swallowing problems (dysphagia)
	  o Tooth decay (cavities)
	
	Mouth problems are more serious if they interfere with eating and drinking because they can lead to dehydration and/or malnutrition.
	
	It's important to call your doctor or nurse if you have pain in your mouth, lips, or throat that makes it difficult to eat, drink, or sleep or if you have a fever of 100.5 °F (38 °C) or higher.
	
	Ways to Prevent Mouth and Dental Problems
	• Get a dental check-up before starting treatment.
	  o Before you start treatment, visit your dentist for a cleaning and check-up. Tell the dentist about your cancer treatment and try to get any dental work completed before starting treatment.
	• Check and clean your mouth daily.
	  o Check your mouth every day for sores or white spots.
	  o Rinse your mouth throughout the day with a solution of warm water, baking soda, and salt.
	  o Gently brush your teeth, gums, and tongue after each meal and before going to bed at night. Use a very soft toothbrush or cotton swabs.
	  o If you are at risk of bleeding, ask if you should floss.
		Your health care team may suggest that you take these and other steps to manage these problems:
		
		For a sore mouth or throat: Choose foods that are soft, wet, and easy to swallow. Soften dry foods with gravy, sauce, or other liquids. Use a blender to make milkshakes or blend your food to make it easier to swallow. Ask about pain medicine, such as lozenges or sprays that numb your mouth and make eating less painful. Avoid foods and drinks that can irritate your mouth; foods that are crunchy, salty, spicy, or sugary; and alcoholic drinks. Don't smoke or use tobacco.
		
		For a dry mouth: Drink plenty of liquids because a dry mouth can increase the risk of tooth decay and mouth infections. Keep water handy and sip it often to keep your mouth wet. Suck on ice chips or sugar-free hard candy, have frozen desserts, or chew sugar-free gum. Use a lip balm. Ask about medicines such as saliva substitutes that can coat, protect, and moisten your mouth and throat. Acupuncture may also help with dry mouth.
		
		For changes to your sense of taste: Foods may seem to have no taste or may not taste the way they used to or food may not have much taste at all. Radiation therapy may cause a change in sweet, sour, bitter, and salty tastes. Chemotherapy drugs may cause an unpleasant chemical or metallic taste in your mouth. If you have taste changes it may help to try different foods to find ones that taste best to you. Trying cold foods may also help. Here are some more tips to consider:
		• If food tastes bland, marinate foods to improve their flavor or add spices to foods.
		• If red meat tastes strange, switch to other high-protein foods such as chicken, eggs, fish, peanut butter.
		• If foods taste salty, bitter, or acidic, try sweetening them.
		• If foods taste metallic, switch to plastic utensils and non-metal cooking dishes.
		• If you have a bad taste in your mouth, try sugar-free lemon drops, gum, or mints.

SIDE EFFECT AND POSSIBLE CAUSE	DESCRIPTION	WAYS TO MANAGE
Nausea and Vomiting Cancer treatments, including, but not limited to chemotherapy	• Nausea is when you feel sick to your stomach, as if you are going to throw up. • Vomiting is when you throw up. • There are different types of nausea and vomiting caused by cancer treatment, including anticipatory, acute, and delayed nausea and vomiting. • Controlling nausea and vomiting will help you to feel better and prevent more serious problems such as malnutrition and dehydration. • Your doctor or nurse will determine what is causing your symptoms and advise you on ways to prevent them. • Medicines called anti-nausea drugs or antiemetics are effective in preventing or reducing many types of nausea and vomiting. The medicine is taken at specific times to prevent and/or control symptoms of nausea and vomiting. These foods and drinks may be easy on your stomach: SOUPS • Clear broth, such as chicken, beef, and vegetable DRINKS • Clear soda, such as ginger ale • Cranberry or grape juice • Oral rehydration drinks, such as Pedialyte® • Tea • Water MAIN MEAL AND SNACKS • Chicken—broiled or baked without the skin • Cream of wheat or rice cereal • Crackers or pretzels • Oatmeal • Pasta or noodles • Potatoes—boiled, without the skin • White rice • White toast FRIUITS and SWEETS • Bananas • Canned fruit such as applesauce, peaches, and pears • Gelatin (Jell-O®) • Popsicles and sherbet • Yogurt (plain or vanilla)	You may be advised to take these steps to feel better: **Take anti-nausea medicine.** Talk with your doctor or nurse to learn when to take your medicine. Most people need to take an anti-nausea medicine even on days when they feel well. Tell your doctor or nurse if the medicine doesn't help. There are different kinds of medicine, and one may work better than another for you. **Drink plenty of water and fluids.** Drinking will help to prevent dehydration, a serious problem that happens when your body loses too much fluid and you are not drinking enough. Try to sip on water, fruit juices, ginger ale, tea, and/or sports drinks throughout the day. **Have enough to eat and drink.** Take small sips of water during the day, if you find it hard to drink a full glass at one time. Eat 5 or 6 small meals during the day, instead of 3 big meals. **Avoid certain foods.** Don't eat greasy, fried, sweet, or spicy foods if you feel sick after eating them. If the smell of food bothers you, ask others to make your food. Try cold foods that do not have strong smells, or let food cool down before you eat it. **Try these tips on treatment days.** Some people find that it helps to eat a small snack before treatment. Others avoid eating or drinking right before or after treatment because it makes them feel sick. After treatment, wait at least 1 hour before you eat or drink. **Learn about complementary medicine practices that may help.** Acupuncture relieves nausea and/or vomiting caused by chemotherapy in some people. Deep breathing, guided imagery, hypnosis, and other relaxation techniques (such as listening to music, reading a book, or meditating) also help some people. *See Eating Hints*

SIDE EFFECT AND POSSIBLE CAUSE	DESCRIPTION	WAYS TO MANAGE
Nerve Problems (Peripheral Neuropathy)	• Some cancer treatments cause peripheral neuropathy, a result of damage to the peripheral nerves. These nerves carry information from the brain to other parts of the body. • Side effects depend on which peripheral nerves (sensory, motor, or autonomic) are affected. Damage to sensory nerves (nerves that help you feel pain, heat, cold, and pressure) can cause: • Tingling, numbness, or a pins-and-needles feeling in your feet and hands that may spread to your legs and arms • Inability to feel a hot or cold sensation, such as a hot stove • Inability to feel pain, such as from a cut or sore on your foot Damage to motor nerves (nerves that help your muscles to move) can cause: • Weak or achy muscles. You may lose your balance or trip easily. It may also be difficult to button shirts or open jars. • Muscles that twitch and cramp or muscle wasting (if you don't use your muscles regularly). • Swallowing or breathing difficulties (if your chest or throat muscles are affected) Damage to autonomic nerves (nerves that control functions such as blood pressure, digestion, heart rate, temperature, and urination) can cause: • Digestive changes such as constipation or diarrhea • Dizzy or faint feeling, due to low blood pressure • Sexual problems: men may be unable to get an erection and women may not reach orgasm • Sweating problems (either too much or too little sweating) • Urination problems, such as leaking urine or difficulty emptying your bladder	*Ways to Prevent or Manage Problems Related to Nerve Changes* You may be advised to take these steps: **Prevent falls.** Have someone help you prevent falls around the house. Move rugs out of your path so you will not trip on them. Put rails on the walls and in the bathroom, so you can hold on to them and balance yourself. Put bathmats in the shower or tub. Wear sturdy shoes with soft soles. Get up slowly after sitting or lying down, especially if you feel dizzy. **Take extra care in the kitchen and shower**. Use potholders in the kitchen to protect your hands from burns. Be careful when handling knives or sharp objects. Ask someone to check the water temperature, to make sure it's not too hot. **Protect your hands and feet**. Wear shoes, both inside and outside. Check your arms, legs, and feet for cuts or scratches every day. When it's cold, wear warm clothes to protect your hands and feet. **Ask for help and slow down.** Let people help you with difficult tasks. Slow down and give yourself more time to do things. **Ask about pain medicine and integrative medicine practices**. You may be prescribed pain medicine. Sometimes practices such as acupuncture, massage, physical therapy, yoga, and others may also be advised to lower pain. Talk with your health care team to learn what is advised for you.

SIDE EFFECT AND POSSIBLE CAUSE	DESCRIPTION	WAYS TO MANAGE
Pain See 1st Column *Different cancer treatments may cause specific types of pain.*	• Cancer itself and the side effects of cancer treatment can sometimes cause pain. • Pain is not something that you have to "put up with." Controlling pain is an important part of your cancer treatment plan. • Pain can suppress the immune system, increase the time it takes your body to heal, interfere with sleep, and affect your mood. Talk with your health care team about pain, especially if: • The pain isn't getting better or going away with pain medicine • the pain comes on quickly • The pain makes it hard to eat, sleep, or perform your normal activities • You feel new pain • You have side effects from the pain medicine such as sleepiness, nausea, or constipation ***Different cancer treatments may cause specific types of pain.*** Patients may have different types of pain depending on the treatments they receive, including: • **Spasms, stinging, and itching** caused by intravenous chemotherapy. • **Mucositis** (sores or inflammation in the mouth or other parts of the digestive system) caused by chemotherapy or targeted therapy. • **Skin pain, rash, or hand-foot syndrome** (redness, tingling, or burning in the palms of the hands and/or the soles of feet) caused by chemotherapy or targeted therapy. • **Pain in joints and muscles** throughout the body caused by paclitaxel or aromatase inhibitor therapy. • **Osteonecrosis** of the jaw caused by bisphosphonates given for cancer that has spread to the bone.	Here are some steps you can take, as you work with your health care team to prevent, treat, or lessen pain: **Keep track of your pain levels.** Each day, write about any pain you feel. Writing down answers to the questions below will help you describe the pain to your doctor or nurse. • What part of your body feels painful? • What does the pain feel like (is it sharp, burning, shooting, or throbbing) and where do you feel the pain? • When does the pain start? How long does the pain last? • What activities (such as eating, sleeping, or other activities) does pain interfere with? • What makes the pain feel better or worse? For example, do ice packs, heating pads, or exercises help? • Does pain medicine help? How much do you take? How often do you take it? • How bad is the pain, on a scale of 1 to 10, where "10" is the most pain and "1" is the least pain? **Take the prescribed pain medicine.** • Take the right amount of medicine at the right time. • Do not wait until your pain gets too bad before taking pain medicine. Waiting to take your medicine could make it take longer for the pain to go away or increase the amount of medicine needed to lower pain. • Do not stop taking the pain medicine unless your doctor advises you to. • Tell your doctor or nurse if the medicine no longer lowers the pain, or if you are in pain, but it's not yet time to take the pain medicine.

| Pain Continued | • **Pain syndromes caused by radiation,** including:
  ○ Pain from brachytherapy.
  ○ Pain from the position the patient stays in during radiation therapy.
  ○ Mucositis.
  ○ Inflammation of the mucous membranes in areas treated with radiation.
  ○ Dermatitis (inflammation of the skin in areas treated with radiation).
  ○ Pain flares (a temporary worsening of pain in the treated area). | **Meet with a pain specialist.** Specialists who treat pain often work together as part of a pain or palliative care team. These specialists may include a neurologist, surgeon, physiatrist, psychiatrist, psychologist, or pharmacist.
• Talk with your health care team to find a pain specialist.
• **Ask about integrative medicine.** Treatments such as acupuncture, biofeedback, hypnosis, massage therapy and physical therapy may also be used to treat pain.

Pain may affect quality of life after treatment ends.

• Pain that is severe or continues after cancer treatment ends increases the risk of anxiety and depression.
• Patients may be disabled by their pain, unable to work, or feel that they are losing support once their care moves from their oncology team back to their primary care team.
• Feelings of anxiety and depression can worsen pain and make it harder to control. |

SIDE EFFECT AND POSSIBLE CAUSE	DESCRIPTION	WAYS TO MANAGE
Skin and Nail Changes *Radiation therapy *Chemotherapy *Biological therapy *Targeted therapy	Cancer treatments may cause a range of skin and nail changes. Talk with your health care team to learn whether or not you will have these changes, based on the treatment you are receiving. **Radiation therapy** can cause the skin on the part of your body receiving radiation therapy to become dry and peel, itch (called pruritus), and turn red or darker. It may look sunburned or tan and be swollen or puffy. **Chemotherapy** • May damage fast growing skin and nail cells. This can cause problems such as skin that is dry, itchy, red, and/or that peels. • Some people may develop a rash or sun sensitivity, causing you to sunburn easily. • Nail changes may include dark, yellow, or cracked nails and/or cuticles that are red and hurt. • Chemotherapy in people who have received radiation therapy in the past can cause skin to become red, blister, peel, or hurt on the part of the body that received radiation therapy; this is called radiation recall. **Biological therapy** may cause itching (pruritus). **Targeted therapy** May cause a dry skin, a rash, and nail problems. These skin problems are more serious and need urgent medical attention: • Sudden or severe itching, a rash, or hives during chemotherapy. These may be signs of an allergic reaction. • Sores on the part of your body where you are receiving treatment that become painful, wet, and/or infected. This is called a moist reaction and may happen in areas where the skin folds, such as around your ears, breast, or bottom.	Depending on what treatment you are receiving, you may be advised to take these steps to protect your skin, prevent infection, and reduce itching: **Use only recommended skin products.** Use mild soaps that are gentle on your skin. Ask your nurse to recommend specific lotions and creams. Ask when and how often to use them. Ask what skin products to avoid. For example, you may be advised to not use powders or antiperspirants before radiation therapy. **Protect your skin**. Ask about lotions or antibiotics for dry, itchy, infected or swollen skin. Don't use heating pads, ice packs, or bandages on the area receiving radiation therapy. Shave less often and use an electric razor or stop shaving if your skin is sore. Wear sunscreen and lip balm or a loose-fitting long-sleeved shirt, pants, and a hat with a wide brim when outdoors. **Prevent or treat dry, itchy skin (pruritus)**. Your doctor will work to assess the cause of pruritus. There are also steps you can take to feel better. Avoid products with alcohol or perfume, which can dry or irritate your skin. Take short showers or baths in lukewarm, not hot, water. Put on lotion after drying off from a shower, while your skin is still slightly damp. Keep your home cool and humid. Eat a healthy diet and drink plenty of fluids to help keep your skin moist and healthy. Applying a cool washcloth or ice to the affected area may also help. Acupuncture also helps some people. **Prevent or treat minor nail problems.** Keep your nails clean and cut short. Wear gloves when you wash the dishes, work in the garden, or clean the house. Check with your nurse about products that can help your nails. If your skin hurts in the area where you get treatment, tell your doctor or nurse. Your skin might have a moist reaction. Most often this happens in areas where the skin folds, such as behind the ears or under the breasts. It can lead to an infection if not properly treated. Ask your doctor or nurse how to care for these areas.

SIDE EFFECT AND POSSIBLE CAUSE	DESCRIPTION	WAYS TO MANAGE
Sleep Problems	• Sleeping well is important for your physical and mental health. A good night's sleep not only helps you to think clearly, it also lowers your blood pressure, helps your appetite, and strengthens your immune system. • Sleep problems such as being unable to fall asleep and/or stay asleep, also called insomnia, are common among people being treated for cancer. Studies show that as many as half of all patients have sleep-related problems. These problems may be caused by the side effects of treatment, medicine, long hospital stays, or stress. • Talk with your health care team if you have difficulty sleeping, so you can get the help you need. • Sleep problems that go on for a long time may increase the risk of anxiety or depression. • Your doctor will do an assessment, which may include a polysomnogram (recordings taken during sleep that show brain waves, breathing rate, and other activities such as heart rate) to correctly diagnose and treat sleep problems. Assessments may be repeated from time to time, since sleeping problems may change over time.	There are steps that you and your health care team can take to help you sleep well again. **Tell your doctor about problems that interfere with sleep**. Getting treatment to lower side effects such as pain or bladder or gastrointestinal problems may help you sleep better. **Cognitive behavioral therapy (CBT) and relaxation therapy** may help. Practicing these therapies can help you to relax. For example, a CBT therapist can help you learn to change negative thoughts and beliefs about sleep into positive ones. Strategies such as muscle relaxation, guided imagery, and self-hypnosis may also help you. **Set good bedtime habits.** Go to bed only when sleepy, in a quiet and dark room, and in a comfortable bed. If you do not fall asleep, get out of bed and return to bed when you are sleepy. Stop watching television or using other electrical devices for a couple of hours before going to bed. Don't drink or eat a lot before bedtime. While it's important to keep active during the day with regular exercise, exercising a few hours before bedtime may make sleep more difficult. **Sleep medicine may be prescribed**. Your doctor may prescribe sleep medicine for a short period if other strategies don't work. The sleep medicine prescribed will depend on your specific problem (such as trouble falling asleep or trouble staying asleep) as well as other medicines you are taking.

SIDE EFFECT AND POSSIBLE CAUSE	DESCRIPTION	WAYS TO MANAGE
Urinary and Bladder Problems *Radiation therapy *Chemotherapy *Immunotherapy *Surgery	*Symptoms of a Urinary Problem* Some urinary or bladder changes may be normal, such as changes to the color or smell of your urine caused by some types of chemotherapy. Your health care team will determine what is causing your symptoms and will advise on steps to take to feel better. Irritation of the bladder lining (radiation cystitis): • Pain or a burning feeling when you urinate • Blood in your urine • Trouble starting to urinate • Trouble emptying your bladder completely • Feeling that you need to urinate urgently or frequently • Leaking a little urine when you sneeze or cough • Bladder spasms, cramps, or discomfort in the pelvic area Urinary tract infection (UTI): • Pain or a burning feeling when you urinate • Urine that is cloudy or red • Fever of 100.5 °F (38 °C) or higher, chills, and fatigue • Pain in your back or abdomen • Difficulty urinating or not being able to urinate In people being treated for cancer, a UTI can turn into a serious condition that needs immediate medical care. Antibiotics will be prescribed if you have a bacterial infection.	*Ways to Prevent or Manage* Here are some steps you may be advised to take to feel better and to prevent problems: **Drink plenty of liquids.** Most people need to drink at least 8 cups of fluid each day, so that urine is light yellow or clear. You'll want to stay away from things that can make bladder problems worse. These include caffeine, drinks with alcohol, spicy foods, and tobacco products. **Prevent urinary tract infections.** Your doctor or nurse will talk with you about ways to lower your chances of getting a urinary tract infection. These may include going to the bathroom often, wearing cotton underwear and loose-fitting pants, learning about safe and sanitary practices for catheterization, taking showers instead of baths, and checking with your nurse before using products such as creams or lotions near your genital area. *Drink more liquids* • Drink liquids such as water, soup, milkshakes, and cranberry juice. Add extra water to the juice. • Ask your doctor or nurse how many cups of liquid you should drink each day. Most people need to drink at least 8 cups a day. • Keep drinking liquids even if you have to go to the bathroom a lot. Liquids help your body to work well. Some liquids can make bladder problems worse. Talk with your doctor or nurse to learn what you should stop drinking or drink less of. These include: • Drinks with caffeine, such as coffee, black tea, and soda. • Drinks with alcohol, such as beer, wine, mixed drinks, and liquor.

LATE SIDE EFFECT	DESCRIPTION	WAYS TO MANAGE
Bone Loss	• Chemotherapy, steroid medicines, hormonal therapy, or radiation therapy may cause thinning of the bones. • With radiation therapy, bone loss will occur only in the part of the body that was treated.	After cancer treatment, you should have regular check-ups. During these visits, your doctor or nurse will do a physical exam and may order tests to check for bone loss. You can help lower your risk of bone loss by: • Not smoking or using other tobacco products • Eating foods that are rich in calcium and vitamin D • Walking, jogging, or doing other weight-bearing exercise • Limiting how much alcohol you drink • If you had radiation to the head and neck, also see Mouth Changes for tips on managing bone loss in your jaw.
Brain Changes	Some chemotherapy drugs and radiation therapy to the brain can cause problems months or years after treatment ends. Late effects may include: • Memory loss • Problems doing math • Problems concentrating • Slow processing of information • Personality changes • Movement problems Radiation to the brain can cause radiation necrosis. This problem may happen when an area of dead tissue forms at the site of the brain tumor. Radiation necrosis can cause movement problems, problems concentrating, slow processing of information, and headaches.	After cancer treatment, you should have regular check-ups. If you have symptoms of brain changes, you will have tests to see whether they are due to the cancer or are late side effects of your treatment. If you have late side effects, your doctor or nurse: • Will talk with you about ways to manage late side effects • May refer you to a physical, occupational, or speech therapist who can help with problems caused by late side effects • May prescribe medicine or suggest surgery to help with the symptoms

LATE SIDE EFFECT	DESCRIPTION	WAYS TO MANAGE
Eye Problems	Chemotherapy, hormone therapy, immunotherapy, and steroid medicines may increase the risk of cataracts. Cataracts are a problem in which the lens of your eye becomes cloudy. Cataracts can cause: • Blurred, cloudy, or double vision • Sensitivity to light • Trouble seeing at night Some chemotherapy drugs can cause dry eye syndrome. This is a problem in which your eyes do not produce enough tears. • Symptoms include feeling as if your eyes are dry or have something in them.	If you are at risk for cataracts, you should have regular visits with an ophthalmologist (a medical doctor who treats eye problems). • If cataracts become serious, they can be treated with surgery. • In this type of surgery, an eye surgeon will remove the clouded lens and replace it with a plastic lens. You will usually have local anesthesia and be able to go home the same day. If you develop dry eye syndrome, your doctor may prescribe regular treatment with eye drops or ointments.
Hearing Loss	• Watch for signs of hearing loss. Let your doctor know right away if you notice changes in your hearing. • Treatment with certain chemotherapy drugs (in particular, cisplatin and high doses of carboplatin) and high doses of radiation to the brain can cause hearing loss.	• See an audiologist. An audiologist is a professional trained in hearing disorders. • If you had a cancer treatment that can cause hearing loss, you should have at least one visit with an audiologist after you have finished treatment. • Depending on the type and dose of cancer treatment that you received, you may need to see an audiologist more often.

LATE SIDE EFFECT	DESCRIPTION	WAYS TO MANAGE

Heart Problems	Certain cancer drugs, chemotherapy, and radiation therapy to the chest may cause heart problems.
	Examples of drugs that tend to cause heart problems include:
	• Trastuzumab
	• Doxorubicin
	• Daunorubicin (Cerubidine)
	• Epirubicin (Ellence)
	• Cyclophosphamide (Neosar)
	
	Heart problems caused by cancer treatment may include:
	• A weakening of the heart muscle, which is known as congestive heart failure.
	   ○ It can cause shortness of breath, dizziness, and swollen hands or feet.
	• Coronary artery disease, which occurs when the small blood vessels that supply blood and oxygen to the heart become narrow.
	   ○ It can cause chest pain or shortness of breath.
	   ○ This problem is more common in those who had high doses of radiation therapy to the chest.
		After cancer treatment, you should have regular check-ups. If you have heart problems, your doctor or nurse might suggest that you:
		
		Eat a heart-healthy diet: A heart-healthy diet includes a variety of fruits, vegetables, and whole grains. It also includes lean meats, poultry, fish, beans, and fat-free or low-fat milk or milk products. Your doctor will probably recommend that you follow a diet low in salt, because salt can cause extra fluid to build up in your body, making heart problems worse. *The American Heart Association* has many tips for heart-healthy eating.
		
		Watch fluid intake: Drinking too much fluid can worsen heart problems, so it's important for people who have heart failure to drink the correct amounts and types of fluid. Talk with your doctor about what amounts and types of fluid you should have each day. Let your doctor know right away if you have sudden weight gain. This could mean extra fluid is building up. Also, if you have heart failure, you shouldn't drink alcohol.
		
		Lose weight if you're overweight or obese: Carrying extra weight can put added strain on your heart. Work with your health care team to lose weight safely.
		
		Exercise: The right type and amount of exercise can help keep you and your heart healthy. Talk with your doctor about which activities you can safely do. Exercise can help you become more fit and stay as active as possible.
		
		Quit smoking and avoid using illegal drugs: Talk with your doctor about programs and products that can help you quit smoking. Also, try to avoid secondhand smoke. Smoking and drugs can make heart failure worse and harm your health.
		
		Get enough rest: *See Sleep Problems above under SIDE EFFECT AND POSSIBLE CAUSE.*
		
		Take medicines prescribed by your doctor: Your doctor may prescribe medicines based on the type of heart problem you have, how severe it is, and your response to certain medicines.

LATE SIDE EFFECT	DESCRIPTION	*NON-DRUG TREATMENT FOR HOT FLASHES AND NIGHT SWEATS IN PATIENTS WITH CANCER*	*DRUG TREATMENT FOR HOT FLASHES AND NIGHT SWEATS IN PATIENTS WITH CANCER*
Hot Flashes and Night Sweats	In patients with cancer, hot flashes and night sweats may be caused by the tumor, its treatment, or other conditions. Sweating happens with disease conditions such as fever and may occur without disease in warm climates, during exercise, and during hot flashes in menopause. Sweating helps balance body temperature by allowing heat to evaporate through the skin. Hot flashes and night sweats are common in patients with cancer and in cancer survivors. They are more common in women but can also occur in men. Many patients treated for breast cancer and prostate cancer have hot flashes. Menopause in women can have natural, surgical, or chemical causes. Chemical menopause in women with cancer is caused by certain types of chemotherapy, radiation, or hormone therapy with androgen (a male hormone).	**Treatments that help patients cope with stress and anxiety may help manage hot flashes.** Treatments that change how patients deal with stress, anxiety, and negative emotions may help manage hot flashes. These are called psychological interventions. Psychological interventions help patients gain a sense of control and develop coping skills to manage symptoms. Staying calm and managing stress may lower levels of a hormone called serotonin that can trigger hot flashes. Psychological interventions may help hot flashes and related problems when used together with drug treatment. **Hypnosis may help relieve hot flashes.** Hypnosis is a trance-like state that allows a person to be more aware, focused, and open to suggestion. Under hypnosis, the person can concentrate more clearly on a specific thought, feeling, or sensation without becoming distracted. In hypnosis, a therapist helps the patient to deeply relax and focus on cooling thoughts. This may lower stress levels, balance body temperature, and calm the heart rate and breathing rate. **Comfort measures may help relieve night sweats related to cancer.** Comfort measures may be used to treat night sweats related to cancer. Since body temperature goes up before a hot flash, doing the following may control body	**Hot flashes may be controlled with estrogen replacement therapy.** Hot flashes during natural or treatment-related menopause can be controlled with estrogen replacement therapy. However, many women are not able to take estrogen replacement (for example, women who have or had breast cancer). Hormone replacement therapy that combines estrogen with progestin may increase the risk of breast cancer or breast cancer recurrence. **Other drugs may be useful in some patients.** Studies of non-estrogen drugs to treat hot flashes in women with a history of breast cancer have reported that many of them do not work as well as estrogen replacement or have side effects. Megestrol (a drug like progesterone), certain antidepressants, anticonvulsants, and clonidine (a drug used to treat high blood pressure) are non-estrogen drugs used to control hot flashes. Some antidepressants may change how other drugs, work in the body.

Hot Flashes and Night Sweats *Continued*	Treatment for breast cancer and prostate cancer can cause menopause or menopause-like effects, including severe hot flashes. Certain types of drugs can cause night sweats. Drugs that may cause night sweats include the following: • Tamoxifen. • Aromatase inhibitors. • Opioids. • Tricyclic antidepressants • Steroids.	temperature and help control symptoms: • Wear loose-fitting clothes made of cotton. • Use fans and open windows to keep air moving. • Practice relaxation training and slow, deep breathing. **Herbs and dietary supplements should be used with caution.** Most studies of soy and black cohosh show they are no better than a placebo in reducing hot flashes. *Soy contains estrogen -like substances; the effect of soy on the risk of breast cancer growth or recurrence is not clear.* Studies of ground flaxseed to treat hot flashes have shown mixed results. Claims are made about several other plant-based and natural products as remedies for hot flashes. These include dong quai, milk thistle, red clover, licorice root extract, and chaste tree berry. Since little is known about how these products work or whether they affect the risk of breast cancer, women should be cautious about using them. **Acupuncture has been studied in the treatment of hot flashes.** Pilot studies of acupuncture and randomized clinical trials that compare true acupuncture and sham (inactive) treatment have been done in patients with hot flashes and results are mixed. A review of many studies combined showed that acupuncture had slight or no effects in breast cancer patients with hot flashes. (See the Vasomotor symptoms section in the PDQ health professional summary on Acupuncture for more information.) .	Side effects of drug therapy may include the following: • Antidepressants used to treat hot flashes over a short period of time may cause nausea, drowsiness, dry mouth, and changes in appetite. • Anticonvulsants used to treat hot flashes may cause drowsiness, dizziness, and trouble concentrating. • Clonidine may cause dry mouth, drowsiness, constipation, and insomnia. Patients may respond in different ways to drug therapy. It is important that the patient's health care providers know about all medicines, dietary supplements, and herbs the patient is taking. If one medicine does not improve symptoms, switching to another medicine may help.

LATE SIDE EFFECT	DESCRIPTION	WAYS TO MANAGE
Joint Changes	• Radiation therapy, some chemotherapy drugs, and steroids can cause scar tissue, weakness, and bone loss. • These problems can lead to loss of motion in joints, such as your jaw, shoulders, hips, or knees. • If you receive radiation therapy, these problems will occur only in the part of the body that was treated.	It is important to be aware of early signs of joint problems so these can be addressed before they worsen. These signs include: • Trouble opening your mouth wide • Pain when you make certain movements, such as reaching over your head or putting your hand in a back pocket Talk with your doctor or nurse. He or she may refer you to a physical therapist, which will assess your joint problems and give you exercises to do. Physical therapy exercises can decrease pain, increase strength, and improve movement.
Lung Problems	• Chemotherapy and radiation therapy to the chest may damage the lungs. • Cancer survivors who received both chemotherapy and radiation therapy to the chest may have a higher risk of lung damage. • Lung damage can cause shortness of breath, wheezing, fever, dry cough, congestion, and feeling tired. • Tell your doctor if you have any of these symptoms.	**Oxygen therapy:** If you have serious trouble breathing, your doctor may prescribe oxygen therapy. Oxygen is most often given through nasal prongs or a mask that fits over your mouth and nose. In some cases, you might receive oxygen through a ventilator. **Lose weight if you're overweight or obese:** Excess weight can make it hard to breathe. Work with your doctor and health care team to lose weight safely. **Exercise:** Talk with your doctor about which activities you can safely do. Exercise can help you become more fit and stay as active as possible. **Quit smoking and avoid using illegal drugs:** Talk with your doctor about programs and products that can help you quit smoking. Also, try to avoid secondhand smoke. Smoking and drugs can worsen lung problems and harm your health. For help to quit smoking, visit *Smokefree.gov* or call toll-free, 1-800-QUIT-NOW (1-800-784-8669). **Take medicines prescribed by your doctor:** Your doctor can prescribe medicines to help you relax when it is hard to breathe, relieve discomfort, and treat pain. **Some people with lung problems take steroid pills.** Steroids can interfere with the way the body uses specific nutrients, including calcium, potassium, sodium, protein, and vitamins C and D. If you take steroid pills for lung problems, it is very important to eat a balanced diet. A healthy diet that includes foods from each food group can make up for some of the effects of steroid therapy.

LATE SIDE EFFECT	DESCRIPTION	WAYS TO MANAGE
Mouth Changes	• Radiation therapy to your head or neck and some chemotherapy drugs can cause late side effects in your mouth. • Problems may include dry mouth, cavities, or bone loss in the jaw.	**Visit your dentist** You may be asked to have your teeth checked every 1 to 2 months for at least 6 months after radiation treatment ends. During this time, your dentist will look for changes in your mouth, teeth, and jaw. **Exercise your jaw** Your doctor or nurse may suggest that you open and close your mouth 20 times as far as you can without causing pain, three times a day, even if your jaw isn't stiff. **Stimulate saliva** Your doctor or nurse may suggest that you drink 8 to 10 cups of liquid per day. Keep a water bottle handy so you can sip throughout the day. You may also find sucking on sugarless candy or chewing gum helpful. **Take good care of your teeth and gums** Floss and use a mouthwash with fluoride every day. Brush your teeth after meals and before you go to bed. Also, avoid mouthwashes that contain alcohol. **Explore your treatment options** Ask your dentist to contact your radiation oncologist before you have dental or gum surgery. There may be other treatment options besides surgery. Also, do not have teeth pulled from the part of your mouth that received radiation.
Second Primary Cancer	• Cancer treatment can sometimes cause a new cancer many years after you have finished treatment. • When a new primary cancer occurs in a person with a history of cancer, it is known as a second primary cancer. • Second primary cancers do not occur very often, but they can happen.	• Talk with your doctor about the types of second cancers you may be at risk for. • Have regular check-ups for the rest of your life to check for cancer—the one you were treated for and any new cancer that may occur. Your doctor can suggest tests you may need to look for a new cancer and how often you should have them. • Tell your doctor if you have any new symptoms or problems.

NIH (NCI)
https://www.cancer.gov/about- cancer/treatment/side-effects

Eating Hints: Before, during, and after Cancer Treatment
by the *National Cancer Institute*

Clear Liquids
This list may help if you have appetite loss, constipation, diarrhea, or vomiting.

Soups	• Bouillon • Clear, fat-free broth • Consommé
Drinks	• Clear apple juice • Clear carbonated beverages • Fruit-flavored drinks; Fruit punch • Sports drinks • Water • Weak, caffeine-free tea
Sweets	• Fruit ices made without fruit pieces or milk • Gelatin • Honey • Jelly • Popsicles
Meal replacements and supplements	• Clear nutrition supplements (such as Resource® Breeze) and Carnation® Instant Breakfast® Juice

Full-Liquid Foods
This list may help if you have appetite loss, vomiting, or weight loss.

Cereals	• Refined hot cereals (such as Cream of Wheat®, Cream of Rice®, instant oatmeal, and grits)	
Soups	• Breakfast® Juice • Bouillon • Broth • Soup that has been strained or put through a blender	
Drinks	• Carbonated drinks • Coffee • Fruit drinks • Fruit punch • Milk, Milkshakes	• Smoothies • Sports drinks • Tea • Tomato juice, Vegetable juice • Water
Desserts and snacks	• Custard (soft or baked) • Frozen yogurt • Fruit purees that are watered down • Gelatin • Honey • Ice cream with no chunks (such as nuts or cookie pieces)	• Jelly • Pudding • Sherbet • Sorbet • Syrup • Yogurt (plain or vanilla) • Ice milk
Meal replacements and supplements	• Instant breakfast drinks (such as Carnation® Instant Breakfast®) • Liquid meal replacements (such as Ensure® and Boost®) • Clear nutrition supplements (such as Resource® Breeze, Carnation® Instant Breakfast® Juice, and Ensure® Clear)	

Foods and Drinks that Are Easy on the Stomach	
This list may help if you have nausea or once your vomiting is under control.	
Soups	• Clear broth (such as chicken, vegetable, or beef) • All kinds (strain or puree, if needed), except those made with foods that cause gas, such as dried beans and peas, broccoli, or cabbage
Drinks	• Clear carbonated drinks that have lost their fizz • Cranberry or grape juice • Fruit-flavored drinks • Fruit punch • Milk • Sports drinks • Tea • Vegetable juices • Water
Main meals and snacks	• Avocado • Potatoes, without skins, boiled or baked • Beef, tender cuts only • Pretzels • Cheese, hard, mild types, such as American • Refined cold cereals, such as corn flakes, Rice Krispies®, Rice Chex®, and Corn Chex® • Cheese, soft or semi-soft, such as cottage cheese or cream cheese Refined hot cereals, such as Cream of Wheat® • Chicken or turkey, broiled or baked without skin • Saltine crackers • Eggs • Tortillas, white flour • Fish, poached or broiled • Vegetables, tender, well-cooked • Noodles • White bread • Pasta, plain • White rice • Peanut butter, creamy, and other nut butters • White toast
Desserts	• Angel food cake • Bananas • Canned fruit, such as applesauce, peaches, and pears • Custard • Frozen yogurt • Gelatin • Ice cream; Ice milk • Lemon drop candy • Popsicles • Pudding • Sherbet; Sorbet • Yogurt (plain or vanilla)
Meal replacements and supplements	• Instant breakfast drinks (such as Carnation® Instant Breakfast®) • Liquid meal replacements (such as Ensure®) • Clear nutrition supplements (such as Resource® Breeze, Carnation® Instant Breakfast® juice, and Ensure®Clear)

Low-Fiber Foods This list may help if you have diarrhea.	
Main meals	• Chicken or turkey (skinless and baked, broiled, or grilled) • Cooked refined cereals (such as Cream of Rice®, instant oatmeal, and grits) • Eggs • Fish • Noodles • Potatoes, without skins (boiled or baked) • White bread • White rice
Fruits and vegetables	• Carrots, cooked • Canned fruit, such as peaches, pears, and applesauce • Fruit juice • Mushrooms • String beans, cooked • Vegetable juice
Sweets and snacks	• Angel food cake • Animal crackers • Custard • Gelatin • Ginger snaps • Graham crackers • Saltine crackers • Sherbet • Sorbet • Vanilla wafers • Yogurt (plain or vanilla)
Fats	• Oil • Salad dressing (without seeds) • Butter • Mayonnaise

High-Fiber Foods	
This list may help if you have constipation or weight gain.	
Main meals	• Bran muffins • Bran or whole-grain cereals • Cooked dried or canned peas and beans, such as lentils or pinto, black, red, or kidney beans • Peanut butter and other nut butters • Soups with vegetables and beans, such as lentil and split pea • Whole-grain cereals, such as oatmeal and shredded wheat • Whole-wheat bread; Whole-wheat pasta
Fruits and vegetables	• Apples • Berries, such as blueberries, blackberries, and strawberries • Broccoli • Brussels sprouts • Cabbage • Corn • Dried fruit, such as apricots, dates, prunes, and raisins • Green leafy vegetables, such as spinach, lettuce, kale, and collard greens • Peas • Potatoes with skins • Spinach • Sweet potatoes; Yams
Snacks	• Bran snack bars • Granola • Nuts • Popcorn • Seeds, such as pumpkin or sunflower • Trail mix

High Protein Foods		
It is important to increase your protein to assist with energy and healing.		
Drinks	• Whole Milk • Milkshakes • Smoothies made with Milk or Yogurt	
Main Meals and Snacks	• Bean Burger • Beans and Peas • Beef, Chicken, Fish, Turkey • Cheese, including cottage and cream • Custard and Pudding • Eggs • Hummus (chickpea spread)	• Nuts, seeds, wheat germ • Peanut butter and other nut butters • Soups with beans, lentils or peas • Soups, such as chicken or cream • Sour Cream • Yogurt, including frozen
Meal Replacement and Protein Supplements If requiring *Soy Free*, please read ingredients	• Liquid Meal Replacement, such as Ensure®, Boost® or other protein drinks • Use "instant breakfast powder" in milk drinks and desserts • Protein Powders - Mix with ice cream, milk, and fruit flavoring for a high-protein milkshake or smoothie • Powdered Milk – Add to foods, such as milkshakes, smoothies, scrambled eggs	

Foods and Drinks that Are Easy to Chew and Swallow
This list may help if you have dry mouth, sore mouth, sore throat, or trouble swallowing.

Main meals	• Baby food • Casseroles • Chicken salad • Cooked refined cereals, such as Cream of Wheat®, Cream of Rice®, instant oatmeal, and grits • Cottage cheese • Eggs, soft boiled or scrambled • Egg salad • Macaroni and cheese • Mashed potatoes • Peanut butter, creamy • Pureed cooked foods • Soups • Stews • Tuna salad • Custard
Desserts and Snacks	• Flan • Fruit, pureed or baby food • Gelatin • Ice cream • Milkshakes • Puddings • Sherbet • Smoothies • Soft fruits, such as bananas or applesauce • Sorbet • Yogurt, plain or vanilla
Meal replacements and supplements	• Instant breakfast drinks, such as Carnation® Instant Breakfast® • Liquid meal replacements, such as Ensure® • Clear nutrition supplements, such as Resource® Breeze, Carnation® Instant Breakfast® juice, and Ensure® Clear

HOME EXERCISE GUIDE - TOC

Quick Summary this Section

Safety First
- Benefits / Before Starting a Routine
- Averages, Body Temperature
- Respiration, Blood Pressure, Heart Rate
- How to Monitor Intensity of Heart Rate
- Temperature – Heat and Cold
- Dehydration; Altitude

Components of a Conditioning Program
- Warm up/cool down
- Duration, Frequency, Intensity & Movement Patterns
- Breathing – Diaphragmatic, Pursed lip and with Exercise
- Equipment That May be Needed

Self-Tests:
- Prior to starting program

Exercise Worksheets:
- Exercises below with:
  - Exercise name and number for section
    - Reps, Sets, How many times a day and how long a stretch should be held (Ex. 20 seconds)

EXERCISE Flexibility (Stretching)	EXERCISE NUMBER	PAGE	REPS	SETS	X DAY	HOLD
PRAYER STRETCH and LATERAL	53					

Exercises:
- Myofascial release
- Flexibility / Stretches / ROM
- Core / Abdominal
- Strengthening - Upper and Lower Extremity
- Balance > Lower Extremity Standing Exercises
- Agility
- Endurance/Aerobic Capacity
- Calories
- Worksheet with room for notes under each section

EXERCISE Core / Stability / Balance	EXERCISE NUMBER	NOTES
PRONE BALL	27	

References

PHYSICAL AND PSYCHOLOGICAL BENEFITS OF KEEPING PHYSICALLY FIT

- Contributes positively to maintaining a healthy weight, building and maintaining healthy bone density, muscle strength, joint mobility, reducing surgical risks, and strengthening the immune system.
- Helps to prevent or treat serious and life-threatening chronic conditions such as high blood pressure, obesity, heart disease, Type 2 diabetes, insomnia, and depression.
- Endurance exercise before meals lowers blood glucose more than the same exercise after meals.
- It also improves mental health, helps prevent depression, helps to promote or maintain positive self-esteem, and can even augment an individual's sex appeal or body image.

(Physical Exercise - Wikipedia)

Before starting a routine here are some factors to consider

AGE	Men over 45 and women over 55 should have medical evaluation before starting a vigorous exercise program. If you will be participating in low to moderate exercise, it is suggested that those with, or have signs and symptoms of cardiopulmonary disease, set up a medical evaluation.
MEDICAL AND PHYSICAL CONDITION	It is very important for you to be aware of any medical or physical problems that may impede your performance. **If you have any of the following issues, please see a medical doctor and/or physical therapist to address issues before starting an exercise program:** - Cardiac issues - Pulmonary issues - Arthritis - Joint pain - Back pain - Diabetes - Acute or Chronic issues, such as, but not limited to, Parkinson's, Stroke, Autoimmune Diseases, Metabolic Disease or Orthopedic disorders/joint replacements.

VITAL SIGN AVERAGES

Adult (resting)	
Body Temperature	98.6 Fahrenheit under tongue.
Respiration	12-20 breaths per minute

Blood Pressure
 	
Systolic/Diastolic
	120/80.
	Systolic is when the heart pumps blood to the body / Diastolic is blood that remains in arteries when the heart relaxes.
	Pre-hypertension: 120-139/80-89.
	Hypertension:
	    Stage I 140-159/90-99
	    Stage II over 160/100

Resting pulse	**Men**: 70 beats per minute. **Women:** 75 beats per minute.

HOW to MONITOR EXERCISE INTENSITY

Ways to monitor heart rate (HR):

Talk Test Method	This is a simple, subjective method for the beginner to determine your comfort zone while exercising. Are you able to breathe and talk comfortably throughout the workout without gasping for air? If not, reduce your activity level, catch your breath, and resume at a slower pace.
Heart Rate monitor or Watch	This is a device you wear on your wrist or chest, which allows you to measure your heart rate in real time. These devices range in price at about $50.00 for just a basic HR monitor or higher with other bells and whistles. Some of the popular manufacturers are Fitbit, Apple Watch, Garmin and Samsung Galaxy among others. (See *Target Heart Rate*)
Rate of Perceived Exertion	This method was designed by Dr. Gunnar Borg and is often called the Borg Scale (revised). It rates what you feel your level of exertion is from a scale of 1-10, one being at rest and ten at maximal exertion. A rate of 5-7 is recommended, somewhere between somewhat hard and very hard. Like the talk test method, this is subjective and should be used with HR monitoring.
Training Heart Rate	Measuring Heart Rate: Place your first and second finger over the pulse site and gently apply pressure. Palpate the number of beats for a full minute or 30 sec x 2, 15 sec x 4 or 6 sec x 10. If you have in irregular heartbeat, it is suggested counting the full 60 seconds. Do not use the thumb, as this has its own pulse.
	Take your pulse after you've been exercising for at least five minutes. An easy way to check your pulse without interrupting your workout too much is to take a quick 6-second count and then multiply that number by 10 to get your heart rate in beats per minute (BPM). Make sure your pulse is within your target heart rate zone (*see below*). You can then increase or decrease your intensity based on your heart rate. You can also wear a heart rate monitor.

Radial: Wrist following line from base of thumb.	Carotid: Side of larynx.

Target heart rate range (THR)	**Beginner or low fitness level**: 50-60%
	Intermediate or average fitness level: 60-70%
	Advanced or high fitness level: 75-85%
Percent of maximal heart rate	220 - Age = predicted maximum heart rate (HR). To get the desired exercise intensity, multiply the predicted maximal HR by the percentage. For example, a woman who is 40 years old of Intermediate fitness level would use the following equation at a 70% target heart rate: 220 – 40 (age) =180 predicted maximal HR. 180 x 0.70 (THR) = 126 BPM - desired exercise HR.
Karvonen Formula	Percentage of Heart-rate reserve. This formula factors in the resting HR as well, which will make the target heart rate higher than just the percentage of maximal heart rate. To figure this out, take the predicted maximal heart rate as above with a resting HR prior to exercise. Maximal HR – resting heart rate (RHR) = heart rate reserve; multiply by intensity + RHR + Target HR. See example under Percentage of maximal HR. Rest heart rate = 80. 220 – 40 (age) =180 (as above) – 80 (RHR) = 100 x 0.70 (THR) = 70 + 80 = 150 Target HR.

TEMPERATURE – HEAT and COLD

HEAT

Avoid exercise in the hottest part of the day, as well as in humid weather. People need to sweat to regulate internal body temperature and must evaporate to dissipate heat. During hot, humid weather, sweat cannot evaporate, and therefore cannot cool the body down. It is also important to drink plenty of cool water during exercise, about 7-10 oz. every 10-20 minutes during exercise (see *Dehydration*).

Heat cramps:	• Severe cramps that begin in hands, feet or calves • Hard, tense muscles
Heat exhaustion: Requires immediate medical attention, although not usually life threatening	• Fatigue • Nausea • Headache • Excessive thirst • Muscle aches and cramps • Confusion or anxiety • Weakness • Severe sweats that can be accompanied by cold, clammy skin • Slow heartbeat (decreased pulse rate) • Dizziness or fainting • Agitation
Heat Stroke: Can occur suddenly, with or without warning from heat exhaustion. Obtain immediate medical attention, as this can be *fatal*	• Nausea and vomiting • Headache • Increased body temperature, but DECREASED sweating. • Hot, flushed, DRY skin • Dizziness • Fatigue • Rapid heart rate • Shortness of breath • Decreased urination or may have blood in the urine. • Confusion or loss of consciousness • Convulsions

COLD

It is just as important to drink plenty of water when exercising in the cold weather secondary to increased urine production.　Be sure to dress in layers to help self-regulate body temperature.　This simply involves taking off or putting back on clothing as dictated by the changing weather conditions. Choose clothing that will keep moisture out and away from the skin, such as Gortex® brand. Clothing that stays wet because of sweat will decrease your body temperature.

Hypothermia-Mild: A body temperature that is below normal. People with hypothermia are usually not aware of their condition due to confusion or being overly focused on their current activity. Hypothermia may or may not include shivering in the early stages	• Confusion • Lack of coordination • Fatigue • Nausea or vomiting • Dizziness
Hypothermia	• Shivering • Slurred speech • Mumbling • Clumsiness • Difficulty speaking • Stumbling • Poor decision making • Drowsiness • Weak pulse • Shallow breathing • Progressive loss of consciousness

DEHYDRATION

Excessive loss of body fluid (which can include water and solutes, usually sodium or electrolytes). It is also important to drink plenty of cool water during exercise, about 7-10 oz. every 10-20 minutes during exercise. During exercise, sports drinks may be necessary to keep an electrolyte balance as well.

Dehydration-Mild: About 2% of water depletion	• Thirst • Decreased urine volume • Abnormally dark urine • Unexplained tiredness • Irritability • Lack of tears when crying • Headache • Dry mouth • Dizziness when standing due to orthostatic hypotension • May cause insomnia.
Moderate: About 5% -6% of water depletion	• Grogginess or sleepiness • Headache • Nausea • May feel tingling in limbs (parenthesis)
Severe: About 10% -15% of water depletion	• Muscles may become spastic • Skin may shrivel and wrinkle (decreased skin turgor) • Vision may dim • Urination will be greatly reduced and may become painful • Delirium may begin.
Over 15% of water depletion	• Usually, fatal.

COMPONENTS OF A CONDITIONING PROGRAM

WARM UP and COOL DOWN

Warming up and cooling down are very important parts of the exercise routine. There are physical and psychological benefits to both these components that can be as simple as a slow walk before and after your exercise program.

Benefits of warming up	Benefits of cooling down
<ul><li>Increases the temperature in the muscles, which increases the speed of contraction and relaxation.</li><li>Reduces premature lactic acid build up and fatigue during high level exercises.</li><li>Increases speed of nerve impulse conduction.</li><li>Increases elasticity of connective tissues</li><li>Increases muscle metabolism and oxygen consumption that enhances aerobic performance.</li><li>Alert for potential muscle injury that may arise during higher intensities.</li><li>Increases endorphins.</li><li>Allows the heart rate to get to a workable rate for beginning exercise.</li><li>Increases production of synovial fluid located between the joints to reduce friction.</li><li>Psychological warm up to mentally focus on training and competition.</li></ul>	<ul><li>Prevents venous blood pooling at the extremities, which reduces chance of dizziness or fainting.</li><li>Reduces the potential for Delayed Onset Muscle Soreness (DOMS).</li><li>Aids in removing waste products in muscles, such as lactic acid.</li><li>Reduces the level of adrenaline and other exercise hormones in the blood to lower the chance of post-exercise disturbances in cardiac rhythm.</li><li>Allows the heart to return back safely to resting rate.</li></ul>

Start out every routine with a warmup first. Here are some suggestions

- Walking or outside
- Running up and down some stairs
- Jumping jacks
- Running in place
- Dynamic stretching

Equipment

- Treadmill
- Stationary or Recumbent bike
- Stair climber or Elliptical
- Mini trampoline

Duration, Frequency, Intensity and Movement Patterns

Intensity: How *much* mental and physical *effort* it takes to sustain an activity.	This can be done using the target heart rate range THR (optimum exercise intensity levels through beats per minute, talk test or rate of perceived exertion.
Duration: How *long* the training lasts.	The higher the intensity, the shorter the duration. The American College of Sports Medicine guidelines recommends all healthy adults aged 18–65 yr should participate in moderate intensity aerobic physical activity for a minimum of 30 min on five days per week, or vigorous intensity aerobic activity for a minimum of 20 min on three days per week.
Frequency: How *often* the training occurs.	Training should be performed at least every other day or three days a week. Cardiac/aerobic conditioning can be done daily, although you may want to vary exercises. Regarding strength training, it is important to give each muscle group 48 hours to recover. Alternate upper and lower body with isolated abdomen/core exercises every other day. For those working out several days a week, find a schedule that works for you as long as you give each muscle group 48 hours of recovery time.
Movement Patterns and Examples Basic movements that help to increase overall body strengthening	<ul><li>Bend and Lift: Squats, Dead Lifts and Leg presses<ul><li>Picking up item off floor</li></ul></li><li>Single Leg: Step ups, Single leg stance, Lunges<ul><li>Walking up steps</li></ul></li><li>Push: Shoulder press, Bench press, Push up<ul><li>Pushing Shopping cart or Lawn mower</li></ul></li><li>Pull: Lat pull downs, Seated rows<ul><li>Vacuuming, Raking</li></ul></li><li>Rotational<ul><li>Shoveling snow</li></ul></li></ul>

Diaphragmatic Breathing

- Lie either on your back with your knees bent or sit up
- Inhale through your nose; as you do so, allow your stomach to rise. Limit movement in your chest. Attempt to push your bottom ribs out to the side as you breathe in.
- Exhale through your mouth; as you do so, allow your stomach to fall. Limit movement in your chest.
- Repeat for at least 10 cycles.

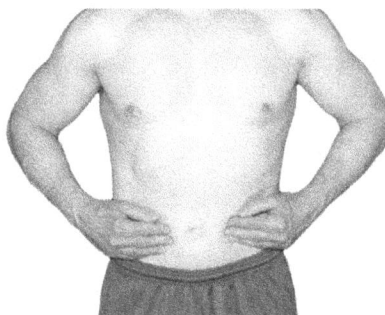

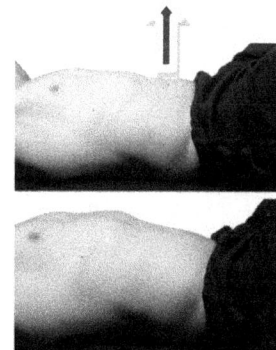

Pursed Lip Breathing

(PLB) is a breathing technique that consists of inhaling through the nose with the mouth closed and then exhaling through tightly pressed (pursed) lips. This technique is frequently in those with cardiac or respiratory issues.   *"Smell the Roses then Blow Out the Candle".*

Breathing with Exercise

Exhale on the exertion. For example, exhale when you are lying on your back and pushing a weight up or when bending your arm doing a bicep curl,. Inhale as you bring the weight slowly to your chest or when you straighten your arm with a bicep curl..

ANATOMY

ANATOMICAL POSITIONS and PLANES

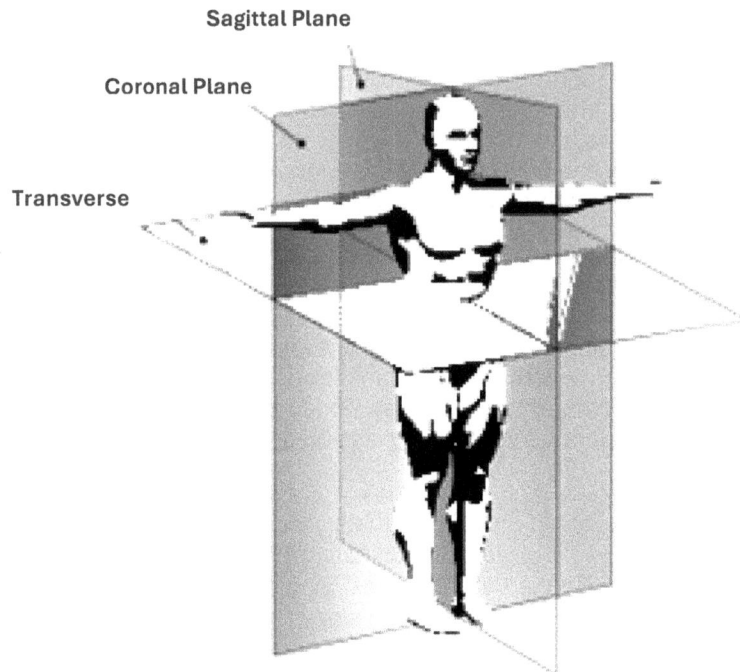

Anterior – Towards the front of the body.

Posterior – Towards the back of the body.

Distal – Away from the body or any point of reference, or from the point of attachment or origin.

Proximal – Closer to the body or any point of reference, or to the point of attachment or origin.

Medial – Situated towards the midline of the body.

Lateral – Position farther from the midline of the body.

Inferior – Away from the head or lower surface of a structure.

Superior – Towards the head or situated above.

Transverse /Axial / Horizontal plane is parallel to the ground, which separates the superior from the inferior or the head from the feet.

Coronal / Frontal/Frontal plane is perpendicular to the ground, which separates the anterior from the posterior or the front from the back

Sagittal / Lateral plane is a Y-Z plane, perpendicular to the ground, which separates left from right.

Upper Extremity (UE): Shoulders, Chest, Arms, Hands, etc

Lower Extremity (LE): Hips, Legs, Ankle Foot , etc

ANATOMICAL DIRECTIONS

Range of Motion (ROM): The distance and direction a joint can move between the flexed and extended position (*see flexion and extension below*). This can also be the act of attempting to increase the distance through therapeutic exercise and/or stretching for physiological gain.

Flexion - Bending movement that decreases the angle between two parts. Bending the knee or elbow are examples of flexion. Flexion of the hip or shoulder moves the limb forward (towards the front of the body).

Extension - The opposite of flexion; a straightening movement that increases the angle between body parts. The knees are extended when standing up. When straightening the arm, the elbow is extended. Extension of the hip or shoulder moves the limb backward (towards the back of the body).

Hyperextension – Extending the joint beyond extension.

Abduction - A lateral movement that pulls a structure or part away from the midline of the body. Raising the arms to the sides is an example of abduction.

Adduction - A medial movement that pulls a structure or part towards the midline of the body, or towards the midline of a limb. Dropping the arms to the sides, or bringing the knees together, are examples of adduction.

Internal rotation (or *medial rotation*). Inward rotary movement around the axis of the bone. Internal rotation of the shoulder or hip would point the toes or the flexed forearm inwards (towards the midline).

External rotation (or *lateral rotation*). External rotary movement around the axis of the bone. It would turn the toes or the flexed forearm outwards (away from the midline).

Elevation - Movement in a superior direction. Shrugging or bringing the shoulders up is an example of elevation.

Depression - Movement in an inferior direction, the opposite of elevation. Pushing the shoulders down is an example of depression.

Pronation - Internal rotation the hand or foot to face downward or posterior. Pronating the foot is a combination of eversion and abduction.

Supination - External rotation of the hand or foot to face upward or anterior. Raising the inside or medial margin of the foot.

Dorsiflexion – Movement at the ankle of the foot superiorly towards the shin. The up position of tapping the foot.

Plantarflexion – Movement at the ankle of the foot inferiorly away from the shin. Pointing the foot downward.

Eversion – Moving the sole of the foot away from the median plane or outward.

Inversion - Moving the sole of the foot towards the median plane or inward.

Ipsilateral – Same side of the body

Contralateral – Opposite side of the body

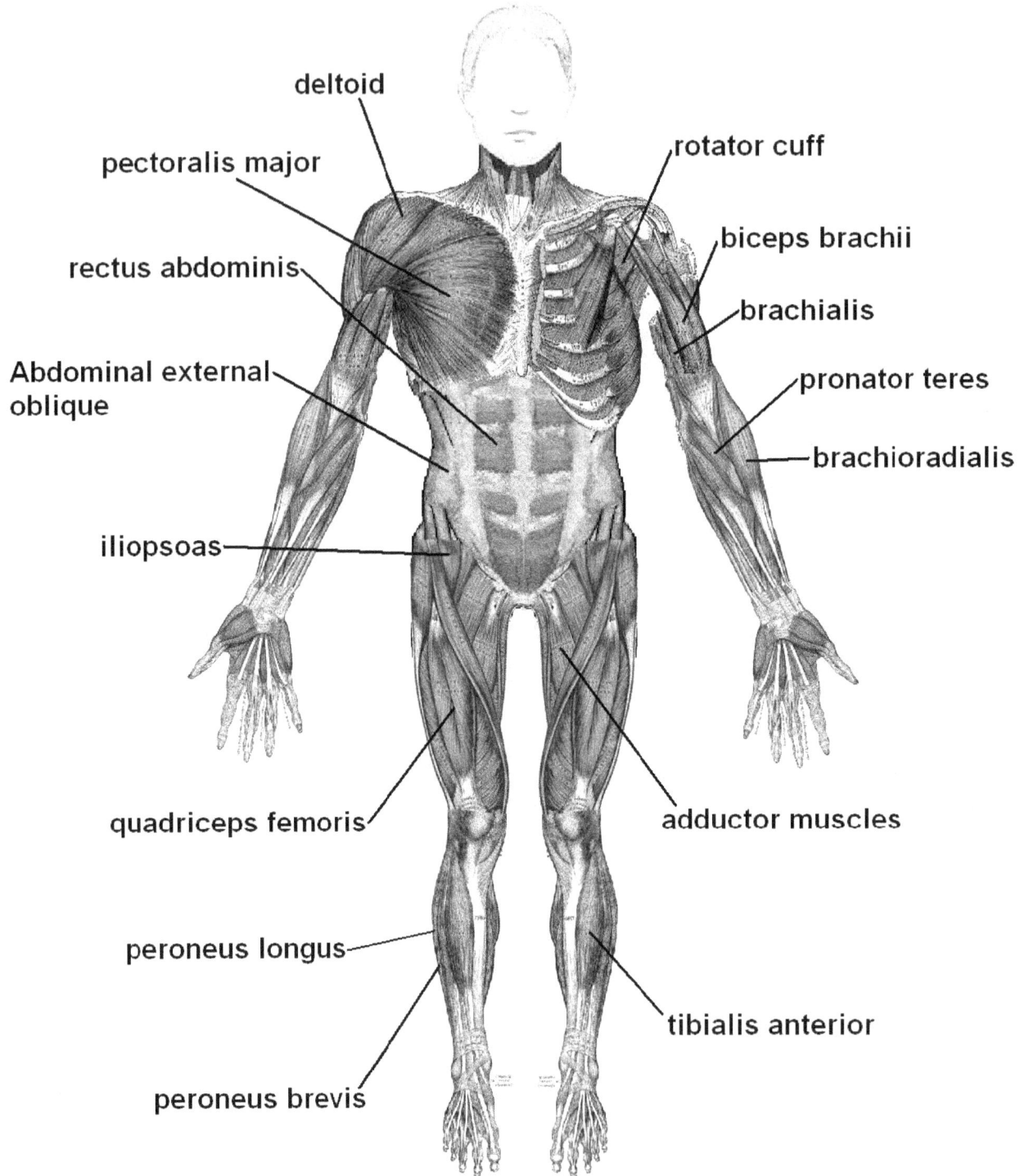

MUSCLES

Grey's Anatomy

ANTERIOR

deltoid

pectoralis major

rectus abdominis

Abdominal external oblique

iliopsoas

quadriceps femoris

peroneus longus

peroneus brevis

rotator cuff

biceps brachii

brachialis

pronator teres

brachioradialis

adductor muscles

tibialis anterior

Muscle Name (AKA)	Joint Action
Pectoralis major	Shoulder flexion, adduction, internal rotation
Deltoid (anterior)	Shoulder abduction, flexion, internal rotation
Rotator cuff (SITS) Supraspinatus Infraspinatus Teres minor Subscapularis	Shoulder: Supraspinatus: Abduction Infraspinatus: External rotation Teres minor: External rotation Subscapularis: Internal rotation
Biceps brachii	Elbow flexion; Forearm supination
Brachialis	Elbow flexion
Pronator teres	Elbow flexion; Forearm pronation
Brachioradialis	Elbow flexion
Tensor fasciae latae	Hip flexion, medial rotation & abduction
Gracilis*	Hip adduction & internal rotation;Knee flexion & internal rotation
Adductor muscles Adductor magnus, longus & brevis	Hip adduction
Tibialis anterior	Ankle dorsiflexion; foot inversion
Peroneus brevis	Ankle plantarflexion; Foot eversion
Peroneus longus	Ankle plantarflexion; Foot eversion
Rectus femoris (quadriceps femoris)	Hip extension (esp. when knee is extended); Knee flexion
Vastus medialis	Knee extension (esp. when hip is flexed)
Vastus lateralis	Knee extension (esp. when hip is flexed)
Sartorius	Hip flexion & external rotation; Knee flexion & internal rotation
Pectineus	Hip adduction
Iliopsoas, Psosas, Iliacus	Hip flexion & external rotation
Abdominal external oblique	Trunk lateral flexion
Rectus abdominis	Trunk flexion & lateral flexion
Abdominal internal oblique	Trunk lateral flexion

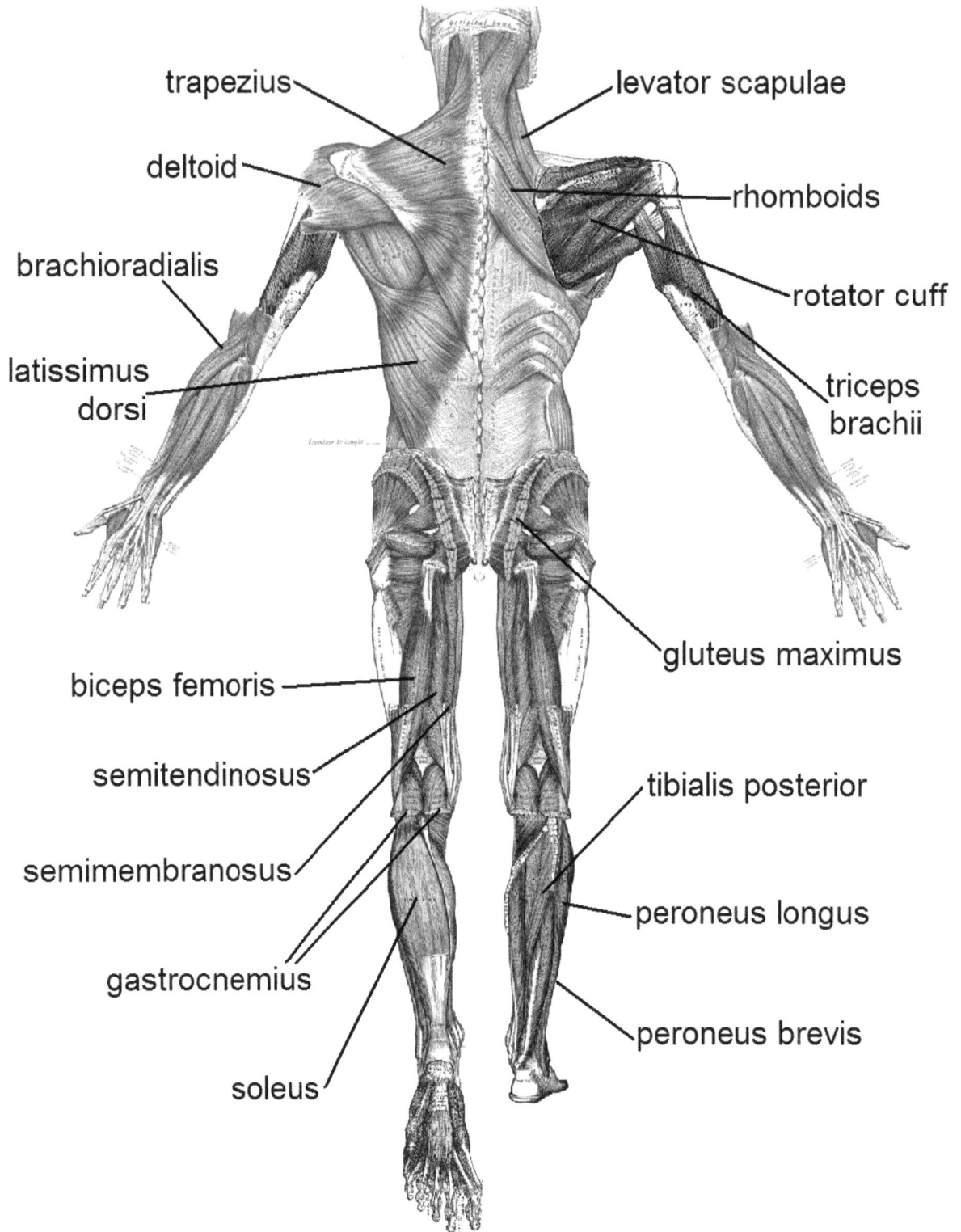

MUSCLES

Grey's Anatomy

POSTERIOR

trapezius

levator scapulae

deltoid

rhomboids

brachioradialis

rotator cuff

latissimus dorsi

triceps brachii

gluteus maximus

biceps femoris

semitendinosus

tibialis posterior

semimembranosus

peroneus longus

gastrocnemius

peroneus brevis

soleus

Muscle Name (AKA)	Joint Action
Deltoid (posterior)	Shoulder abduction, extension, external rotation
Trapezius	Scapula or Shoulder girdle:, Upper traps: Scapula elevation. Middle traps: Scapula adduction. Lower traps: Scapula depression
Levator scapulae	Scapula elevation
Rhomboids	Scapula adduction & elevation
Triceps brachii	Elbow extension
Gluteus medius	Hip abduction
Gluteus maximus	Hip extension & external rotation
Tibialis, posterior	Inversion, stabilization, assists with plantarflexion
Soleus	Ankle plantarflexion
Gastrocnemius	Knee flexion; Ankle plantarflexion
Semimembranosus	Hip extension & internal rotation; Knee flexion & internal rotation
Semitendinosus	Hip extension & internal rotation; Knee flexion & internal rotation
Biceps femoris (long head)	Hip extension & internal rotation; Knee flexion & external rotation
Latissimus dorsi	Shoulder extension, adduction, internal rotation
Erector spinae, Longissimus, Spinalis, Iliocostalis	Trunk extension, hyperextension & lateral flexion Deep muscle that originate in the posterior iliac crest & sacrum running up the spine and inserts in the transverse process of ribs
Pes anserine, Gracilis, Sartorius, Semimembranosus, Semitendinosus	Internal rotation of tibia when knee is flexed

SKELETON

ANTERIOR (FRONT)

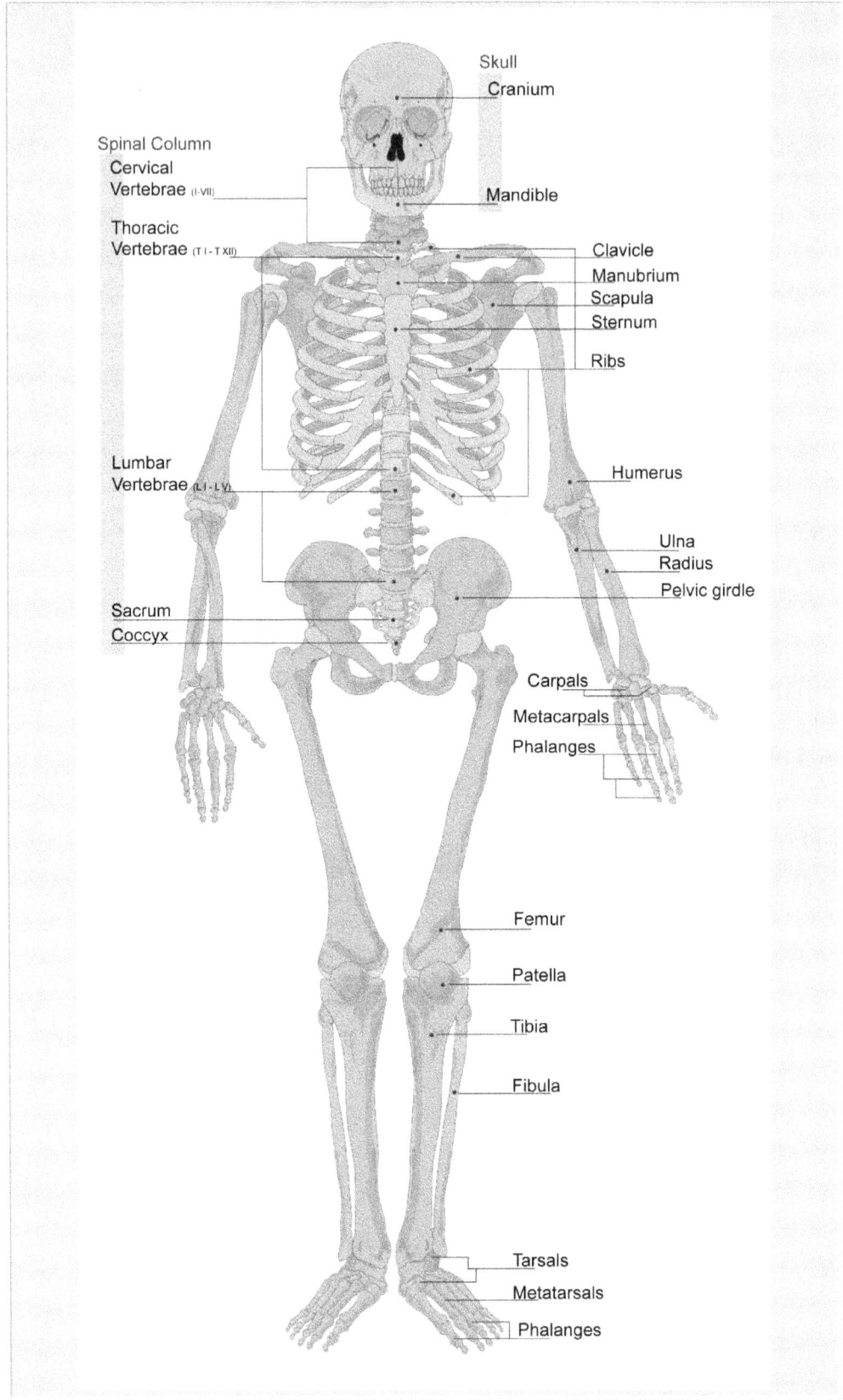

Skull
Cranium

Spinal Column
Cervical
Vertebrae (I-VII)

Mandible

Thoracic
Vertebrae (T I - T XII)

Clavicle
Manubrium
Scapula
Sternum

Ribs

Lumbar
Vertebrae (L I - L V)

Humerus

Ulna
Radius

Pelvic girdle

Sacrum
Coccyx

Carpals

Metacarpals

Phalanges

Femur

Patella

Tibia

Fibula

Tarsals

Metatarsals

Phalanges

SKELETON

POSTERIOR (BACK)

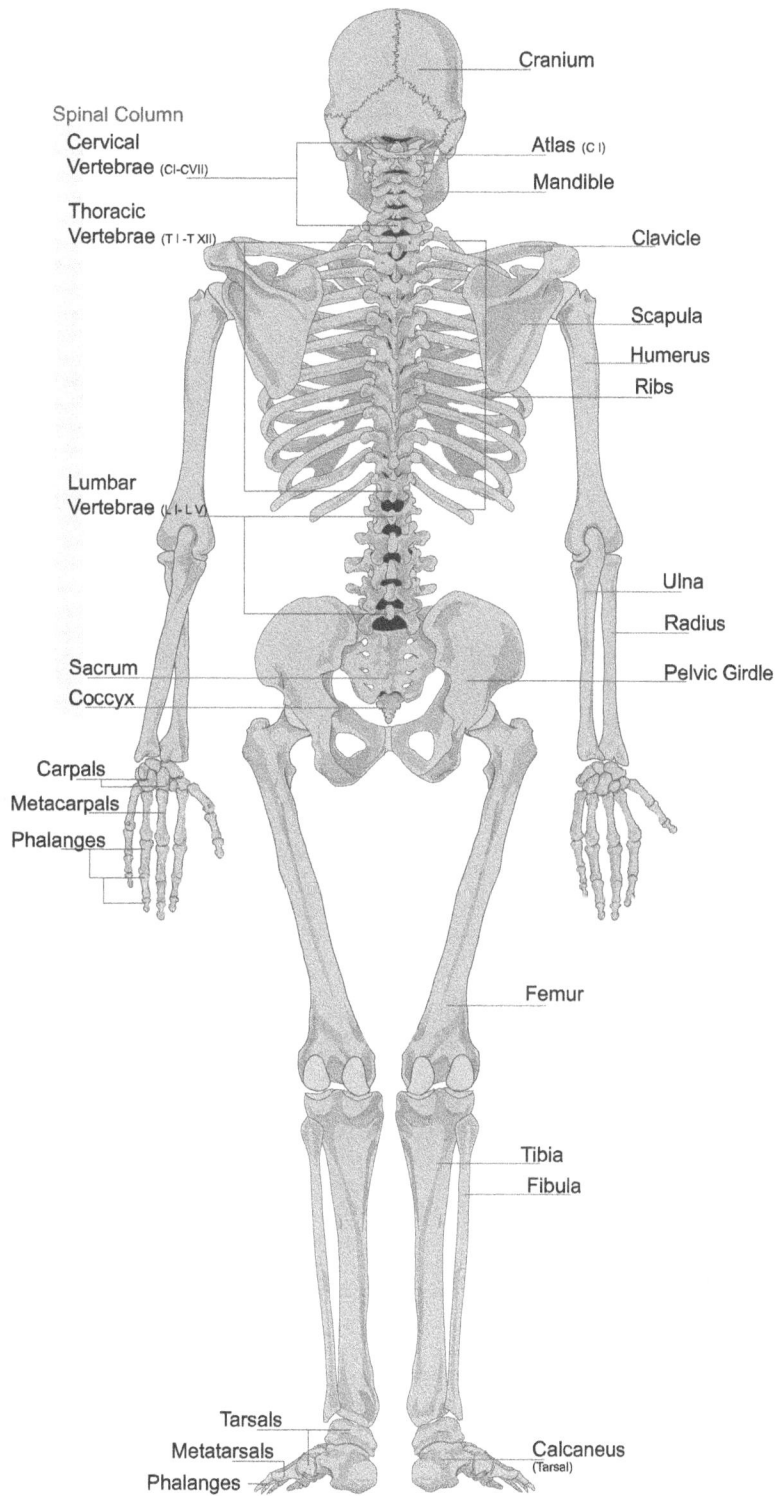

Cranium

Spinal Column

Cervical
Vertebrae (CI-CVII)

Thoracic
Vertebrae (T I -T XII)

Atlas (C I)

Mandible

Clavicle

Scapula

Humerus

Ribs

Lumbar
Vertebrae (LI-LV)

Ulna

Radius

Sacrum

Coccyx

Pelvic Girdle

Carpals

Metacarpals

Phalanges

Femur

Tibia

Fibula

Tarsals

Metatarsals

Phalanges

Calcaneus
(Tarsal)

Average Joint Range of Motion

Anatomical Positions – Upper Extremity

Joint UPPER EXTREMITY	Movement	Normal Range of Motion (degrees)	Plane
Elbow	Flexion	150	Sagittal
	Extension	0 (neutral)	Sagittal
	Hyperextension	< 10	Sagittal
Shoulder	Flexion	180	Sagittal
	Extension	0 (neutral)	Sagittal
	Hyperextension	60	Sagittal
	Adduction (Add)	0 (neutral)	Frontal
	Abduction (Abd)	180	Frontal
	Horizontal Add/Flexion	130	Transverse
	Horizontal Abd	0 (to neutral)	Transverse
	Horizontal Extension	45	Transverse
	Internal rotation	70	Sagittal
	External rotation	90	Sagittal
Radioulnar	Pronation	90	Transverse
	Supination	90	Transverse

Average Joint Range of Motion

Anatomical Positions – Lower Extremity

Joint LOWER EXTREMITY	Movement	Normal Range of Motion (degrees)	Plane
Knee	Flexion	135	Sagittal
	Extension	0 (neutral)	Sagittal
	Hyperextension	10	Sagittal
Hip	Flexion	120	Sagittal
	Extension	0 (neutral)	Sagittal
	Hyperextension	< 20	Sagittal
	Adduction (Add)	0 (neutral)	Frontal
	Abduction (Abd)	50	Frontal
	Internal rotation	40	Transverse
	External rotation	50	Transverse
Ankle	Dorsiflexion	20	Sagittal
	Plantarflexion	50	Sagittal

EQUIPMENT used in this Book.

Don't buy a lot of equipment before knowing what your goals are.

Stability / Exercise Ball Bosu

These can replace an exercise bench if you do not have the space. It is also used for many of the core strengthening exercises

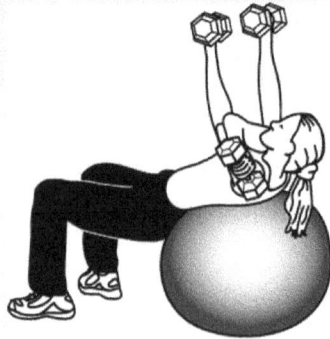

Should be inflated so that when you sit on it you are at a 90-degree angle.

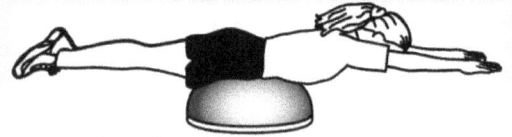

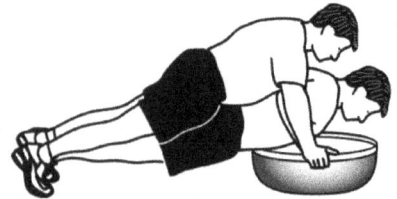

Dumbbells

Kettle Bell
(optional)

Dowel with/without weight

These will be needed for your strength exercises. See *Strengthening* section on for resistance.

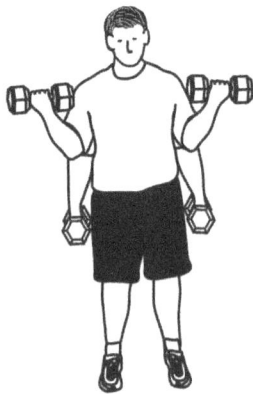

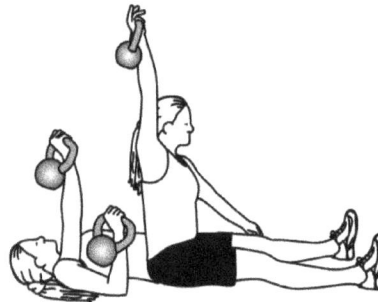

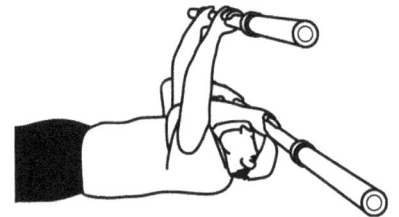

Resistance bands

In different weights/ resistance.

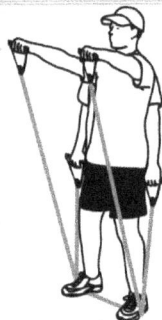

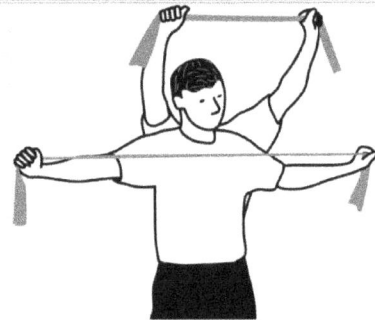

Agility Equipment

Cone hurdles, Speed hurdles, Agility ladder/rings/pole s, Bosu, Stair step, Jump rope.

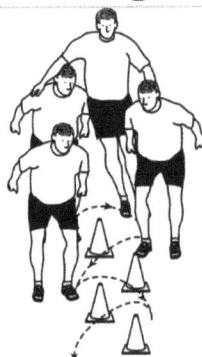

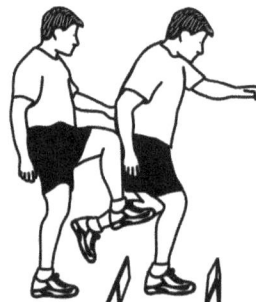

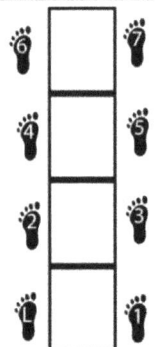

Balance Equipment

Can include **Foam rollers** *(also see Myofascial below)*

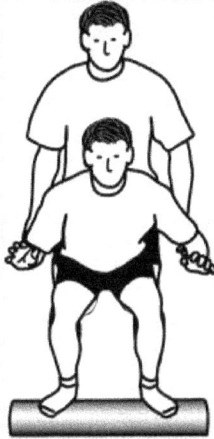

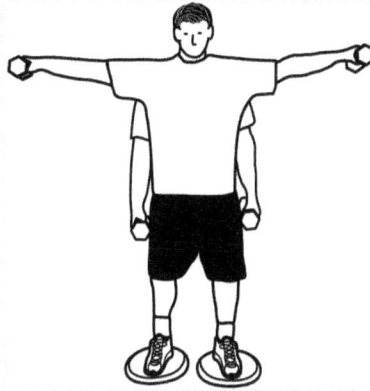

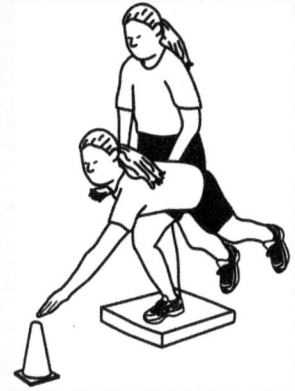

Balance discs
Balance pad
Cones
Stepper
Bosu

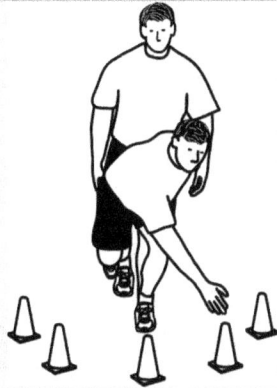

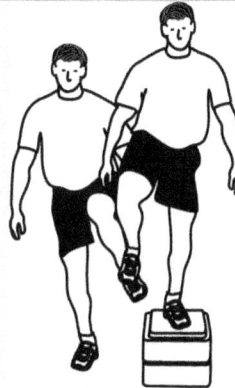

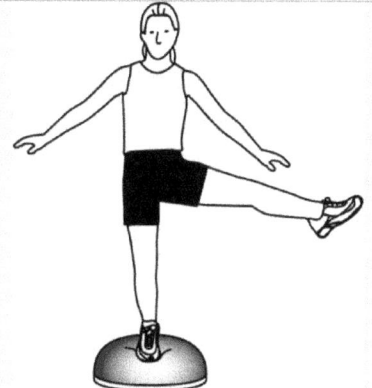

Exercise Bench (Optional)

The type really depends on what you will use it for. You can get a plain bench just for support (as above you can use a stability ball) or you can get all the bells and whistles. Some have pieces for leg extensions and curls, as well as arm pieces for butterflies. If you do not already have one, I suggest waiting until you start your exercise program and see what you feel you will need to advance.

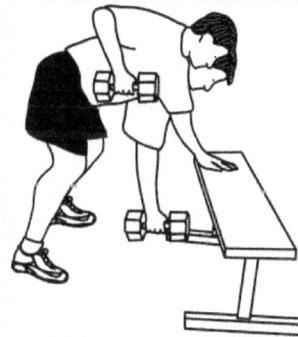

Examples For Myofascial

Massage Ball

Foam/Textured Rollers (also see balance)

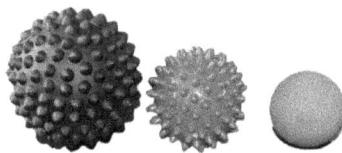

Full Rollers

Half Roller with Flat Bottom

Not Shown

- **Exercise mat for floor exercises**
- **Ankle Weights**
- **Bed, couch or high table/mat**
- **Chair with/without arms - High or Low**

- **10-inch play ball**
- **Pillow**
- **Towel roll**
- **Strap for stretches**

SELF TESTS

Before starting the exercise program, it is a good idea to see where your baseline is. Taking the following tests will help guide you in the level you will need to start, and help progress by retaking the test periodically. *It is suggested to get a partner to help with both timing and safety, especially with balance tests.* The first 6 tests are modified versions starting at age 60 but are great for adults of any age. Tests 7-10 will help determine how quickly you can advance your balance program.

As with the exercises in this book, these tests should also be performed by those that are otherwise healthy with no chronic or acute ailments OR with supervision of a qualified health coach/personal trainer/physical therapist.

Tests 1-6 should be conducted in the following order if you are doing them at the same time.

A general warm up should be done prior to tests (*see Warm up/Cool down*).

- Stop immediately if any adverse reactions, such as nausea, dizziness, blurred vision, pain of any kind, chest pain, confusion or loss of muscle control.
- Stay hydrated, and do not proceed with testing on days with high temperature/humidity or any other conditions where you would not normally exercise.
- Practice each test several times before attempting to get an accurate score.
- It is advised that you have a second person to time the tests and make sure you are following proper form. Make sure your partner also understands the precautions and goals of these tests.

1. 30 second chair stand - Lower body strength
    - Needed for stair climbing, walking getting up out of tub/chair/car and reduce the risk of falls
2. 30 second arm curl test – Upper body strength
    - Needed to lift and carry everyday items, such as groceries and toolbox
3. 2-minute step test – Aerobic endurance
    - Needed for activities that require endurance, such as walking distance, grocery shopping and climbing stairs
4. Chair sit and reach – Lower body flexibility
    - Needed for normal gait patterns, correct posture, getting in/out of car/tub
5. Back stretch test – Shoulder flexibility
    - Needed to do various activities, such as combing hair and putting on overhead garments
6. 8 foot get up and go – Agility and dynamic balance
    - Needed for pretty much anything you do that requires getting up and walking, such as go to kitchen, bathroom or answering phone.
7. Narrow stance – Balance progression
8. Staggered stance – Balance progression
9. Tandem stance – Balance progression
10. One leg standing – Balance progression

TEST AND PURPOSE	PICTURE	EQUIPMENT NEEDED	EXPLANATION	RESULTS
30 Second Chair Stand Assess lower body strength *May not want to perform if any chronic pain or back issues. *If you are tall and have had a recent hip replacement skip this or use taller chair.		Straight back or folding chair (~17 inch height) against wall. Stopwatch, wrist watch or clock within view with second hand	*Sit with feet flat on the floor and arms crossed over the chest. *Get up to a full stand and then sit back down. ** Start the time – Immediately repeat as many *full stands* as you can in 30 seconds. *If you cannot stand with hands over chest, try pushing off on your thighs or get a chair with arms and push off arms. If using assist, make sure you note this for progression.*	**Normal Range repetitions** *Age* / *Men* / *Women* 60-64 / 14-19 / 12-17 65-69 / 12-18 / 11-16 70-74 / 12-17 / 10-15 75-79 / 11-17 / 10-15 80-84 / 10-15 / 9-14 85-89 / 8-14 / 8-13 90-94 / 7-12 / 4-11

Normal Range repetitions (30 Second Chair Stand):

Age	Men	Women
60-64	14-19	12-17
65-69	12-18	11-16
70-74	12-17	10-15
75-79	11-17	10-15
80-84	10-15	9-14
85-89	8-14	8-13
90-94	7-12	4-11

TEST AND PURPOSE	PICTURE	EQUIPMENT NEEDED	EXPLANATION	RESULTS
30 Second Arm Curl Test Upper body strength		Straight back or folding chair without arms. Can be done in standing. Stopwatch or clock within view with second hand Women: 5 lb dumbbell Men: 8 lb dumbbell Can use a wrist weight if arthritis and cannot hold a dumbbell	*Sit with feet flat on the floor towards the edge seat towards dominant side. **Start with the arm extended by your side holding dumbbell in the dominant hand. *Bend elbow with palm facing you keeping the upper arm next to the body (elbow pressed into your side). *Return to starting position. *Keep the wrist straight – do not flex or extend the wrist. **Start the time – Immediately repeat as many arm curls as you can in 30 seconds *with proper form.* *If you cannot hold the suggested weight with proper form, use a lighter weight. Make sure you note this for progression.*	**Normal Range repetitions**

Normal Range repetitions (30 Second Arm Curl Test):

Age	Men	Women
60-64	16-22	13-19
65-69	15-21	12-18
70-74	14-21	12-17
75-79	13-19	11-17
80-84	13-19	10-16
85-89	11-17	10-15
90-94	10-14	8-13

TEST AND PURPOSE	PICTURE	EQUIPMENT NEEDED	EXPLANATION	RESULTS
2 Minute Step Test Aerobic endurance		Wall for support and to mark step height. Sturdy chair to hold on opposite side if unsteady. Stopwatch or clock within view with second hand	*For accuracy, may need a second person to judge step height and count. *Step with side next to wall. Bring knee up mid-thigh between the knee and the hip. Mark the wall with tape at this height. This will be your minimum step height. *Practice marching in place to this step height. **Start the time – Immediately start marching (not jogging) for 2 minutes. Count the number of *full steps* (both legs) that come up to step height. Every time the right knee reaches proper step height; this is counted as one step. *If shortness of breath, extreme fatigue or unable to continue to step height, stop test and this is your baseline. * If unable to get to step height, but able to complete 2 minutes. Make sure you note this for progression. *If unsteady, hold onto chair on opposite side for support.	**Normal Range steps** See table below.

Normal Range steps

Age	Men	Women
60-64	87-115	75-107
65-69	86-116	73-107
70-74	80-110	68-101
75-79	73-109	68-100
80-84	71-103	60-90
85-89	59-91	55-85
90-94	52-86	44-72

TEST AND PURPOSE	PICTURE	EQUIPMENT NEEDED	EXPLANATION	RESULTS
Chair Sit And Reach Lower body flexibility, *primarily hamstrings* *Do not do if recent hip replacement or severe osteoporosis. *Stretch to discomfort, not pain.		Chair (~17 inch height). Make sure chair is secure and does not tip forward. 18 inch ruler or yardstick	*Sit on the edge chair – you should feel the middle of the thigh at the edge of the chair. *Bend one leg with foot flat on floor. *Straighten the target leg in front with heel on the floor and foot flexed up. *Reach forward with one hand over the other and middle fingers even. *Exhale as you bend forward at the hips and reach forward towards or past the toes. Keep the extended knee straight and adjust if it bends. *Practice a few times on both legs to see which one you would prefer for testing. Do two tests and measure as below. **Measure tips of middle fingers to the tip of the shoe (closest to ½ inch). ***The midpoint at the toe of the shoe is considered zero (0), and is scored as such if you reach this point. ***If the reach is short, score this as a minus (-) ***If the reach is past this point, score this as a plus (+)	**Normal Range inches** <table><tr><td>Age</td><td>Men</td><td>Women</td></tr><tr><td>60-64</td><td>-2.5 +4.0</td><td>-0.5 + 5.0</td></tr><tr><td>65-69</td><td>-3.0 +3.0</td><td>-0.5 + 4.5</td></tr><tr><td>70-74</td><td>-3.0 +3.0</td><td>-1.0 + 4.0</td></tr><tr><td>75-79</td><td>-4.0 +2.0</td><td>-1.5 + 3.5</td></tr><tr><td>80-84</td><td>-5.5 +1.5</td><td>2.0 + 3.0</td></tr><tr><td>85-89</td><td>-5.5 +0.5</td><td>-2.5 + 2.5</td></tr><tr><td>90-94</td><td>-6.5 -0.5</td><td>-4.5 + 1.0</td></tr></table>

TEST AND PURPOSE	PICTURE	EQUIPMENT NEEDED	EXPLANATION	RESULTS
Back Stretch Test Shoulder flexibility *Do not do if any upper back, shoulder or neck injuries		18-inch ruler or yardstick	*Will need second person to measure. *Stand and place the target arm over the same shoulder, palm down with fingers extended. Reach down the middle of the back. *Place the opposite arm around the back, palm up reaching up the middle of the back towards other hand. Try to touch middle fingers together or overlap if possible. *Do not overlap fingers and pull.* *Practice a few times on both arms to see which one you would prefer for testing. Do two tests and measure as below. **Measure the distance between tips of middle fingers or overlap. ***If the middle fingers do not touch, score this as a minus (-) ***If the middle fingers just touch, score this as a zero (0) ***If the middle fingers overlap, score this as a plus (+)	**Normal Range inches** <table><tr><td>Age</td><td>Men</td><td>Women</td></tr><tr><td>60-64</td><td>-6.5 +0.0</td><td>-3.0 + 1.5</td></tr><tr><td>65-69</td><td>-7.5 -1.0</td><td>-3.5 + 1.5</td></tr><tr><td>70-74</td><td>-8.0 -1.0</td><td>-4.0 + 1.0</td></tr><tr><td>75-79</td><td>-9.0 -2.0</td><td>-5.0 + 0.5</td></tr><tr><td>80-84</td><td>-9.5 -2.0</td><td>-5.5 + 0.0</td></tr><tr><td>85-89</td><td>-9.5 -3.0</td><td>-7.0 -1.0</td></tr><tr><td>90-94</td><td>-10.5 -4.0</td><td>-8.0 -1.0</td></tr></table>

TEST AND PURPOSE	PICTURE	EQUIPMENT NEEDED	EXPLANATION	RESULTS		
8 Foot Get Up And Go Agility and dynamic balance *If unsteady, have someone by your side in case you lose your balance.	 8 feet →	Chair against wall (~17-inch height) Cone or another marker to walk around Stopwatch or clock within view with second hand *Put chair against wall and cone 8 feet in front. Measure from front of chair to back of cone (side facing chair).	*This is done better with a partner watching the clock or a stopwatch. *Sit on chair, back straight, feet flat on floor, one foot slightly in front, torso leaning slightly forward and hands resting on thighs. **Start the time – Immediately get up and walk around the cone (either side) and return to chair. Stopwatch immediately when seated. **Try 2-3x and record the fastest time within 10th /second. *Can use a cane or walker or start from standing position. Make sure you note this for progression.	**Normal Range seconds**		
				Age	Men	Women
				60-64	5.6-3.8	6.0-4.4
				65-69	5.9-4.3	6.4-4.8
				70-74	6.2-4.4	7.1-4.9
				75-79	7.2-4.6	7.4-5.2
				80-84	7.6-5.2	8.7-5.7
				85-89	8.9-5.5	9.6-6.2
				90-94	10.0-6.2	11.5-7.3

TEST AND PURPOSE	PICTURE	EQUIPMENT NEEDED	EXPLANATION	RESULTS
Narrow Stance Balance progression		Wall, counter or chair within arm's reach for support if needed Stopwatch or clock within view with second hand	Keep your feet together and stand for up to one minute. *Time stops if loss of balance with need to hold on to support.	One minute: Normal *Progress to Staggered Stance Test* *Less than 30 seconds: Continue balance program with wider stance and progress to narrow stance using support. *(See Balance)*
Staggered Stance Balance progression		Wall, counter or chair within arm's reach for support if needed Stopwatch or clock within view with second hand	Stand with one foot in front of the other and slightly off to the side. Stand for up to one minute. Repeat on other side for comparison *Time stops if loss of balance with need to hold on to support.	One minute: Normal *Progress to Tandem Stance Test* *Less than 30 seconds: Continue balance program using support. *(See Balance)*
Tandem Stance Balance progression		Wall, counter or chair within arm's reach for support if needed Stopwatch or clock within view with second hand	Stand with one foot directly in back of the other – toe should be touching the opposite heel. Hold for up to one minute. Repeat on other side for comparison *Time stops if loss of balance with need to hold on to support.	One minute: Normal *Progress to One Leg Standing Balance* *Less than 30 seconds: Continue balance program using support. *(See Balance)*
Single Leg Stance Balance progression		Wall, counter or chair within arm's reach for support if needed Stopwatch or clock within view with second hand	Stand on one leg for up to one minute. Repeat on other side for comparison *Time stops if loss of balance with need to hold on to support or if opposite foot taps the floor	One minute: Normal *Less than 30 seconds: Continue balance program using support. *(See Balance)*

HOME EXERCISE GUIDE

EXERCISE Myofascial Release	EXERCISE NUMBER	PAGE	REPS	SETS	X DAY	HOLD
ANTERIOR CHEST - BALL	1					
ANTERIOR CHEST - FOAM ROLL	2					
LATISSIMUS DORSI – BALL	3					
LATISSIMUS DORSI - FOAM ROLL	4					
TRICEP – FOAM ROLL	5					
OCCIPITAL RELEASE - FOAM ROLL	6					
THORACIC MOBILIZATION – SUPINE - FOAM ROLL	7					
THORACIC MOBILIZATION – STANDING - FOAM ROLL	8					
LUMBAR – STANDING – BALL - can do with foam roll	9					
LUMBAR – SUPINE – FOAM ROLLER	10					
HIP FLEXORS - BALL	11					
HIP FLEXORS – FOAM ROLL	12					
QUADRICEPS – BILATERAL - FOAM ROLL	13					
QUADRICEP – SINGLE - FOAM ROLL	14					
GLUTE /PIRIFORMIS - FOAM ROLL	15					
HIP ADDUCTORS – FOAM ROLL	16					
HAMSTRING – BILATERAL - FOAM ROLL	17					
HAMSTRING – SINGLE – FOAM ROLL	18					
CALVES – BILATERAL - FOAM ROLL	19					
CALVES – SINGLE - FOAM ROLL	20					
ILIOTIBIAL BAND (IT Band) - FOAM ROLL	21					
ILIOTIBIAL BAND (IT Band) - BALL	22					
PLANTAR FASCIA ROLLING – BALL	23					
PLANTAR FASCIA ROLLING - COLD SODA CAN	24					

HOME EXERCISE GUIDE

EXERCISE Flexibility (Stretching)	EXERCISE NUMBER	PAGE	REPS	SETS	X DAY	HOLD
INVERSION	1					
EVERSION	2					
ANTERIOR TIBIALIS	3					
PLANTARFLEXION	4					
DORSIFLEXION - STRAP	5					
DORSIFLEXION - FLOOR ASSISTED	6					
STANDING CALF STRETCH - GASTROC	7					
STANDING CALF STRETCH - GASTROC – HAND ON KNEE	8					
GASTROCNEMIUS STAIR STRETCH	9					
STANDING CALF STRETCH - SOLEUS	10					
HAMSTRING STRETCH – TOWEL, BAND, STRAP or BELT	11					
HAMSTRING STRETCH – TOWEL, BAND, STRAP or BELT	12					
HAMSTRING STRETCH - TABLE, BED OR COUCH	13					
HAMSTRING / KNEE EXTENSION STRETCH - SEATED	14					
HAMSTRING STRETCH - STANDING	15					
TOE TOUCH – STANDING - NARROW or WIDE BOS	16					
HEEL SLIDES - SELF ASSISTED	17					
HEEL SLIDES - LONG SIT ASSISTED - TOWEL, BAND, STRAP or BELT	18					
HEEL SLIDES - SUPINE	19					
KNEE BENDS - EXERCISE BALL	20					
KNEE FLEXION – SELF ASSISTED - PRONE	21					
KNEE FLEXION – BELT ASSISTED - PRONE	22					
HEEL SLIDES - SELF ASSISTED	23					
HEEL SLIDES - SEATED	24					
KNEE FLEXION – SCOOT FORWARD - SEATED	25					

HOME EXERCISE GUIDE

EXERCISE Flexibility (Stretching)	EXERCISE NUMBER	PAGE	REPS	SETS	X DAY	HOLD
KNEE FLEXION – STAIR OR STEP	26					
PIRIFORMIS STRETCH	27					
PIRIFORMIS STRETCH - EXERCISE BALL	28					
PIRIFORMIS STRETCH - LONG SIT	29					
PIRIFORMIS STRETCH – STANDING	30					
HIP FLEXOR STRETCH - SIDE OF BALL or CHAIR	31					
HIP FLEXOR STRETCH - STANDING	32					
HIP FLEXOR STRETCH - HALF KNEEL	33					
RUNNER'S STRETCH - MODIFIED	34					
HIP FLEXOR STRETCH – SUPINE	35					
HIP FLEXOR STRETCH – SUPINE - 2	36					
QUAD STRETCH - SIDELYING	37					
QUAD STRETCH - STANDING	38					
KNEE FALL OUT STRETCH or FROG STRETCH	39					
BUTTERFLY STRETCH	40					
HIP ADDUCTOR STRECH – KNEELING	41					
HIP ADDUCTOR STRECH - STANDING	42					
HIP EXTERNAL ROTATION STRETCH - SUPINE	43					
HIP INTERNAL ROTATION STRETCH - SEATED	44					
IT BAND STRETCH - STANDING	45					
IT BAND STRETCH -- SIDELYING	46					
NECK ROTATION and SIDE BENDS	47					
NECK FLEXION AND EXTENSION	48					
TRUNK FLEXION - SEATED	49					
LOW BACK STRETCH - SEATED	50					
LOW BACK STRETCH – STANDING - STRAIGHT & LATERAL	51					
LOW BACK STRETCH – RAIL OR DOORKNOB	52					

HOME EXERCISE GUIDE

EXERCISE Flexibility (Stretching)	EXERCISE NUMBER	PAGE	REPS	SETS	X DAY	HOLD
PRAYER STRETCH and LATERAL	53					
PRAYER STRETCH - EXERCISE BALL	54					
CAT AND CAMEL	55					
KNEE TO CHEST STRETCH - SINGLE and BILATERAL	56					
PRONE ON ELBOWS	57					
PRESS UPS	58					
TRUNK ROTATION STRETCH – SINGLE LEG	59					
LOWER TRUNK ROTATIONS – BILATERAL	60					
TRUNK ROTATION - SEATED	61					
TRUNK ROTATION - STANDING or SEATED – DOWEL	62					
LATERAL TRUNK STRETCH - SINGLE, SEATED or STANDING	63					
LATERAL TRUNK STRETCH - BILATERAL SEATED or STANDING	64					
FLEXION - SUPINE - DOWEL	65					
WALL WALK	66					
FLEXION - TABLE SLIDE	67					
FLEXION - TABLE SLIDE - BALL	68					
EXTERNAL ROTATION - SUPINE – DOWEL *INTERNAL ROTATION ON OPPOSITE ARM*	69					
EXTERNAL ROTATION - 90-90 - DOWEL	70					
EXTERNAL ROTATION – SEATED – DOWEL *INTERNAL ROTATION ON OPPOSITE ARM*	71					
EXTERNAL ROTATION – STANDING – DOWEL *INTERNAL ROTATION ON OPPOSITE ARM*	72					
ABDUCTION - TABLE SLIDE - BALL	75					
ABDUCTION WITH DOWEL	76					
LYING DOWN EXTENSION - TABLE or BED	77					
WAND EXTENSION - STANDING	78					
CHEST STRETCH – SEATED, STANDING, or SUPINE	79					

EXERCISE **Flexibility (Stretching)**	EXERCISE NUMBER	PAGE	REPS	SETS	X DAY	HOLD
TRICEP STRETCH - STRAP or TOWEL	82					
POSTERIOR SHOULDER/DELTOID RELEASE	83					
POSTERIOR CAPSULE STRETCH	84					

EXERCISE Core / Stability	EXERCISE NUMBER	PAGE	REPS	SETS	X DAY	HOLD
ABDOMINAL BRACING TRAINING	1					
ABDOMINAL BRACING - SUPINE	2					
PELVIC TILT - SUPINE	3					
PELVIC TILT - KNEELING	4					
BRIDGING	5					
BRIDGE - BOSU	6					
BRIDGING WITH PILLOW SQUEEZE	7					
BRIDGING WITH PILLOW SQUEEZE - BOSU	8					
BRACE SUPINE MARCHING / BRIDGE LEG UP	9					
BRIDGE LEG UP - BOSU -	10					
SINGLE LEG BRIDGE	11					
BRIDGE SINGLE LEG - BOSU	12					
BRIDGING CROSSED LEG	13					
BRIDGING CROSSED LEG – BOSU	14					
BRIDGING CROSSED LEG - ARMS UP	15					
BRIDGING CROSSED LEG - ARMS UP - BOSU	16					
BRIDGE - ELASTIC BAND	17					
BRIDGING - ABDUCTION - ELASTIC BAND	18					
FLOOR BRIDGE - EXERCISE BALL	19					
FLOOR BRIDGE ALTERNATE LEG LIFT - EXERCISE BALL	20					
BRIDGE UPPER BACK - EXERCISE BALL	21					
BRIDGE UPPER BACK - SINGLE LEG - EXERCISE BALL	22					
QUADRUPED ALTERNATE ARM	23					
QUADRUPED ALTERNATE LEG	24					
QUADRUPED ALTERNATE ARM AND LEG	25					
BIRD DOG ELBOW TOUCHES	26					

HOME EXERCISE GUIDE

EXERCISE Core / Stability	EXERCISE NUMBER	PAGE	REPS	SETS	X DAY	HOLD
PRONE BALL	27					
PRONE BALL - ALTERNATE ARM	28					
PRONE BALL - ALTERNATE LEG	29					
PRONE BALL - ALTERNATE ARM AND LEG	30					
MODIFIED PLANK	31					
MODIFIED PLANK - ALTERNATE LEG	32					
FULL PLANK	33					
PLANK - ALTERNATE ARMS	34					
PLANK - ALTERNATE LEGS	35					
PLANK - EXERCISE BALL	36					
PRONE ON ELBOWS	37					
PRESS UPS	38					
SKYDIVER	39					
PRONE SUPERMAN - BOSU	40					
TRUNK EXTENSION - BOSU	41					
TRUNK EXTENSION - HANDS CROSSED IN FRONT - BOSU	43					
SUPERMAN - ARMS BACK- EXERCISE BALL	44					
SUPERMAN – BOTH ARMS IN FRONT - EXERCISE BALL	45					
SUPERMAN – ONE ARM FORWARD / ONE ARM BACK - EXERCISE BALL	46					
LATERAL PLANK MODIFIED	47					
LATERAL PLANK MODIFIED- BOSU	48					
LATERAL PLANK - 1 KNEE 1 FOOT	49					
LATERAL PLANK - 1 KNEE 1 FOOT – BOSU	50					
LATERAL PLANK	51					
LATERAL PLANK - BOSU	52					

EXERCISE Core / Stability	EXERCISE NUMBER	PAGE	REPS	SETS	X DAY	HOLD
LEAN BACK	53					
LEAN BACK - BOSU	54					
LEAN BACK WITH ARMS OUT	55					
LEAN BACK WITH ARMS OUT - BOSU	56					
LEAN BACK WITH TWIST	57					
LEAN BACK WITH TWIST – BOSU	58					
CRUNCHY FROG	59					
SEATED BIKE - FORWARD AND BACKWARDS	60					
CRUNCH – ARMS OUT	61					
CRUNCH – ARMS OUT - BOSU	62					
CRUNCH – ARMS IN BACK OF HEAD	63					
CRUNCH – ARMS IN BACK OF HEAD - BOSU	64					
OBLIQUE CRUNCH	65					
OBLIQUE CRUNCH - BOSU	66					
90 DEGREE CRUNCH	67					
BALL CRUNCH – Can put legs on seat of chair	68					
CURL UPS – ARMS ON LEGS - EXERCISE BALL	69					
CURL UPS- ARMS CROSSED IN FRONT - EXERCISE BALL	70					
CURL UPS – ARMS BEHIND HEAD - EXERCISE BALL	71					
SUPINE CRUNCH TOUCH - EXERCISE BALL	72					
LOWER ABDOMINAL CRUNCH – WITH or WITHOUT BALL	73					
HIGH MARCH CRUNCH	74					
STANDING SIDE CRUNCH	75					
STANDING BIKE CRUNCH	76					

EXERCISE Lower Extremity - Lying & Seated Strengthening and Range of Motion	EXERCISE NUMBER	PAGE	REPS	SETS	X DAY	HOLD
INVERSION – SEATED - ELASTIC BAND	1					
INVERSION – SEATED - ELASTIC BAND - 2	2					
EVERSION – SEATED - ELASTIC BAND	3					
EVERSION – SEATED - ELASTIC BAND - 2	4					
ANKLE PUMPS - SEATED	5					
ANKLE PUMPS – SUPINE or FEET UP ON STOOL	6					
DORSIFLEXION – SEATED - ELASTIC BAND	7					
DORSIFLEXION – SEATED - ELASTIC BAND - 2	8					
PLANTARFLEXION - STRAP	9					
PLANTARFLEXION - SEATED – ELASTIC BAND	10					
HEEL SLIDES - SUPINE	11					
HEEL SLIDES - RESISTED EXTENSION – ELASTIC BAND	12					
QUAD SET –ISOMETRIC	13					
QUAD SET WITH TOWEL UNDER HEEL - ISOMETRIC	14					
SHORT ARC QUAD (SAQ) – SELF ASSISTED	15					
SHORT ARC QUAD - (SAQ)	16					
KNEE EXTENSION - SELF ASSISTED	17					
PARTIAL ARC QUAD - LOW SEAT	18					
LONG ARC QUAD (LAQ) – LOW SEAT (90 deg)	19					
LONG ARC QUAD (LAQ) – LOW SEAT - ANKLE WEIGHTS	20					
LONG ARC QUAD (LAQ) - HIGH SEAT	21					
LONG ARC QUAD (LAQ) - HIGH SEAT - ANKLE WEIGHTS	22					
LONG ARC QUAD - ELASTIC BAND – HAND HELD	23					
LONG ARC QUAD - ELASTIC BAND	24					

EXERCISE Lower Extremity - Lying & Seated Strengthening and Range of Motion	EXERCISE NUMBER	PAGE	REPS	SETS	X DAY	HOLD
HAMSTRING CURLS - PRONE - ASSISTED	25					
HAMSTRING CURLS - PRONE	26					
HAMSTRING CURLS - - PRONE - WEIGHTS	27					
HAMSTRING CURLS – PRONE - ELASTIC BAND	28					
HAMSTRING CURLS – ELASTIC BAND	29					
HAMSTRING CURLS – ELASTIC BAND - 2	30					
HAMSTRING CURLS ON BALL	31					
HAMSTRING CURLS - SINGLE LEG - EXERCISE BALL	32					
HIP FLEXION ISOMETRIC	33					
HIP FLEXION ISOMETRIC BILATERAL	34					
HIP FLEXION – ISOMETRIC	35					
STRAIGHT LEG RAISE (SLR)	36					
STRAIGHT LEG RAISE (SLR) – ANKLE WEIGHTS	37					
STRAIGHT LEG RAISE (SLR) - ELASTIC BAND	38					
SEATED MARCHING	39					
SEATED MARCHING - ELASTIC BAND	40					
HIP EXTENSION - PRONE	41					
HIP EXTENSION – PRONE – ANKLE WEIGHTS	42					
HIP EXTENSION – PRONE – ELASTIC BAND	43					
HIP EXTENSION – QUADRUPED	44					
HIP ABDUCTION - SUPINE	45					
HIP ABDUCTION - SUPINE – ANKLE WEIGHTS	46					
HIP ABDUCTION – SUPINE - ELASTIC BAND	47					
HIP ABDUCTION / CLAMS– SUPINE - ELASTIC BAND	48					
MODIFIED HIP ABDUCTION – SIDELYING	49					

EXERCISE Lower Extremity - Lying & Seated Strengthening and Range of Motion	EXERCISE NUMBER	PAGE	REPS	SETS	X DAY	HOLD
HIP ABDUCTION – SIDELYING	50					
HIP ABDUCTION – SIDELYING - WEIGHTS	51					
HIP ABDUCTION – SIDELYING - ELASTIC BAND	52					
CLAM SHELLS	53					
SIDELYING CLAM - ELASTIC BAND	54					
HIP ABDUCTION - FIRE HYDRANT - QUADRUPED	55					
HIP ABDUCTION - FIRE HYDRANT – QUADRUPED - ELASTIC BAND	56					
HIP ABDUCTION - SEATED - STRAIGHT LEG	57					
HIP ABDUCTION - SEATED - STRAIGHT LEG – ANKLE WEIGHT	58					
HIP ABDUCTION - SINGLE- SEATED	59					
HIP ABDUCTION - SINGLE- SEATED – ELASTIC BAND	60					
HIP ABDUCTION - BILATERAL- SEATED	61					
HIP ABDUCTION - BILATERAL- SEATED - ELASTIC BAND	62					
HIP ADDUCTION SQUEEZE – SUPINE – KNEES BENT	63					
HIP ADDUCTION SQUEEZE – SUPINE – LEGS STRAIGHT	64					
HIP ADDUCTION - SIDELYING	65					
INTERNAL ROTATION - HEEL SQUEEZE - ISOMETRIC	67					
HIP INTERNAL ROTATION - SUPINE	68					
REVERSE CLAMS - SIDELYING	69					
REVERSE CLAMS - SIDELYING - ELASTIC BAND	70					
HIP INTERNAL ROTATION - SEATED	71					
HIP INTERNAL ROTATION - ELASTIC BAND	72					
HIP EXTERNAL ROTATION - SUPINE	73					

EXERCISE Lower Extremity - Lying & Seated Strengthening and Range of Motion	EXERCISE NUMBER	PAGE	REPS	SETS	X DAY	HOLD
HIP EXTERNAL ROTATION - ELASTIC BAND	74					
HIP ROTATIONS – BILATERAL - SIDELYING	75					
HIP ROTATION - SEATED - BALL and ELASTIC BAND	76					
PRESS – BILATERAL – ELASTIC BAND	77					
PRESS – SINGLE LEG – ELASTIC BAND	78					
HIP HIKE - STANDING	79					
HIP HIKE – KNEELING	80					
GLUTE SETS - PRONE	81					
GLUTE SET - SUPINE	82					
GLUTE SQUEEZE - SITTING	83					
GLUTE SCULPT (MAX/MEDIUS)	84					

HOME EXERCISE GUIDE

EXERCISE Upper Extremity Strengthening and Range of Motion	EXERCISE NUMBER	PAGE	REPS	SETS	X DAY	HOLD
ELBOW FLEXION EXTENSION - SUPINE	1					
ELBOW FLEXION / EXTENSION - GRAVITY ELIMINATED	2					
BICEPS CURLS – ALTERNATING	3					
BICEPS CURL - SELF FIXATION – ELASTIC BAND	4					
SEATED BICEPS CURLS - ALTERNATING	5					
SEATED BICEPS CURLS - BILATERAL	6					
CONCENTRATION CURLS – SITTING	7					
PREACHER CURL ON BALL	8					
BICEPS CURLS	9					
BICEPS CURLS - RADIOBRACHIALIS - HAMMER CURL	10					
BICEPS CURLS - BRACHIALIS	11					
BICEPS CURLS – ROTATE OUTWARD	12					
BICEPS CURLS – ONE ARM - ELASTIC BAND	13					
BICEPS CURLS – BILATERAL - ELASTIC BAND	14					
BICEPS CURLS - RADIOBRACHIALIS - HAMMER CURL – ONE ARM - ELASTIC BAND	15					
BICEPS CURLS - RADIOBRACHIALIS - HAMMER CURL – BILATERAL - ELASTIC BAND	16					
BICEPS CURLS – BRACHIALIS - ONE ARM - ELASTIC BAND	17					
BICEPS CURL – BRACHIALIS – BILATERAL - ELASTIC BAND	18					
TRICEPS - SELF FIXATION - ELASTIC BAND	19					
OVERHEAD TRICEPS - SELF FIXATION –SEATED OR STANDING - ELASTIC BAND	20					
TRICEP EXTENSION – SITTING OR STANDING - WEIGHT	21					
TRICEP EXTENSION – SITTING OR STANDING – BILATERAL - WEIGHT	22					
ELBOW EXTENSION - BALL	23					

EXERCISE **Upper Extremity** **Strengthening and Range of Motion**	EXERCISE NUMBER	PAGE	REPS	SETS	X DAY	HOLD
ELBOW EXTENSION - SKULL CRUSHER - BALL	24					
TRICEPS - ELASTIC BAND	25					
TRICEPS - BENT OVER	26					
CHAIR DIPS / PUSH UPS	27					
DIPS OFF CHAIR	28					
PENDULUM SHOULDER FORWARD/BACK	29					
PENDULUM SHOULDER – SIDE TO SIDE	30					
PENDULUM SHOULDER CIRCLES	31					
PENDULUMS - SUPINE	32					
ISOMETRIC FLEXION	33					
SHOULDER FLEXION – SIDELYING	34					
FLEXION – SUPINE - SINGLE OR BILATERAL	35					
FLEXION – SUPINE – SINGLE OR BILATERAL - WEIGHT	36					
FLEXION – SUPINE - DOWEL	37					
FLEXION – SUPINE - DOWEL - Weight	38					
FLEXION - SELF FIXATION – ELASTIC BAND	39					
FLEXION – ELASTIC BAND	40					
FLEXION - STANDING - PALMS DOWN / OVERHAND DOWEL	41					
FLEXION - STANDING - PALMS UP / UNDERHAND DOWEL	42					
FLEXION – PALMS FACING INWARD	43					
FLEXION – PALMS DOWN	44					
V RAISE	45					
V RAISE – WEIGHTS	46					
MILITARY PRESS – DOWEL	47					
MILITARY PRESS - FREE WEIGHTS	48					

EXERCISE Upper Extremity Strengthening and Range of Motion	EXERCISE NUMBER	PAGE	REPS	SETS	X DAY	HOLD
ISOMETRIC EXTENSION	49					
PRONE EXTENSION - EXERCISE BALL	50					
SHOULDER EXTENSION - STANDING	51					
SHOULDER EXTENSION - STANDING - WEIGHTS	52					
EXTENSION – STANDING – DOWEL	53					
EXTENSION - SELF FIXATION - ELASTIC BAND	54					
EXTENSION - ELASTIC BAND	55					
EXTENSION - BILATERAL - ELASTIC BAND	56					
INTERNAL ROTATION – ISOMETRIC	57					
INTERNAL ROTATION - ISOMETRIC- ELEVATED	58					
INTERNAL ROTATION - SIDELYING	59					
INTERNAL ROTATION - ELASTIC BAND	60					
INTERNAL / EXTERNAL ROTATION - STANDING – DOWEL	61					
INTERNAL ROTATION – DOWEL	62					
EXTERNAL ROTATION - ISOMETRIC	63					
EXTERNAL ROTATION - ISOMETRIC – ELEVATED	64					
EXTERNAL ROTATION WITH TOWEL - SIDELYING	65					
EXTERNAL ROTATION – 90/90 - WEIGHTS	66					
EXTERNAL ROTATION - BILATERAL - ELASTIC BAND	67					
EXTERNAL ROTATION - ELASTIC BAND	68					
ADDUCTION – ISOMETRIC	69					
ADDUCTION - ELASTIC BAND	70					
ABDUCTION – ISOMETRIC	71					
HORIZONTAL ABDUCTION - DOWEL	72					

EXERCISE Upper Extremity Strengthening and Range of Motion	EXERCISE NUMBER	PAGE	REPS	SETS	X DAY	HOLD
HORIZONTAL ABDUCTION/ADDUCTTION - SUPINE	73					
HORIZONTAL ABDUCTION/ADDUCTTION - SUPINE -WEIGHT	74					
ABDUCTION - SIDELYING	75					
HORIZONTAL ABDUCTION - SIDELYING	76					
ABDUCTION – WEIGHT	77					
ABDUCTION – ELASTIC BAND	78					
HORIZONTAL ABDUCTION – BILATERAL - ELASTIC BAND	79					
90/90 ABDUCTION - WEIGHT	80					
LATERAL RAISES	81					
LATERAL RAISES – LEAN FORWARD	82					
LATERAL RAISES – LEAN FORWARD - ARM ROTATION	83					
FRONTAL RAISE – WEIGHTS	84					
UPRIGHT ROW – WEIGHTS	85					
UPRIGHT ROW – ELASTIC BAND	86					
SHRUGS	87					
SHRUGS - WEIGHTS	88					
SHOULDER ROLLS	89					
SHOULDER ROLLS - WEIGHTS	90					
SCAPULAR RETRACTIONS - BILATERAL	91					
SCAPULAR RETRACTION – SINGLE ARM	92					
ELASTIC BAND SCAPULAR RETRACTIONS WITH MINI SHOULDER EXTENSIONS	93					
PRONE RETRACTION	94					
SCAPULAR PROTRACTION - SUPINE - BILATERAL	95					
SCAPULAR PROTRACTION - SUPINE - WEIGHT	96					

EXERCISE Upper Extremity Strengthening and Range of Motion	EXERCISE NUMBER	PAGE	REPS	SETS	X DAY	HOLD
SCAPULAR PROTRACTION - SUPINE - ELASTIC BAND	97					
SCAPULAR PROTRACTION / TABLE PLANK	98					
CHEST PRESS – SEATED or STANDING - ELASTIC BAND	99					
CHEST PRESS – BALL, FLOOR or BENCH- WEIGHTS	100					
DOWEL PRESS – STANDING	101					
CHEST PRESS – STANDING or SEATED	102					
BENT OVER ROWS	103					
ROWS – PRONE	104					
ROWS - ELASTIC BAND	105					
WIDE ROWS - ELASTIC BAND	106					
LOW ROW – ELASTIC BAND	107					
HIGH ROW – ELASTIC BAND	108					
FLY'S – FLOOR - WEIGHT	109					
FLY'S – BALL or BENCH – WEIGHT	110					
WALL PUSH UPS	111					
WALL PUSH UP - BALL	112					
WALL PUSH UP - Triceps uneven	113					
WALL PUSH UP - Hands inverted	114					
WALL PUSH UP - Narrow	115					
WALL PUSH UP – Wide	116					
PUSH UPS - BALL	117					
PUSH UP - MODIFIED	118					
PUSH UP	119					
PUSH UP -DIAMOND	120					
PUSH UP – MODIFIED - BOSU - UNSTABLE	121					

EXERCISE **Upper Extremity** **Strengthening and Range of Motion**	EXERCISE NUMBER	PAGE	REPS	SETS	X DAY	HOLD
PUSH UP – BOSU - UNSTABLE	122					
PUSH UP – MODIFIED – INVERTED BOSU - UNSTABLE	123					
PUSH UP – INVERTED BOSU - UNSTABLE	124					

HOME EXERCISE GUIDE

EXERCISE Balance / Standing Exercises	EXERCISE NUMBER	PAGE	REPS	SETS	X DAY	HOLD
WIDE BOS DECREASING TO NARROW BOS	1					
NARROW BOS	2					
ARM MOVEMENT	3					
TRUNK ROTATION	4					
EYES SHUTS	5					
HEAD TURNS	6					
READING ALOUD	7					
BALANCE PAD	8					
SPLIT STANCE – SEMI TANDEM	9					
SPLIT STANCE - Progression	10					
TANDEM- SHARPENED ROMBERG STANCE	11					
TANDEM STANCE - Progression	12					
SINGLE LEG STANCE (SLS)	13					
SINGLE LEG STANCE (SLS) - Progression	14					
SLS – LEG FORWARD	15					
SLS – LEG BACKWARDS	16					
SLS – LEG FORWARD / OPPOSITE ARM UP	17					
SLS – LEG BACKWARDS / OPPOSITE ARM UP	18					
SLS - REACH FORWARD	19					
SLS - REACH TWIST	20					
SINGLE LEG TOE TAP	21					
SINGLE LEG STANCE - CLOCKS	22					
BALL ROLLS - HEEL TOE	23					
BALL ROLLS - LATERAL	24					
SQUAT	25					
SIT TO STAND	26					

HOME EXERCISE GUIDE

EXERCISE Balance / Standing Exercises	EXERCISE NUMBER	PAGE	REPS	SETS	X DAY	HOLD
SQUATS – WALL WITH BALL	27					
SQUATS WITH WEIGHTS	28					
MINI SQUAT - UNSTABLE SUPPORT - FOAM PAD	29					
SQUATS - SINGLE LEG	30					
SIDE TO SIDE WEIGHT SHIFT	31					
FORWARD AND BACKWARDS WEIGHT SHIFTS	32					
SPLIT STANCE WEIGHT SHIFT SIDE TO SIDE	33					
SPLIT STANCE WEIGHT SHIFT FORWARD AND BACKWARDS	34					
WALL FALLS - FORWARD - BALANCE DRILL	35					
WALL FALLS - LATERAL - BALANCE DRILL	36					
WALL FALLS - BACKWARDS - BALANCE DRILL	37					
WALL FALLS - SINGLE LEG - FORWARD - BALANCE DRILL	38					
WALL FALLS - SINGLE LEG - LATERAL - BALANCE DRILL	39					
WALL FALLS - SINGLE LEG - MEDIAL - BALANCE DRILL	40					
WALL FALLS - SINGLE LEG - BACKWARDS - BALANCE DRILL	41					
FALL LATERAL - STEP RECOVERY	42					
FALL FORWARD - STEP RECOVERY	43					
FALL BACKWARD - STEP RECOVERY	44					
TOE TAP ABDUCTION	45					
HIP ABDUCTION - STANDING	46					
HIP EXTENSION – STANDING	47					
HIP FLEXION - STANDING – STRAIGHT LEG RAISE	48					
HIP / KNEE FLEXION - SINGLE LEG	49					
STANDING MARCHING	50					

EXERCISE	EXERCISE NUMBER	PAGE	REPS	SETS	X DAY	HOLD
Balance / Standing Exercises						
HAMSTRING CURL	51					
TOE RAISES	52					
TOE RAISES IR AND ER	53					
ONE LEGGED TOE RAISE	54					
SINGLE LEG BALANCE FORWARD	55					
SINGLE LEG BALANCE LATERAL	56					
SINGLE LEG BALANCE RETRO	57					
SINGLE LEG STANCE RETROLATERAL	58					
SQUAT	59					
SINGLE LEG SQUAT	60					
LUNGE – STATIC	61					
LUNGE FORWARD/BACKWARD	62					
FOUR CORNER MARCHING IN PLACE	63					
FOUR CORNER MARCHING IN PLACE WITH HEAD TURNS	64					
WALKING ON HEELS FORWARD AND BACKWARDS	65					
WALKING ON TOES FORWARD AND BACKWARDS	66					
TANDEM STANCE AND WALK – FORWARD AND BACKWARDS	67					
RUNNING MAN	68					
HOP STICK - FORWARD	69					
HOP STICK - BACKWARDS	70					
MINI LATERAL LUNGE	71					
SIDE STEPPING	72					
HOP STICK - LATERAL	73					
SINGLE LEG DEAD LIFT	74					

EXERCISE	EXERCISE NUMBER	PAGE	REPS	SETS	X DAY	HOLD
Balance / Standing Exercises						
CONE TAPS - SINGLE LEG STANCE	75					
CONE TAPS - SINGLE LEG STANCE - UNSTABLE	76					
FIGURE 8 AROUND CONES	77					
FIGURE 8 AROUND CONES – FOOT OR HAND TAP	78					
BALANCE DOUBLE LEG STANCE - WIDE	79					
BALANCE DOUBLE LEG STANCE - NARROW	80					
TANDEM STANCE	81					
TANDEM WALK	82					
SINGLE LEG STANCE - ABDUCTION	83					
SINGLE LEG STANCE - ABDUCTION	84					
SINGLE LEG STANCE – FORWARD KICK	85					
SINGLE LEG STANCE – HAMSTRING CURL	86					
SINGLE LEG SQUAT – LEG FORWARD	87					
SINGLE LEG SQUAT – LEG BACKWARDS	88					
TOE TAP OR HEEL PLACEMENT	89					
PULL UP FOOT TOUCHES ON STEP	90					
ALTERNATING SUSTAINED FOOT TOUCHES ON STEP	91					
STEP UP AND OVER	92					
FORWARD SWING THROUGH STEP	93					
SIDE STEPPING - *REPEAT STEPS 89-93 from a side approach.*	94					

HOME EXERCISE GUIDE

EXERCISE Agility/Reactivity/Speed	EXERCISE NUMBER	PAGE	REPS	SETS	X DAY	HOLD
Four Square Drills	1					
Dots	2					
Ladder Drills	3					
Box Drills	4					
Cones	5					
Hurdles	6					

Myofascial Release

Myofascial release (MFR, self-myofascial release) is an alternative medicine therapy that claims to treat skeletal muscle immobility and pain by relaxing contracted muscles, improving blood and lymphatic circulation, and stimulating the stretch reflex in muscles.

Fascia is a thin, tough, elastic type of connective tissue that wraps most structures within the human body, including muscle. Fascia supports and protects these structures. Osteopathic theory proposes that this soft tissue can become restricted due to psychogenic disease, overuse, trauma, infectious agents, or inactivity, often resulting in pain, muscle tension, and corresponding diminished blood flow. (Wikipedia - *https://en.wikipedia.org/wiki/Myofascial_release*)

Possible Benefits of Myofascial Release

- Muscle relaxation
- Improves muscular and joint range of motion
- Reduces muscle soreness and improves tissue recovery
- Encourages the flow of lymph.
- Improves neuromuscular efficiency.
- Reduces adhesions and scar tissue.
- Releases trigger point (sensitivity and pain) – brings in blood flow and nutrient exchange.
- Maintains normal functional muscular length / Provides optimal length-tension relationship.
- Corrects muscle imbalances

USE

- Roll on foam roller or ball until you find the sore spot or trigger point. When you find this point, stop and rest on it or decrease the range to this particular area and hold for 10-20 seconds.
- Apply pressure to muscle area only. Try not to roll over bones, joints or directly on the spine (you can use a ball over the muscles on the side of the spine).
- Use this as a part of your warmup for particular areas you are exercising that day (for instance the hamstrings, calves and quadricep on leg strengthening day)
- You can use this technique on additional days for trouble areas and can even devote a dedicated session for whole body myofascial release.

Equipment Needed: FOAM ROLLER and/or TEXTURED or SOFT MASSAGE BALL

CAUTION

Do not Roll over Tumors or Lymph Nodes – *See Lymphedema*

EXERCISE Myofascial Release	EXERCISE NUMBER	NOTES
ANTERIOR CHEST - BALL	1	
ANTERIOR CHEST - FOAM ROLL	2	
LATISSIMUS DORSI – BALL	3	
LATISSIMUS DORSI - FOAM ROLL	4	
TRICEP – FOAM ROLL	5	
OCCIPITAL RELEASE - FOAM ROLL	6	
THORACIC MOBILIZATION – SUPINE - FOAM ROLL	7	
THORACIC MOBILIZATION – STANDING - FOAM ROLL	8	
LUMBAR – STANDING – BALL - can do with foam roll	9	
LUMBAR – SUPINE – FOAM ROLLER	10	
HIP FLEXORS - BALL	11	
HIP FLEXORS – FOAM ROLL	12	
QUADRICEPS – BILATERAL - FOAM ROLL	13	
QUADRICEP – SINGLE - FOAM ROLL	14	
GLUTE /PIRIFORMIS - FOAM ROLL	15	
HIP ADDUCTORS – FOAM ROLL	16	
HAMSTRING – BILATERAL - FOAM ROLL	17	
HAMSTRING – SINGLE – FOAM ROLL	18	
CALVES – BILATERAL - FOAM ROLL	19	
CALVES – SINGLE - FOAM ROLL	20	
ILIOTIBIAL BAND (IT Band) - FOAM ROLL	21	
ILIOTIBIAL BAND (IT Band) - BALL	22	
PLANTAR FASCIA ROLLING – BALL	23	
PLANTAR FASCIA ROLLING - COLD SODA CAN	24	

Myofascial Release

_____ Reps _____ Sets _____X Day _____Hold	_____ Reps _____ Sets _____X Day _____Hold

1	Notes:	2	Notes:

ANTERIOR CHEST - BALL

Face towards the wall and place small ball at the outside of chest. Bend knees up and down to find the target point and hold.

ANTERIOR CHEST - FOAM ROLL

Lie face down so that a foam roll is under the upper part of your arm and chest. Using your other arm and legs, roll forward and back across this area.

_____ Reps _____ Sets _____X Day _____Hold	_____ Reps _____ Sets _____X Day _____Hold

3	Notes:	4	Notes:

LATISSIMUS DORSI – BALL

Turn with your target side towards the wall and place small ball on the side under the shoulder. Bend knees up and down to find the target point and hold.

LATISSIMUS DORSI - FOAM ROLL

Lie on your side so that a foam roll is under the upper part of your arm and back. Using your other arm and legs, roll forward and back across this area.

_____ Reps _____ Sets _____X Day _____Hold

5 | Notes:

TRICEP – FOAM ROLL

In a sidelying position, place your tricep on the foam roll. Use the opposite arm and your body to help roll out the arm on the foam roll.

_____ Reps _____ Sets _____X Day _____Hold

6 | Notes:

OCCIPITAL RELEASE - FOAM ROLL

Lie on your back and put a foam roll under the back of your head. Turn your head slowly from side to side.

_____ Reps _____ Sets _____X Day _____Hold

7 | Notes:

THORACIC MOBILIZATION – SUPINE - FOAM ROLL

Lie on a foam roller. While supporting your neck, roll up and down your mid-back.

_____ Reps _____ Sets _____X Day _____Hold

8 | Notes:

THORACIC MOBILIZATION – STANDING - FOAM ROLL

Stand with a foam roll behind your upper back. Slowly perform mini-squats and allow the foam roller to roll up and down your back for a self-massage.

	_____ Reps _____ Sets _____ X Day _____ Hold
9	Notes:

LUMBAR – STANDING – BALL - can do with foam roll

Place small ball in lower back on the side of the spine. DO NOT roll directly over the spine. Slowly perform mini-squats and allow the ball to roll up and down your back for a self-massage.
*Can use foam roll behind lower back and follow above directions.

	_____ Reps _____ Sets _____ X Day _____ Hold
10	Notes:

LUMBAR – SUPINE – FOAM ROLLER

Lie on a foam roll under the lower back. While supporting your upper body, roll up and down your lower back.

	_____ Reps _____ Sets _____ X Day _____ Hold
11	Notes:

HIP FLEXORS - BALL

Ball under hip flexor

Lie on your stomach and place small ball under hip flexor. Roll up and down ball making small movements and hold on the target muscle.

	_____ Reps _____ Sets _____ X Day _____ Hold
12	Notes:

HIP FLEXORS – FOAM ROLL

Lie on your stomach and place foam roll under both hip flexors. Roll up and down avoiding rolling directly over hip bones.

	_____ Reps _____ Sets _____ X Day _____ Hold
13	**Notes:**

QUADRICEPS – BILATERAL - FOAM ROLL

Lie face down so that a foam roll is under the top of your thighs. Using your arms propped on your elbows, roll forward and back across this area.

	_____ Reps _____ Sets _____ X Day _____ Hold
14	**Notes:**

QUADRICEP – SINGLE - FOAM ROLL

Lie face down so that a foam roll is under the top of your target thigh. Cross your other leg over the top of your target leg. Using your arms propped on your elbows, roll forward and back across this area.

	_____ Reps _____ Sets _____ X Day _____ Hold
15	**Notes:**

GLUTE /PIRIFORMIS - FOAM ROLL

Sit on a foam roll and cross your affected leg on top of your other knee. Lean slightly towards your target side. Using your arms and unaffected leg roll forward and back across your buttock area.

	_____ Reps _____ Sets _____ X Day _____ Hold
16	**Notes:**

HIP ADDUCTORS – FOAM ROLL

Lie on your stomach supported by arms and lace your inner thigh on the roller. Roll and compress the target thigh muscle.

_____ Reps _____ Sets _____ X Day _____ Hold

17   Notes:

HAMSTRING – BILATERAL - FOAM ROLL

Sit on a foam roll under both thighs. Using your arms, roll forward and back across this area

_____ Reps _____ Sets _____ X Day _____ Hold

18   Notes:

HAMSTRING – SINGLE – FOAM ROLL

Sit on a foam roll under thigh. Using your arms, roll forward and back across this area.

_____ Reps _____ Sets _____ X Day _____ Hold

19   Notes:

CALVES – BILATERAL - FOAM ROLL

Sit with the foam roll under your both your calves. Lift your body up with your arms and roll forward and back across your calf area. Try turning toes in and out to access the inside and outside of calf areas. Do not roll in the crease of your knee.

_____ Reps _____ Sets _____ X Day _____ Hold

20   Notes:

CALVES – SINGLE - FOAM ROLL

Sit with the foam roll under your target calf and cross your other leg on top. Lift your body up with your arms and roll forward and back across your calf area. Do not roll in the crease of your knee.

_____ Reps _____ Sets _____X Day _____Hold		_____ Reps _____ Sets _____X Day _____Hold

21 | Notes: | **22** | Notes:

ILIOTIBIAL BAND (IT Band) - FOAM ROLL

Lie on your side with a foam roll under your bottom thigh.
Use your arms and unaffected leg and then roll up and
down the foam roll along the outside of your thigh.

ILIOTIBIAL BAND (IT Band) - BALL

Lie on your side or sit in chair. Hold small ball and
move along the outside of the thigh.   Hold on the
target muscle.

_____ Reps _____ Sets _____X Day _____Hold		_____ Reps _____ Sets _____X Day _____Hold

23 | Notes: | **24** | Notes:

PLANTAR FASCIA ROLLING – BALL

Sit and place ball under foot. Roll plantar fascia over ball
back and forth.

PLANTAR FASCIA ROLLING - COLD SODA CAN

Sit and place cold soda can under foot. Roll plantar
fascia over can back and forth.

Flexibility (Stretching)

Range of motion within a joint across various planes of motion that can be increased with stretching. This is needed to prevent decreased range of motion in a joint. Joint mobility can be inhibited by body habitués, genetics, connective tissue elasticity, skin that surrounds the joint, or the joint itself.

Some of the benefits of stretching: *(ACE Personal Training Manual)*	• Increased physical efficiency and performance. • Decreased risk of injury by decreasing resistance in various tissues. • Increased blood supply and nutrients to joint structures. • Improved nutrient exchange by increasing the quantity and decreasing the thickness of synovial fluid in the joint. • Increased neuromuscular coordination. • Improved muscular balance and postural awareness. • Reduced muscular tension. *(Bryant & Daniel, Ace Personal Training Manual, 2003, pg 306-307)*
Things to remember when stretching	• It is always better to stretch a warm muscle (*see Warm up and Cool down*) when the tissue temperature is above normal. Think of putting an elastic band in the freezer compared to heating it before stretching. Which do you think will get a better stretch? • Static stretching is best for the type for beginning athletes. Static stretching is a slow, gradual lengthening of the connective tissue (tendon, muscles and ligaments) through a full range of motion to the point of discomfort – not pain. This stretch should be held for at least 30 seconds, but no longer than two minutes. • Dynamic stretching consists of controlled leg and arm swings that take you to the limits of your range of motion. This type of stretching is appropriate to perform part of a warmup and/or cool down. • Ballistic stretching is a rapid, bouncing movement that may be appropriate in some sports. The problem is that there is also a high-risk factor for injury and should only be done with a professional's guidance. • Again, always remember to warm up before stretching. Repeat all stretches 2-3 times and hold for 15-30 seconds up to 60 seconds) unless otherwise indicated. • Some evidence shows that static stretching may be more beneficial at the end of the exercise program when there is more certainty that the muscles have warmed up. • Dynamic stretching may be more beneficial at the beginning of the exercise program as part of your warmup. This can also be done at the end as part of the cool down.

EXERCISE Flexibility (Stretching)	EXERCISE NUMBER	NOTES
INVERSION	1	
EVERSION	2	
ANTERIOR TIBIALIS	3	
PLANTARFLEXION	4	
DORSIFLEXION - STRAP	5	
DORSIFLEXION - FLOOR ASSISTED	6	
STANDING CALF STRETCH - GASTROC	7	
STANDING CALF STRETCH - GASTROC – HAND ON KNEE	8	
GASTROCNEMIUS STAIR STRETCH	9	
STANDING CALF STRETCH - SOLEUS	10	
HAMSTRING STRETCH – TOWEL, BAND, STRAP or BELT	11	
HAMSTRING STRETCH – TOWEL, BAND, STRAP or BELT	12	
HAMSTRING STRETCH - TABLE, BED OR COUCH	13	
HAMSTRING / KNEE EXTENSION STRETCH - SEATED	14	
HAMSTRING STRETCH - STANDING	15	
TOE TOUCH – STANDING - NARROW or WIDE BOS	16	
HEEL SLIDES - SELF ASSISTED	17	
HEEL SLIDES - LONG SIT ASSISTED - TOWEL, BAND, STRAP or BELT	18	
HEEL SLIDES - SUPINE	19	
KNEE BENDS - EXERCISE BALL	20	
KNEE FLEXION – SELF ASSISTED - PRONE	21	
KNEE FLEXION – BELT ASSISTED - PRONE	22	
HEEL SLIDES - SELF ASSISTED	23	
HEEL SLIDES - SEATED	24	
KNEE FLEXION – SCOOT FORWARD - SEATED	25	

EXERCISE Flexibility (Stretching)	EXERCISE NUMBER	NOTES
KNEE FLEXION – STAIR OR STEP	26	
PIRIFORMIS STRETCH	27	
PIRIFORMIS STRETCH - EXERCISE BALL	28	
PIRIFORMIS STRETCH - LONG SIT	29	
PIRIFORMIS STRETCH – STANDING	30	
HIP FLEXOR STRETCH - SIDE OF BALL or CHAIR	31	
HIP FLEXOR STRETCH - STANDING	32	
HIP FLEXOR STRETCH - HALF KNEEL	33	
RUNNER'S STRETCH - MODIFIED	34	
HIP FLEXOR STRETCH – SUPINE	35	
HIP FLEXOR STRETCH – SUPINE - 2	36	
QUAD STRETCH - SIDELYING	37	
QUAD STRETCH - STANDING	38	
KNEE FALL OUT STRETCH or FROG STRETCH	39	
BUTTERFLY STRETCH	40	
HIP ADDUCTOR STRECH – KNEELING	41	
HIP ADDUCTOR STRECH - STANDING	42	
HIP EXTERNAL ROTATION STRETCH - SUPINE	43	
HIP INTERNAL ROTATION STRETCH - SEATED	44	
IT BAND STRETCH - STANDING	45	
IT BAND STRETCH -- SIDELYING	46	
NECK ROTATION and SIDE BENDS	47	
NECK FLEXION AND EXTENSION	48	
TRUNK FLEXION - SEATED	49	
LOW BACK STRETCH - SEATED	50	
LOW BACK STRETCH – STANDING - STRAIGHT & LATERAL	51	
LOW BACK STRETCH – RAIL OR DOORKNOB	52	

EXERCISE Flexibility (Stretching)	EXERCISE NUMBER	NOTES
PRAYER STRETCH and LATERAL	53	
PRAYER STRETCH - EXERCISE BALL	54	
CAT AND CAMEL	55	
KNEE TO CHEST STRETCH - SINGLE and BILATERAL	56	
PRONE ON ELBOWS	57	
PRESS UPS	58	
TRUNK ROTATION STRETCH – SINGLE LEG	59	
LOWER TRUNK ROTATIONS – BILATERAL	60	
TRUNK ROTATION - SEATED	61	
TRUNK ROTATION - STANDING or SEATED – DOWEL	62	
LATERAL TRUNK STRETCH - SINGLE, SEATED or STANDING	63	
LATERAL TRUNK STRETCH - BILATERAL SEATED or STANDING	64	
FLEXION - SUPINE - DOWEL	65	
WALL WALK	66	
FLEXION - TABLE SLIDE	67	
FLEXION - TABLE SLIDE - BALL	68	
EXTERNAL ROTATION - SUPINE – DOWEL *INTERNAL ROTATION ON OPPOSITE ARM*	69	
EXTERNAL ROTATION - 90-90 - DOWEL	70	
EXTERNAL ROTATION – SEATED – DOWEL *INTERNAL ROTATION ON OPPOSITE ARM*	71	
EXTERNAL ROTATION – STANDING – DOWEL *INTERNAL ROTATION ON OPPOSITE ARM*	72	
ABDUCTION - TABLE SLIDE - BALL	75	
ABDUCTION WITH DOWEL	76	
LYING DOWN EXTENSION - TABLE or BED	77	
WAND EXTENSION - STANDING	78	
CHEST STRETCH – SEATED, STANDING, or SUPINE	79	

EXERCISE Flexibility (Stretching)	EXERCISE NUMBER	NOTES
TRICEP STRETCH - STRAP or TOWEL	82	
POSTERIOR SHOULDER/DELTOID RELEASE	83	
POSTERIOR CAPSULE STRETCH	84	

Stretching / Range of Motion (ROM)

Inversion

	_____ Reps _____ Sets _____X Day _____Hold
1	Notes:

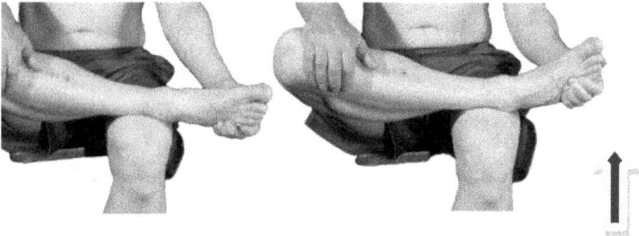

INVERSION

Sit and cross your legs so that the target leg is on top. Hold your foot and pull upwards until a stretch is felt along the side of your ankle.

Eversion

	_____ Reps _____ Sets _____X Day _____Hold
2	Notes:

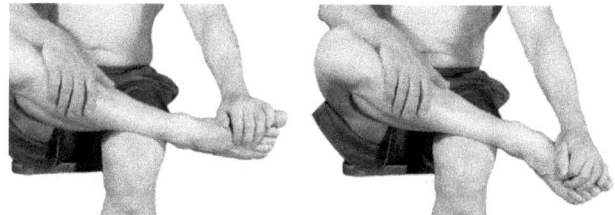

EVERSION

Sit and cross your legs so that the target leg is on top. Hold your foot and push downward until a stretch is felt along the inner side of your ankle.

Anterior Tibialis (Ant Tib)

	_____ Reps _____ Sets _____X Day _____Hold
3	Notes:

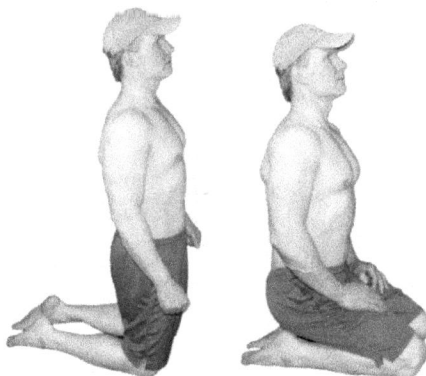

ANTERIOR TIBIALIS

Kneel upright and slowly sit back onto legs forcing heels down towards floor. Sit back until stretch is felt.

Plantarflexion (PF) _DF not shown_

	_____ Reps _____ Sets _____X Day _____Hold
4	Notes:

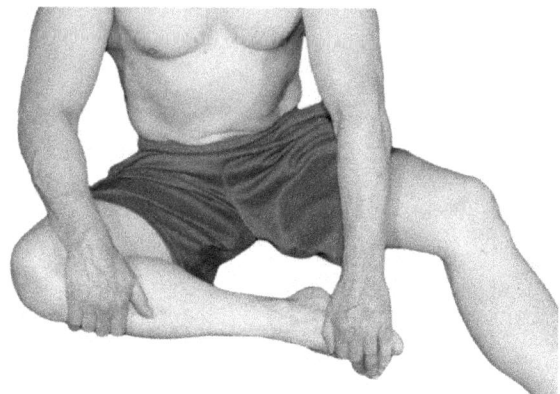

PLANTARFLEXION

Sit and place your affected foot on a firm surface. Use one hand bend the ankle downward as shown.

DORSIFLEXION – _Not shown_
Sit and place your affected foot on a firm surface. Use one hand under foot to push up towards shin (see #5 for movement)

Dorsiflexion (DF)

	_____ Reps _____ Sets _____ X Day _____ Hold		_____ Reps _____ Sets _____ X Day _____ Hold
5	**Notes:** *Lymphedema: Do not wrap band around UE or LE	**6**	**Notes:**

DORSIFLEXION - STRAP

Sit with heel on floor and leg straight. Place belt/strap on forefoot and pull back until stretch is felt.

DORSIFLEXION - FLOOR ASSISTED

Sit and slide your foot back towards under the chair until a stretch is felt at the ankle.

Gastroc/Soleus

	_____ Reps _____ Sets _____ X Day _____ Hold		_____ Reps _____ Sets _____ X Day _____ Hold
7	**Notes:**	**8**	**Notes:**

Target Leg

STANDING CALF STRETCH - GASTROC

Stand in front of a wall, chair, or other sturdy object. Step forward with one foot and maintain your toes on both feet to be pointed straight forward. Keep the leg behind you with a straight knee during the stretch. Lean forward as you allow your front knee to bend until a stretch is felt along the back of your leg. Move closer or further away from the wall to control the stretch of the back leg.

Target Leg

STANDING CALF STRETCH - GASTROC – HAND ON KNEE

Step forward with one foot and place hand on thigh. Maintain your toes on both feet to be pointed straight forward. Keep the leg behind you with a straight knee during the stretch. Lean forward as you allow your front knee to bend until a stretch is felt along the back of your leg. You can adjust the bend of the front knee to control the stretch.

_____ Reps _____ Sets _____ X Day _____ Hold		_____ Reps _____ Sets _____ X Day _____ Hold

9	Notes:	10	Notes:

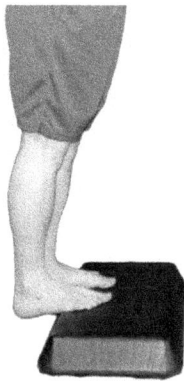

GASTROCNEMIUS STAIR STRETCH

Stand with the middle of your foot on the edge of the stairs while holding onto the railing. Slowly drop heels off until you feel a stretch in the back of your legs keeping your knees straight.

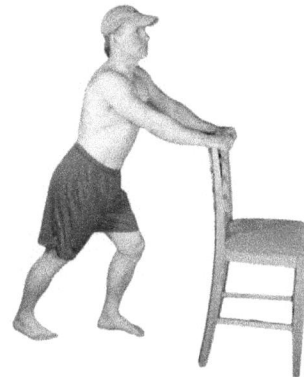

STANDING CALF STRETCH - SOLEUS

Stand in front of a wall, chair or other sturdy object. Step forward with one foot and maintain your toes on both feet to be pointed straight forward. Keep the leg behind you with a slightly bent knee during the stretch. Lean forward towards the wall and support yourself with your arms as you allow your front knee to bend until a gentle stretch is felt along the back of your leg. *Move closer or further away from the wall to control the stretch of the back leg. You can also adjust the bend of the front knee to control the stretch.

Hamstring / Knee Extension

_____ Reps _____ Sets _____ X Day _____ Hold		_____ Reps _____ Sets _____ X Day _____ Hold

11	Notes: *Lymphedema: Do not wrap band around UE or LE	12	Notes: *Lymphedema: Do not wrap band around UE or LE

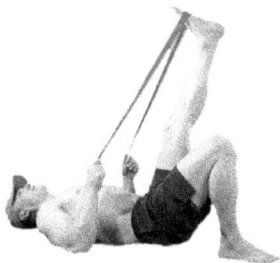

HAMSTRING STRETCH – TOWEL, BAND, STRAP or BELT

Lie down on your back and hook a towel/strap under your foot and draw up your leg until a stretch is felt under your leg/calf area. Keep your knee in a straightened position during the stretch. To increase stretch move strap to forefoot and flex foot.

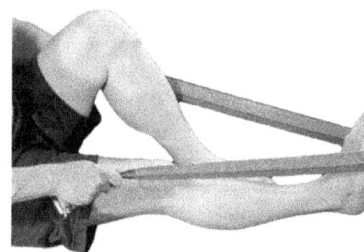

HAMSTRING STRETCH – TOWEL, BAND, STRAP or BELT

While pushing down on thigh above knee cap with opposite hand, pull on towel/ strap to lift heel from floor. Keep thigh flat. To increase stretch move strap to forefoot and flex foot and/or lean forward at the hip.

	_____ Reps _____ Sets _____X Day _____Hold
13	Notes:

HAMSTRING STRETCH - TABLE, BED OR COUCH

Sit on a raised flat surface where you can prop your target leg up on it such as a treatment table, couch or bed. While keeping your knee straight, slowly lean forward and reach your hands towards your foot until a gentle stretch is felt along the back of your knee/thigh. Hold and then return to starting position and repeat. Allow gravity to stretch your knee towards a more straightened position.
* Can use strap, towel or belt around forefoot as in #12

	_____ Reps _____ Sets _____X Day _____Hold
14	Notes:

HAMSTRING / KNEE EXTENSION STRETCH - SEATED

Sit and tighten your top thigh muscle to press the back of your knee downward towards the ground. You should feel a gentle stretch in the back of your knee.

* To increase stretch put strap to forefoot, flex foot and lean forward at the hip.

	_____ Reps _____ Sets _____X Day _____Hold
15	Notes:

HAMSTRING STRETCH - STANDING

Stand and rest your foot on a stool/box/step with your knee straight. Gently lean forward at the hips until a stretch is felt behind your knee/thigh. Keep your back straight. *To increase stretch, flex your foot at the ankle, and/or put strap to forefoot and flex foot. If on stair, you can put foot on 2nd or 3rd step.

	_____ Reps _____ Sets _____X Day _____Hold
16	Notes:

TOE TOUCH – STANDING - NARROW or WIDE BOS

Stand and bend forward at waist keep legs straight and reach for toes. Can perform with either narrow or wide base of support.

Knee Flexion

	_____ Reps _____ Sets _____ X Day _____ Hold	
17	**Notes:**	

HEEL SLIDES - SELF ASSISTED

Lie on your back with knees straight and slide the target heel towards your buttock as you bend your knee. Use the unaffected leg to assist the bending. Hold a gentle stretch in this position and then return to original position.

	_____ Reps _____ Sets _____ X Day _____ Hold	
18	**Notes:** *Lymphedema: Do not wrap band around UE or LE	

HEEL SLIDES - LONG SIT ASSISTED - TOWEL, BAND, STRAP or BELT

Sit with legs straight. Can place a small hand towel under your heel to help slide. Loop a band around your foot and pull your knee into a bend position as your foot slides towards your buttock. Hold a gentle stretch and then return back to original position.

	_____ Reps _____ Sets _____ X Day _____ Hold	
19	**Notes:**	

HEEL SLIDES - SUPINE

Lie on your back with knees straight and slide the target heel towards your buttock as you bend your knee. Hold a gentle stretch in this position and then return to original position.

	_____ Reps _____ Sets _____ X Day _____ Hold	
20	**Notes:**	

KNEE BENDS - EXERCISE BALL

Lie on your back and place your heels on an exercise ball. Roll it closer to your buttocks as your knees and hips bend as shown. Hold and then return to original position. *If you have limited range in one knee, use the other leg to help increase range of motion.

	_____ Reps _____ Sets _____X Day _____Hold		_____ Reps _____ Sets _____X Day _____Hold
21	Notes:	**22**	Notes: *Lymphedema: Do not wrap band around UE or LE

KNEE FLEXION – SELF ASSISTED - PRONE

Lie face down and bend your target knee with the assistance of your unaffected leg.

KNEE FLEXION – BELT ASSISTED - PRONE

Lie face down with a strap looped around your target side ankle or foot. Use the belt to pull the knee into a bent position allowing for a stretch.

	_____ Reps _____ Sets _____X Day _____Hold		_____ Reps _____ Sets _____X Day _____Hold
23	Notes:	**24**	Notes:

HEEL SLIDES - SELF ASSISTED

It and slide your heel towards your buttock with the assist of the unaffected leg. Hold a gentle stretch and then return foot forward to original position.

HEEL SLIDES - SEATED – can use towel or paper under foot to help slide

Sit and place your feet on the floor (can put target foot on a towel or paper to help slide if needed). Slowly slide your foot closer towards you. Hold a gentle stretch and then return foot forward to original position.

_____ Reps _____ Sets _____X Day _____Hold	_____ Reps _____ Sets _____X Day _____Hold

25 Notes:

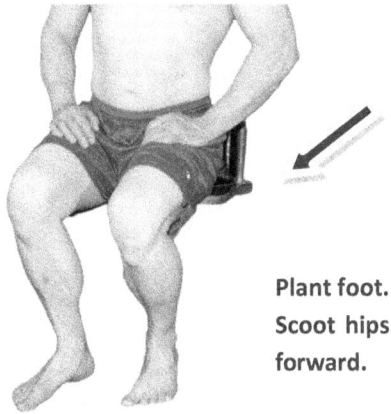

Plant foot.
Scoot hips
forward.

KNEE FLEXION – SCOOT FORWARD - SEATED

Sit and slide your foot back to a bent knee position. Keep your foot planted on the ground and scoot forward until a stretch is felt at the knee. Hold the stretch and then scoot back to original position.

26 Notes:

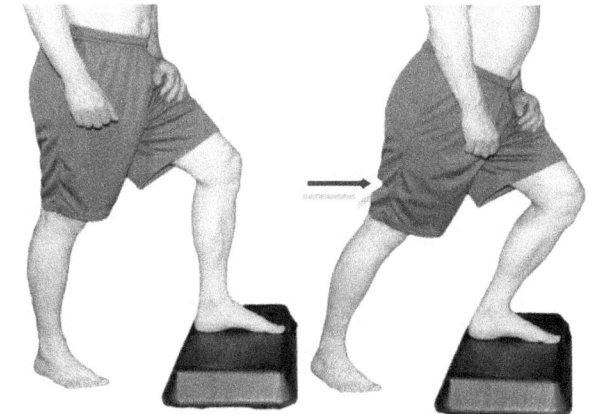

KNEE FLEXION – STAIR OR STEP

Place target foot on stool or step with bent knee. Gently bend forward keeping heel on step. Hold the stretch and then return to original position.

Piriformis

_____ Reps _____ Sets _____X Day _____Hold	_____ Reps _____ Sets _____X Day _____Hold

27 Notes:

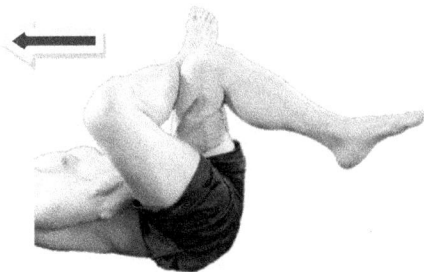

PIRIFORMIS STRETCH

Lie on your back with both knees bent. Cross your target leg on the other knee. Hold your unaffected thigh and pull it up towards your chest until a stretch is felt in the buttock.

28 Notes:

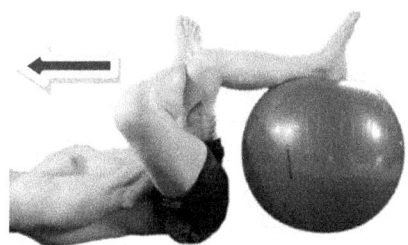

PIRIFORMIS STRETCH - EXERCISE BALL

Lie on your back with one foot placed on the ball. Cross your other leg over the knee of the leg on the ball and gently roll the ball back towards your chest until a stretch is felt in the buttock.

_____ Reps _____ Sets _____X Day _____Hold		_____ Reps _____ Sets _____X Day _____Hold
29	Notes:	**30**	Notes:

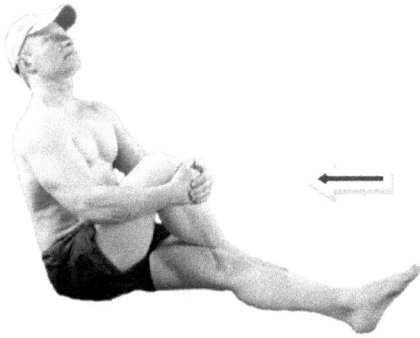

PIRIFORMIS STRETCH - LONG SIT

Sit with one knee straight and the other bent and placed over the opposite knee. Gentle turn your body towards the bend knee side.

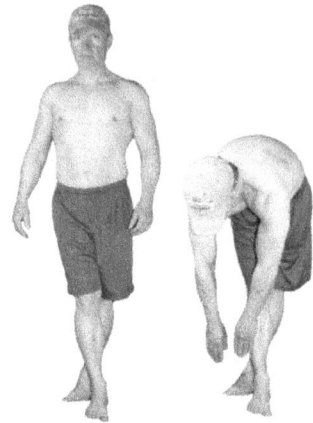

PIRIFORMIS STRETCH – STANDING

Stand with unaffected leg crossed in front of target side. Lean forward reaching for foot on target side until stretch is felt in the buttock.

Hip Flexors

_____ Reps _____ Sets _____X Day _____Hold		_____ Reps _____ Sets _____X Day _____Hold
31	Notes:	**32**	Notes:

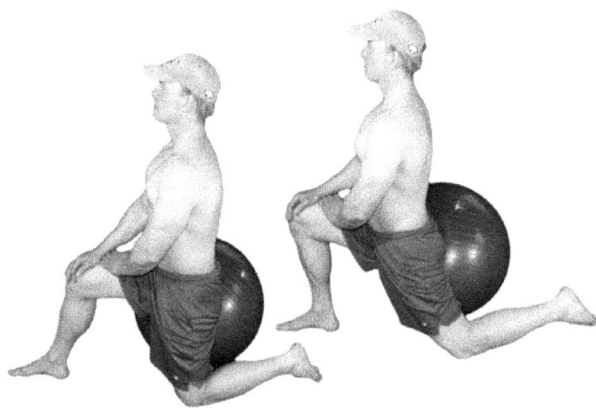

HIP FLEXOR STRETCH - SIDE OF BALL or CHAIR

Sit on edge of chair or ball. Bend your front knee (unaffected side) and lean forward until a stretch is felt along the front of the target hip.

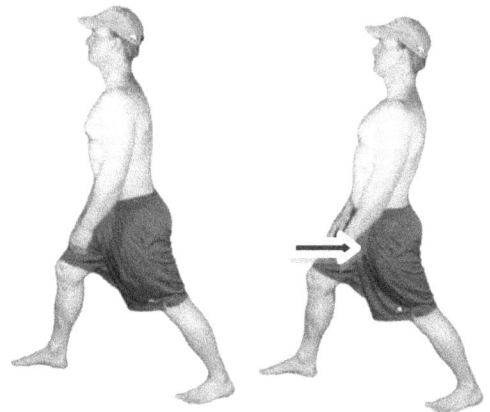

HIP FLEXOR STRETCH - STANDING

Stand and bend one knee forward (unaffected side) and the other in back. Stand up straight leaning slightly backward until a stretch is felt along the front of the target hip.

	_____ Reps _____ Sets _____ X Day _____ Hold
33	Notes:

HIP FLEXOR STRETCH - HALF KNEEL – with or without pad under knee

Begin in a half-kneeling position (you may want to use a pad or pillow for cushion). Bend your front knee (unaffected side) and lean forward until a stretch is felt along the front of the target hip.

	_____ Reps _____ Sets _____ X Day _____ Hold
34	Notes:

RUNNER'S STRETCH - MODIFIED

Stretch target leg in back and bend other knee in front. Bend your front knee (unaffected side) and lean forward until a stretch is felt along the front of the target hip.

	_____ Reps _____ Sets _____ X Day _____ Hold
35	Notes:

HIP FLEXOR STRETCH – SUPINE

Lie on a table, high bed or matt and let the affected leg lower towards the floor until a stretch is felt along the front of your thigh.

	_____ Reps _____ Sets _____ X Day _____ Hold
36	Notes:

HIP FLEXOR STRETCH – SUPINE

Lie on a table, high bed or matt and let the affected leg lower towards the floor until a stretch is felt along the front of your thigh. At the same time, grasp your opposite knee and pull it towards your chest.

Quadriceps (Quad)

	_____ Reps _____ Sets _____X Day _____Hold
37	**Notes:**

QUAD STRETCH - SIDELYING

Lie on your side and reach back holding the top of your foot with bent knee until a stretch is felt.

	_____ Reps _____ Sets _____X Day _____Hold
38	**Notes:**

QUAD STRETCH - STANDING

Stand straight up and bend your knee in back holding your ankle/foot. Gently pull your knee/thigh back in alignment with the standing leg.

Adductor

	_____ Reps _____ Sets _____X Day _____Hold
39	**Notes:**

One Leg

Both Legs

KNEE FALL OUT STRETCH or FROG STRETCH

Lie on your back with one knee bent. Slowly lower your knee to the side as you stretch the inner thigh/hip area. Frog Stretch: Let both knees fall to the side at the same time.

	_____ Reps _____ Sets _____X Day _____Hold
40	**Notes:**

BUTTERFLY STRETCH

Sit on the floor or mat and bend your knees placing the bottom of your feet together. Slowly let your knees lower towards the floor until a stretch is felt at your inner thighs.

_____ Reps _____ Sets _____ X Day _____ Hold		_____ Reps _____ Sets _____ X Day _____ Hold

41 | Notes: | **42** | Notes:

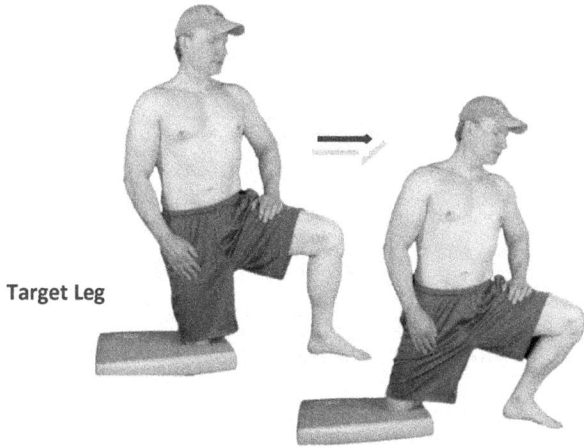

HIP ADDUCTOR STRECH – KNEELING

Kneel down on your target side knee. Place the opposite leg directly out to the side. Lean towards the side as you bend the knee for a stretch to the inner thigh of the target leg.

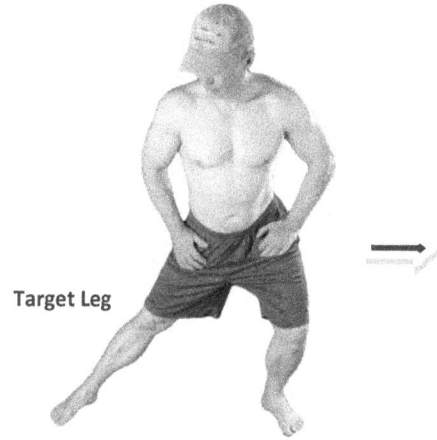

HIP ADDUCTOR STRECH - STANDING

Stand with feet spread wide apart. Slowly bend your knee to allow for a gentle stretch of the opposite leg. Maintain a straight knee on the target leg the entire time. You should feel a stretch on the inner thigh.

External Rotation / Internal Rotation

_____ Reps _____ Sets _____ X Day _____ Hold		_____ Reps _____ Sets _____ X Day _____ Hold

43 | Notes: | **44** | Notes:

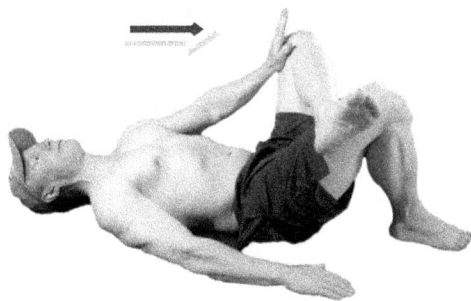

HIP EXTERNAL ROTATION STRETCH - SUPINE

Lie on your back with your leg crossed over your knee. Use your hand and push the crossed knee away from you.

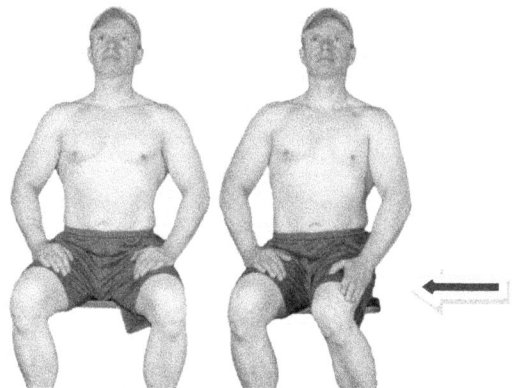

HIP INTERNAL ROTATION STRETCH - SEATED

Sit on a chair with your legs spread apart and feet planted on the ground. Use your hand to draw your knee inward as shown.

Iliotibial Band (IT Band)

	_____ Reps _____ Sets _____X Day _____Hold		_____ Reps _____ Sets _____X Day _____Hold
45	Notes:	**46**	Notes:

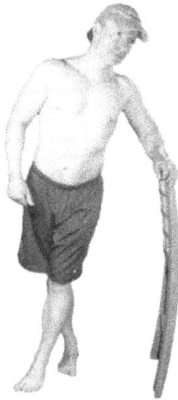

IT BAND STRETCH - STANDING

Stand and cross the target leg behind your unaffected leg. Lean forward and towards the unaffected side while using your arm for balance support.

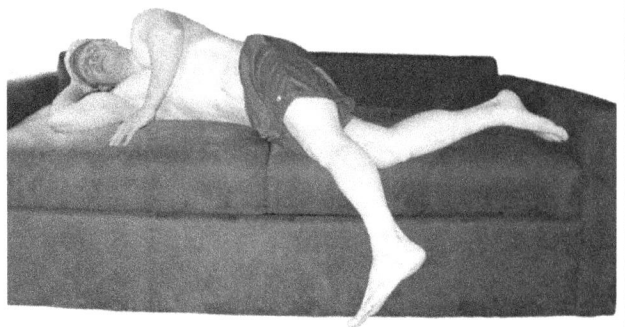

IT BAND STRETCH -- SIDELYING

Lie on bed or couch on unaffected side with target side towards ceiling. Bend lower leg for support. Allow upper leg to drop over side of bed. Keep knee straight and point toe towards floor. May need to roll upper hip backwards in order to feel stretch on side of hip/thigh/knee.

NECK

	_____ Reps _____ Sets _____X Day _____Hold		_____ Reps _____ Sets _____X Day _____Hold
47	Notes:	**48**	Notes:

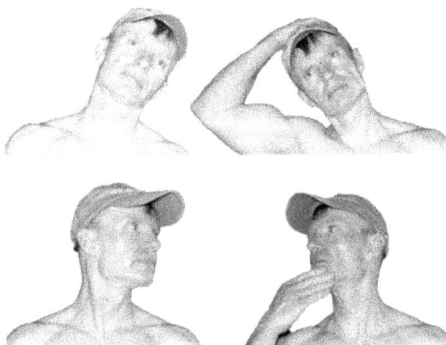

NECK ROTATION and SIDE BENDS

SIDE BENDS: (_Top_) Tilt your head as if you are trying to touch your ear to your shoulder. For extra stretch gently use your hand to increase range and hold.
ROTATION: (_Bottom_) Turn your head to the side as if looking over your shoulder. For an extra stretch gently use your hand on your chin to increase range and hold.

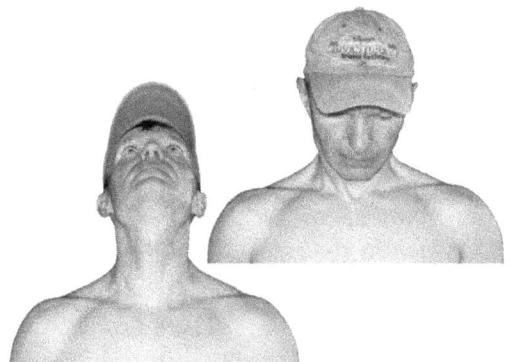

NECK FLEXION AND EXTENSION

EXTENSION: Look up as if you are looking at the sky moving your neck only.
FLEXION: Look down as if you are looking at the floor. For an extra stretch gently put both hands behind your head to move chin towards the chest and hold.

BACK	

_____ Reps _____ Sets _____X Day _____Hold	_____ Reps _____ Sets _____X Day _____Hold
49 Notes:	**50** Notes:

TRUNK FLEXION - SEATED

Sit and cross your arms over your chest. Slowly curl your back forward in order to round your upper back.

LOW BACK STRETCH - SEATED

Sit and slowly bend forward reaching your hands for the floor. Bend your trunk and head forward and down.

_____ Reps _____ Sets _____X Day _____Hold	_____ Reps _____ Sets _____X Day _____Hold
51 Notes:	**52** Notes:

LOW BACK STRETCH – STANDING - STRAIGHT & LATERAL

Stand in front of a table / chair or other surface and bend forward at the waist. Support yourself with your hands on a surface.

Reach to the side for a lateral bend (see #53)

LOW BACK STRETCH – RAIL OR DOORKNOB

Hold onto doorknob, rail or other unmovable surface and pull while moving hips back and hold.

_____ Reps _____ Sets _____X Day _____Hold

53 Notes:

Lateral

Straight

PRAYER STRETCH and LATERAL

STRAIGHT: Start on your hands and knees. Slowly lower your buttocks towards your feet until a stretch is felt along your back and or buttocks.

LATERAL: Start on your hands and knees. Slowly lower your buttocks towards your feet. Lower your chest towards the floor as you reach out towards the side.

_____ Reps _____ Sets _____X Day _____Hold

54 Notes:

PRAYER STRETCH - EXERCISE BALL

Kneel with an exercise ball in front of you. Slowly lean forward and roll the ball forward until a stretch is felt.

*Can do lateral movement as in #53

_____ Reps _____ Sets _____X Day _____Hold

55 Notes:

CAT AND CAMEL

Start on your hands and knees. Raise up your back and arch it towards the ceiling (cat). Return to a lowered position and arch your back the opposite direction (camel).

_____ Reps _____ Sets _____X Day _____Hold

56 Notes:

Both Legs

One Leg

KNEE TO CHEST STRETCH - SINGLE and BILATERAL

BILATERAL: Lie on your back and hold your knees while pulling up towards your chest and hold.
SINGLE: Lie on your back and hold your knee while pulling up towards your chest and hold. Opposite leg can be straight or bent.

Trunk Extension

_____ Reps _____ Sets _____ X Day _____ Hold

57 | Notes:

PRONE ON ELBOWS

Lie on your stomach. Slowly press up and prop yourself up on your elbows. Keep hips on floor/mat.

_____ Reps _____ Sets _____ X Day _____ Hold

58 | Notes:

PRESS UPS

Lie on your stomach. Slowly press up and arch your back using your arms. Keep hips on floor/mat.

Trunk Rotation

_____ Reps _____ Sets _____ X Day _____ Hold

59 | Notes:

TRUNK ROTATION STRETCH – SINGLE LEG

Lie on your back with arms to the sides. Bend one knee and then raise it up and across your body. Allow your trunk to rotate for a gentle stretch to the spine. Hold and then repeat.

_____ Reps _____ Sets _____ X Day _____ Hold

60 | Notes:

LOWER TRUNK ROTATIONS – BILATERAL

Lie on your back with your knees bent and gently move your knees side-to-side.

	_____ Reps _____ Sets _____ X Day _____ Hold
61	Notes:

TRUNK ROTATION - SEATED

Sit up as tall with erect posture. Rotate in one direction, using your hand to press against the opposite thigh to aide in further rotation. Exhale to increase the rotation and stretch. Return to the starting position, maintain an upright posture -repeat in the opposite direction.

	_____ Reps _____ Sets _____ X Day _____ Hold
62	Notes:

TRUNK ROTATION - STANDING or SEATED – DOWEL

Stand or sit holding dowel in hands. Slowly rotate trunk in one direction and then in the opposite direction.

Lateral

	_____ Reps _____ Sets _____ X Day _____ Hold
63	Notes:

LATERAL TRUNK STRETCH - SINGLE
SEATED or STANDING

Raise your arm and bend to the opposite side for a stretch. Hold and repeat with opposite arm.

	_____ Reps _____ Sets _____ X Day _____ Hold
64	Notes:

LATERAL TRUNK STRETCH - BILATERAL
SEATED or STANDING

Clasp hands together and raise arms over head. Bend to one side. Hold and repeat in opposite direction.

Shoulder Flexion

_____ Reps _____ Sets _____X Day _____Hold	_____ Reps _____ Sets _____X Day _____Hold
65 Notes:	**66** Notes:

FLEXION - SUPINE - DOWEL

Lie on your back and hold a dowel/cane. Slowly raise the dowel overhead.

*If you have a weak or injured arm, you can use your unaffected arm to assist with the movement.

WALL WALK

Place your target hand on the wall with the palm facing the wall. Walk your fingers up the wall towards overhead. Slide or walk your hand back down the wall to the starting position.

_____ Reps _____ Sets _____X Day _____Hold	_____ Reps _____ Sets _____X Day _____Hold
67 Notes:	**68** Notes:

FLEXION - TABLE SLIDE

Sit or stand and rest your target arm on a table and gently slide it forward and then back.

FLEXION - TABLE SLIDE - BALL

Stand and rest your target arm on top of a ball on a table. Gently roll the ball forward and then back.

Shoulder External Rotation (ER)

	_____ Reps _____ Sets _____X Day _____Hold
69	**Notes:**

	_____ Reps _____ Sets _____X Day _____Hold
70	**Notes:**

Starting
Position

EXTERNAL ROTATION - SUPINE – DOWEL
INTERNAL ROTATION ON OPPOSITE ARM

Lie on your back holding a dowel/cane with both hands. On the target side, maintain approx. 90-degree bend at the elbow with your arm approximately 30-45 degrees away from your side. Use your other arm to push the dowel/cane to rotate the affected arm back into a stretch. Hold and then return to starting position. Repeat

EXTERNAL ROTATION - 90-90 - DOWEL

Lie on your back and hold a dowel with your elbows out to the side and rested down. Roll your arms back towards overhead until a stretch is felt. Keep elbows bent at a 90-degree angle.

	_____ Reps _____ Sets _____X Day _____Hold
71	**Notes:**

	_____ Reps _____ Sets _____X Day _____Hold
72	**Notes:**

EXTERNAL ROTATION – SEATED – DOWEL
INTERNAL ROTATION ON OPPOSITE ARM

Using the unaffected arm, push the dowel into the hand of the target arm. Keep the arm at a 90-degree angle and push until a stretch is felt. Hold and repeat.

EXTERNAL ROTATION – STANDING – DOWEL
INTERNAL ROTATION ON OPPOSITE ARM

Using the unaffected arm, push the dowel into the hand of the target arm. Keep the arm at a 90-degree angle and push until a stretch is felt. Hold and repeat.

Shoulder Internal Rotation (IR) - *also see #69, 71, 72*

	_____ Reps _____ Sets _____X Day _____Hold		_____ Reps _____ Sets _____X Day _____Hold
73	Notes:	**74**	Notes:

INTERNAL ROTATION – TOWEL OR STRAP

Hold one end of the towel in front and with the target arm behind your back. Gently pull up your target arm behind your back with the assist of a towel.

INTERNAL ROTATION – DOWEL

Hold a dowel/cane behind your back. Slowly pull the target arm towards the center of your back.

Shoulder Abduction

	_____ Reps _____ Sets _____X Day _____Hold		_____ Reps _____ Sets _____X Day _____Hold
75	Notes:	**76**	Notes:

ABDUCTION - TABLE SLIDE - BALL

Stand and rest your target arm on top of a ball on a table and gently roll it to the side and back.

ABDUCTION WITH DOWEL

Hold a dowel/cane in front. Slowly push the dowel of the unaffected arm towards the target arm upward and to the side.

Shoulder Extension

_____ Reps _____ Sets _____X Day _____Hold		_____ Reps _____ Sets _____X Day _____Hold	
77	Notes:	**78**	Notes:

LYING DOWN EXTENSION - TABLE or BED

Lie on your back and gently let target arm drop off table or bed.

WAND EXTENSION - STANDING

Stand and hold a dowel/cane. Use the unaffected arm to help push the target arm back. The elbow should remain straight the entire time.

Chest/Pec Stretch

_____ Reps _____ Sets _____X Day _____Hold		_____ Reps _____ Sets _____X Day _____Hold	
79	Notes:	**80**	Notes:

CHEST STRETCH – SEATED, STANDING, or SUPINE

TOP: Bend arms at a 90-degree angle. Move elbows back until feeling a stretch in front of shoulders/chest.

BOTTOM: Clasp hands in back of head. Move elbows back until feeling a stretch in front of shoulders/chest.

CHEST STRETCH - STEP THROUGH

Stand with arms in doorway at a 90-degree angle. Step through until you feel a stretch through the chest and hold. Keep shoulders down and back. Take another step to increase stretch.

Triceps

	_____ Reps _____ Sets _____ X Day _____ Hold		_____ Reps _____ Sets _____ X Day _____ Hold

81	Notes:	82	Notes: *Lymphedema: Do not wrap band around UE or LE

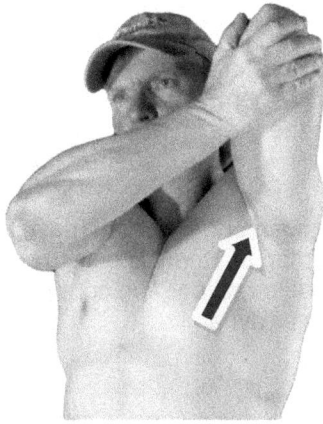

TRICEP STRETCH

With your target elbow bent and shoulder raised, use your other hand and gently push your target elbow back towards overhead until a stretch is felt.

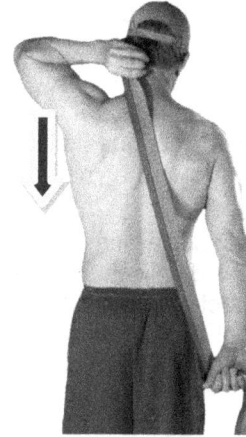

TRICEP STRETCH - STRAP or TOWEL

Hold strap of target arm with your hand above your head. Use the other hand to pull downward on the strap, allowing the elbow to bend until a stretch is in the back of the arm.

Posterior Capsule

	_____ Reps _____ Sets _____ X Day _____ Hold		_____ Reps _____ Sets _____ X Day _____ Hold

83	Notes:	84	Notes:

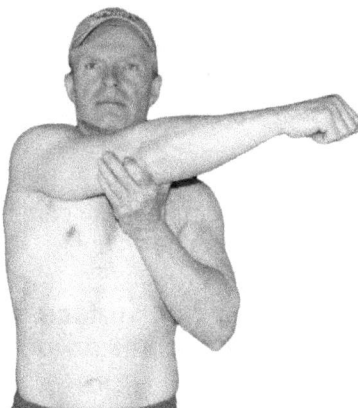

POSTERIOR SHOULDER/DELTOID RELEASE

Bring your target arm across your body. Use the opposite hand to grasp the back of your shoulder and further pull the arm. Hold.

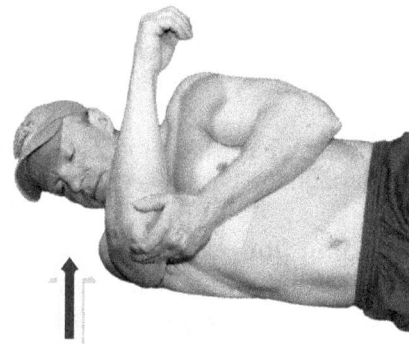

POSTERIOR CAPSULE STRETCH

Lie on your side and grasp the elbow of the arm closest to the floor. Gently pull it upward and across the front of your body.

Core/Stability Training

Core strengthening is the foundation of all the other exercises that follow, especially balance. Core training is not only an important step in conditioning, but also helps other issues, including neurological, orthopedic, weight, or overall weakness

The core includes muscles of the thoraco-lumbar spine (trunk), cervical spine., erector spinae, abdomen, pelvis, shoulder/scapulae, and your lower lats.

Static core functionality is the ability of one's core to align the skeleton to resist a force that does not change. The core is used to stabilize the thorax and the pelvis during dynamic movement. The nature of dynamic movement must consider our skeletal structure (as a lever) in addition to the force of external resistance and consequently incorporates a vastly different complex of muscles and joints versus a static position.

The core is traditionally assumed to originate most full-body functional movement, including most sports. In addition, the core determines to a large part a person's posture. In all, human anatomy is built to take force upon the bones and direct autonomic force, through various joints, in the desired direction. The core muscles align the spine, ribs, and pelvis of a person to resist a specific force, whether static or dynamic.
(Wikipedia: *https://en.wikipedia.org/wiki/Core_(anatomy)*

These muscles work as stabilizers for the entire body. Core training is simply doing specific exercises to develop and strengthen these stabilizer muscles. If any of these core muscles are weakened, it could result in lower back pain or a protruding waistline. Keeping these core muscles strong can do wonders for your posture and help give you more strength in other exercises like running and walking.
(Bodybuilding.com - *https://www.bodybuilding.com/fun/mielke12.htm*)

There is a saying 'form follows function'. This is especially true with core stability and how it affects your balance. Gravity influences all movement, so effective core training must be done against gravity. The rectus abdominus muscle that you are isolating with those crunches flexes the spine/abs only when you are lying on your back or returning the torso to an upright position from hyperextension in standing. "In the upright position, flexion is controlled by eccentric contraction of the back extensors as the lower the weight of the torso in the same direction as gravity". (*Bryant & Green, 2003, p. 84*)

Being able to engage the core with not only your balance exercises but also arm and leg exercises will help prevent injury.

Step 1: First learn to brace the abdomen *(see pictures 1 and 2 on next page)* Think of this as trying to either brace for a punch to the stomach or trying to put on a tight pair of pants (not just sucking in your stomach)

Step 2: After getting a good feel for bracing, try doing a pelvic tilt *(see pictures 3 and 4 on next page)* and then progress to bridging *(see picture 5)*

Step 3: These two basic movements should be done while you progress your abdominal and core training, continuing through the balance section, and to some extent with arm and leg strengthening.

*** When doing floor work, such as crunches, make sure you are on a soft surface, such as a mat, Bosu, stability ball, etc. Pushing your back into a hard surface, such as a wood floor, can do more damage than good to the spine.

*** Breathe – Never hold your breath.

EXERCISE Core / Stability	EXERCISE NUMBER	NOTES
ABDOMINAL BRACING TRAINING	1	
ABDOMINAL BRACING - SUPINE	2	
PELVIC TILT - SUPINE	3	
PELVIC TILT - KNEELING	4	
BRIDGING	5	
BRIDGE - BOSU	6	
BRIDGING WITH PILLOW SQUEEZE	7	
BRIDGING WITH PILLOW SQUEEZE - BOSU	8	
BRACE SUPINE MARCHING / BRIDGE LEG UP	9	
BRIDGE LEG UP - BOSU -	10	
SINGLE LEG BRIDGE	11	
BRIDGE SINGLE LEG - BOSU	12	
BRIDGING CROSSED LEG	13	
BRIDGING CROSSED LEG – BOSU	14	
BRIDGING CROSSED LEG - ARMS UP	15	
BRIDGING CROSSED LEG - ARMS UP - BOSU	16	
BRIDGE - ELASTIC BAND	17	
BRIDGING - ABDUCTION - ELASTIC BAND	18	
FLOOR BRIDGE - EXERCISE BALL	19	
FLOOR BRIDGE ALTERNATE LEG LIFT - EXERCISE BALL	20	
BRIDGE UPPER BACK - EXERCISE BALL	21	
BRIDGE UPPER BACK - SINGLE LEG - EXERCISE BALL	22	
QUADRUPED ALTERNATE ARM	23	
QUADRUPED ALTERNATE LEG	24	
QUADRUPED ALTERNATE ARM AND LEG	25	
BIRD DOG ELBOW TOUCHES	26	

EXERCISE Core / Stability	EXERCISE NUMBER	NOTES
PRONE BALL	27	
PRONE BALL - ALTERNATE ARM	28	
PRONE BALL - ALTERNATE LEG	29	
PRONE BALL - ALTERNATE ARM AND LEG	30	
MODIFIED PLANK	31	
MODIFIED PLANK - ALTERNATE LEG	32	
FULL PLANK	33	
PLANK - ALTERNATE ARMS	34	
PLANK - ALTERNATE LEGS	35	
PLANK - EXERCISE BALL	36	
PRONE ON ELBOWS	37	
PRESS UPS	38	
SKYDIVER	39	
PRONE SUPERMAN - BOSU	40	
TRUNK EXTENSION - BOSU	41	
TRUNK EXTENSION - HANDS CROSSED IN FRONT - BOSU	43	
SUPERMAN - ARMS BACK- EXERCISE BALL	44	
SUPERMAN – BOTH ARMS IN FRONT - EXERCISE BALL	45	
SUPERMAN – ONE ARM FORWARD / ONE ARM BACK - EXERCISE BALL	46	
LATERAL PLANK MODIFIED	47	
LATERAL PLANK MODIFIED- BOSU	48	
LATERAL PLANK - 1 KNEE 1 FOOT	49	
LATERAL PLANK - 1 KNEE 1 FOOT – BOSU	50	
LATERAL PLANK	51	
LATERAL PLANK - BOSU	52	

EXERCISE Core / Stability	EXERCISE NUMBER	NOTES
LEAN BACK	53	
LEAN BACK - BOSU	54	
LEAN BACK WITH ARMS OUT	55	
LEAN BACK WITH ARMS OUT - BOSU	56	
LEAN BACK WITH TWIST	57	
LEAN BACK WITH TWIST – BOSU	58	
CRUNCHY FROG	59	
SEATED BIKE - FORWARD AND BACKWARDS	60	
CRUNCH – ARMS OUT	61	
CRUNCH – ARMS OUT - BOSU	62	
CRUNCH – ARMS IN BACK OF HEAD	63	
CRUNCH – ARMS IN BACK OF HEAD - BOSU	64	
OBLIQUE CRUNCH	65	
OBLIQUE CRUNCH - BOSU	66	
90 DEGREE CRUNCH	67	
BALL CRUNCH – Can put legs on seat of chair	68	
CURL UPS – ARMS ON LEGS - EXERCISE BALL	69	
CURL UPS- ARMS CROSSED IN FRONT - EXERCISE BALL	70	
CURL UPS – ARMS BEHIND HEAD - EXERCISE BALL	71	
SUPINE CRUNCH TOUCH - EXERCISE BALL	72	
LOWER ABDOMINAL CRUNCH – WITH or WITHOUT BALL	73	
HIGH MARCH CRUNCH	74	
STANDING SIDE CRUNCH	75	
STANDING BIKE CRUNCH	76	

Core/Abdominal

Abdominal Bracing – Pelvic Tilt

	_____ Reps _____ Sets _____ X Day _____ Hold
1	**Notes:**

ABDOMINAL BRACING TRAINING

Press your fingertips into your relaxed abdomen lateral of your navel. Tighten and brace your abdomen so that the muscles push your fingertips away from the center of your body. Hold, relax and repeat.
Think of this as trying to either brace for a punch to the stomach or trying to put on a tight pair of pants (not just sucking in your stomach)

	_____ Reps _____ Sets _____ X Day _____ Hold
2	**Notes:**

Starting
Position

ABDOMINAL BRACING - SUPINE

Lie on your back. Tighten your stomach muscles as you draw your navel down towards the floor.

Think of this as trying to either brace for a punch to the stomach or trying to put on a tight pair of pants (not just sucking in your stomach)

	_____ Reps _____ Sets _____ X Day _____ Hold
3	**Notes:**

Starting

Position

PELVIC TILT - SUPINE

Lie on your back with your knees bent. Next, arch your low back and then flatten it repeatedly (bracing as above). Your pelvis should tilt forward and back during the movement. Move through a comfortable range of motion.

	_____ Reps _____ Sets _____ X Day _____ Hold
4	**Notes:**

Starting
Position

PELVIC TILT - KNEELING

Kneel on the floor (you can kneel on a pillow or pad if needed). Arch your lower back and then flatten it repeatedly (bracing as above). Your pelvis should tilt forward and back during the movement. Move through a comfortable range of motion.

Bridging

_____ Reps _____ Sets _____ X Day _____ Hold	_____ Reps _____ Sets _____ X Day _____ Hold

5	Notes:	6	Notes:

Starting

Position

BRIDGING

Lie on your back. Tighten your lower abdominals (as with abdominal bracing), squeeze your buttocks and then raise your buttocks off the floor/bed. Hold and then lower yourself slowly and repeat. Brace the stomach muscles to keep your spine from moving, trying to keep the pelvis level the entire time.

Starting

Position

BRIDGE - BOSU – Can use foam pad, stair step or box

Lie on your back with your feet planted on top of the Bosu and knees bent. Lift up your buttocks as shown. Hold and then lower yourself slowly and repeat.
Brace the stomach muscles to keep your spine from moving, trying to keep the pelvis level the entire time.

_____ Reps _____ Sets _____ X Day _____ Hold	_____ Reps _____ Sets _____ X Day _____ Hold

7	Notes:	8	Notes:

Starting

Position

BRIDGING WITH PILLOW SQUEEZE - Use pillow, ball or rolled towel between knees

Lie on your back and place a pillow, towel roll or ball between your knees and squeeze. Hold this and then tighten your lower abdominals, squeeze your buttocks and raise your buttocks off the floor/bed. Brace the stomach muscles to keep your spine from moving, trying to keep the pelvis level.

Starting

Position

BRIDGING WITH PILLOW SQUEEZE - BOSU - Can use foam pad, stair step or box

Lie on your back with your feet planted on top of the Bosu and knees bent. Place a pillow, towel roll or ball between your knees and squeeze. Lift up your buttocks as shown. Hold and then lower yourself slowly and repeat. Brace the stomach muscles to keep your spine from moving, trying to keep the pelvis level.

	_____ Reps _____ Sets _____ X Day _____ Hold

9 | **Notes:**

Starting
Position

BRACE SUPINE MARCHING / BRIDGE LEG UP

Lie on your back with your knees bent, slowly lift up one foot a few inches and then set it back down. Perform on your other leg. Brace the stomach muscles to keep your spine from moving, trying to keep the pelvis level the entire time.

*To increase challenge, go into bridge position as with #5, then continue march – can bring leg higher to advance

	_____ Reps _____ Sets _____ X Day _____ Hold

10 | **Notes:**

Starting
Position

BRIDGE LEG UP - BOSU - Can use foam pad, stair step or box

Lie on your back with your feet planted on top of the Bosu and knees bent. Slowly lift up one foot a few inches and then set it back down. Next, perform on your other leg. Brace the stomach muscles to keep your spine from moving, trying to keep the pelvis level the entire time. *To increase challenge, go into bridge position as with #6, then continue march – can bring leg higher to advance

	_____ Reps _____ Sets _____ X Day _____ Hold

11 | **Notes:**

Starting
Position

SINGLE LEG BRIDGE

Lie on your back, raise your buttocks off the floor/bed into a bridge position. Straighten a leg so that only one leg is supporting your body. Then, return that leg back to the ground and change to the other side. Brace the stomach muscles to keep your spine from moving, trying to keep the pelvis level the entire time.

	_____ Reps _____ Sets _____ X Day _____ Hold

12 | **Notes:**

Starting
Position

BRIDGE SINGLE LEG - BOSU - can use foam pad, stair step or box

Lie on your back with your feet planted on top of the Bosu and knees bent, lift up your buttocks and then straighten one knee in the air. Return that leg back to the ground and change to the other side. Brace the stomach muscles to keep your spine from moving, trying to keep the pelvis level the entire time.

	_____ Reps _____ Sets _____ X Day _____ Hold
13	**Notes:**

Starting Position

BRIDGING CROSSED LEG

Lie on your back, cross your leg. Tighten your lower abdomen, squeeze your buttocks and raise your buttocks off the floor/bed. Brace the stomach muscles to keep your spine from moving, trying to keep the pelvis level the entire time.

	_____ Reps _____ Sets _____ X Day _____ Hold
14	**Notes:**

Starting Position

BRIDGING CROSSED LEG – BOSU - can use foam pad, stair step or box

Lie on your back with your feet planted on top of the Bosu cross your leg. Tighten your lower abdomen, squeeze your buttocks and raise your buttocks. Brace the stomach muscles to keep your spine from moving, trying to keep the pelvis level the entire time.

	_____ Reps _____ Sets _____ X Day _____ Hold
15	**Notes:**

Starting Position

BRIDGING CROSSED LEG - ARMS UP

Lie on your back, cross your leg and put your hands together as shown. Next, tighten your lower abdomen, squeeze your buttocks and raise your buttocks off the floor/bed. Brace the stomach muscles to keep your spine from moving, trying to keep the pelvis level the entire time.

	_____ Reps _____ Sets _____ X Day _____ Hold
16	**Notes:**

BRIDGING CROSSED LEG - ARMS UP - BOSU - can use foam pad, stair step or box

Lie on your back with your feet planted on top of the Bosu and hands together and leg crossed. Tighten your lower abdomen, squeeze your buttocks and raise your buttocks. Brace the stomach muscles to keep your spine from moving, trying to keep the pelvis level.

_____ Reps _____ Sets _____ X Day _____ Hold

17 Notes:

Starting

Position

BRIDGE - ELASTIC BAND

Lie on your back, hold an elastic band down around your waist for resistance. Tighten your lower abdomen, squeeze your buttocks and then raise your buttocks off the floor/bed. Brace the stomach muscles to keep your spine from moving, trying to keep the pelvis level the entire time.

_____ Reps _____ Sets _____ X Day _____ Hold

18 Notes:

Starting

Position

BRIDGING - ABDUCTION - ELASTIC BAND – can be done with feet on BOSU, foam, stair step or box

Lie on your back, place an elastic band around your knees and pull your knees apart. Hold this and then tighten your lower abdomen, squeeze your buttocks and raise your buttocks off the floor/bed. Brace the stomach muscles to keep your spine from moving, trying to keep the pelvis level the entire time.

_____ Reps _____ Sets _____ X Day _____ Hold

19 Notes:

Starting

Position

FLOOR BRIDGE - EXERCISE BALL

Lie on the floor, place an exercise ball under your lower legs and then raise up your buttocks. Hold and repeat. Brace the stomach muscles to keep your spine from moving, trying to keep the pelvis level the entire time.

_____ Reps _____ Sets _____ X Day _____ Hold

20 Notes:

Starting

Position

FLOOR BRIDGE ALTERNATE LEG LIFT - EXERCISE BALL

Lie on the floor, place an exercise ball under your lower legs and then raise up your buttocks. While holding this position raise up a leg off the ball towards the ceiling then lower back to the ball and alternate to lift the other leg. Brace the stomach muscles to keep your spine from moving, trying to keep the pelvis level.

_____ Reps _____ Sets _____ X Day _____ Hold	_____ Reps _____ Sets _____ X Day _____ Hold
21 Notes:	**22** Notes:

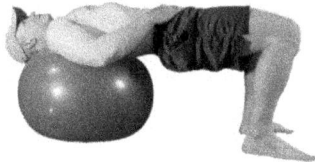

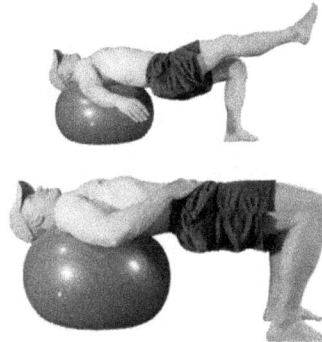

Starting

Position

BRIDGE UPPER BACK - EXERCISE BALL

Start in a seated position on the ball and slowly walk your feet forward so that the ball is on your upper back. Keep your buttocks and pelvis up off the ball and straight with your thighs. Brace the stomach muscles to keep your spine from moving, trying to keep the pelvis level the entire time.
*To increase the challenge, you can do a supine march or perform some arm exercises, such as Fly's or Chest Presses (*See Upper Extremity exercises*)

BRIDGE UPPER BACK - SINGLE LEG - EXERCISE BALL

Start in a seated position on the ball and slowly walk your feet forward so that the ball is on your upper back. Keep your buttocks and pelvis up off the ball and straight with your thighs. Raise up one leg so that you straighten your knee in the air. Return it back to the floor and then switch to raise up the other side. Brace the stomach muscles to keep your spine from moving, trying to keep the pelvis level the entire time.

Quadruped

_____ Reps _____ Sets _____ X Day _____ Hold	_____ Reps _____ Sets _____ X Day _____ Hold
23 Notes:	**24** Notes:

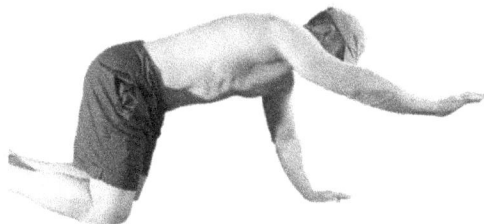

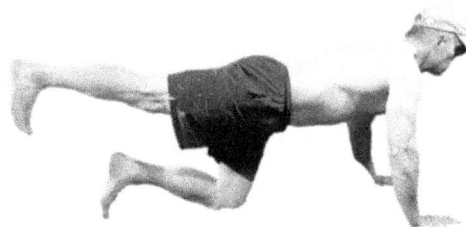

QUADRUPED ALTERNATE ARM

While in a crawling position, slowly raise up an arm out in front of you.

QUADRUPED ALTERNATE LEG

While in a crawling position, slowly draw your leg back behind you as you straighten your knee. Either repeat on same side or alternate.

_____ Reps _____ Sets _____ X Day _____ Hold

25 Notes:

QUADRUPED ALTERNATE ARM AND LEG

While in a crawling position, brace at your abdominals and then slowly lift a leg and opposite arm upwards. Maintain a level and stable pelvis and spine the entire time. Either repeat on same side or alternate.

_____ Reps _____ Sets _____ X Day _____ Hold

26 Notes:

Touch your elbow to your opposite knee

Starting Position

BIRD DOG ELBOW TOUCHES

While in a crawling position, slowly lift your leg and opposite arm upwards. When returning your arm and leg down, do not touch the floor but instead touch your elbow to your opposite knee and lift and straighten them again. Then set them down on the floor. Either repeat on same side or alternate.

_____ Reps _____ Sets _____ X Day _____ Hold

27 Notes:

PRONE BALL

Lie face down over a ball, support your self with your feet and hands.

_____ Reps _____ Sets _____ X Day _____ Hold

28 Notes:

PRONE BALL - ALTERNATE ARM

Lie face down over a ball, support your self with your feet and hands. Next, slowly raise up one arm. Return arm back to floor and then raise up the other arm. Keep alternating arms.

_____ Reps _____ Sets _____X Day _____Hold		_____ Reps _____ Sets _____X Day _____Hold

29	Notes:	30	Notes:

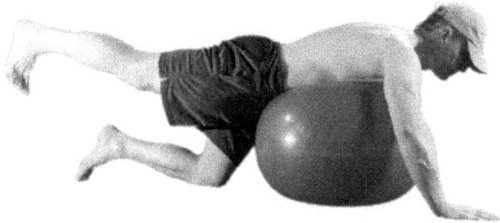

PRONE BALL - ALTERNATE LEG

Lie face down over a ball, support yourself with your arms and legs. Next slowly raise up a leg. Return leg back to floor and then raise up the other leg.

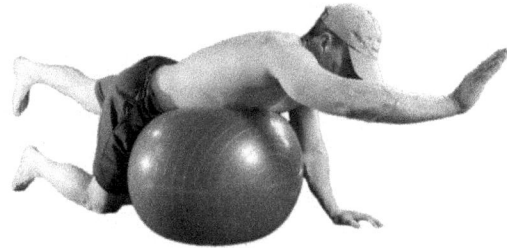

PRONE BALL - ALTERNATE ARM AND LEG

Lie face down over a ball, support yourself with your feet and hands. Next, slowly raise up one arm and opposite leg. Return arm and leg back to floor and then raise up the opposite arm/leg.

Plank

_____ Reps _____ Sets _____X Day _____Hold		_____ Reps _____ Sets _____X Day _____Hold

31	Notes:	32	Notes:

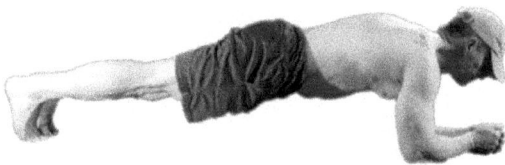

MODIFIED PLANK

Lie face down, lift your body up on your elbows and toes. Try and maintain a straight spine the entire time. Do not allow your low back sag downward.

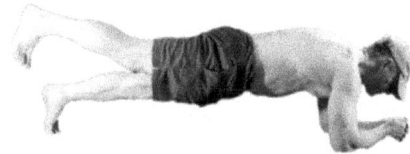

Starting

Position

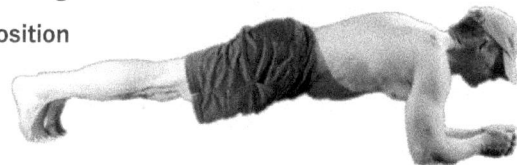

MODIFIED PLANK - ALTERNATE LEG

Lie face down, lift your body up on your elbows and toes. Next, lift one leg off the ground and then set it back down. Then repeat on the other leg. Try and maintain a straight spine the entire time.

_____ Reps _____ Sets _____X Day _____Hold

33 | Notes:

FULL PLANK

Lie face down, lift your body up on your elbows and toes. Straighten your arms in full elbow extension and hold in full plank position. Do not let your back arch down. Try and maintain a straight spine the entire time.

_____ Reps _____ Sets _____X Day _____Hold

34 | Notes:

PLANK - ALTERNATE ARMS

Hold a plank position as previous (#33). Raise one arm out in front of you as shown. Return to the starting position and then raise your other arm out in front of you and repeat.
Try and maintain a straight spine the entire time.

_____ Reps _____ Sets _____X Day _____Hold

35 | Notes:

PLANK - ALTERNATE LEGS

Hold a plank position as previous (#33). Raise one leg off the floor as shown. Return to the starting position and then raise your other leg and repeat. Try and maintain a straight spine the entire time.

_____ Reps _____ Sets _____X Day _____Hold

36 | Notes:

PLANK - EXERCISE BALL

While kneeling on the floor with an exercise ball in front of you, place your elbows and hands on the ball and lift your body up. Try and maintain a straight spine. Do not allow your hips or pelvis on either side to drop.

Back Extension	

	_____ Reps _____ Sets _____ X Day _____ Hold		_____ Reps _____ Sets _____ X Day _____ Hold
37	Notes:	**38**	Notes:

PRONE ON ELBOWS

Lie face down, slowly press up and prop yourself up on your elbows.

PRESS UPS

Lie face down, slowly press up and arch your back using your arms.

	_____ Reps _____ Sets _____ X Day _____ Hold		_____ Reps _____ Sets _____ X Day _____ Hold
39	Notes:	**40**	Notes:

SKYDIVER

Lie face down with arms by your side. Next, lift your upper body, lower legs, thighs, and arms off the ground at the same time as shown. You can place a pillow under your stomach/hips for comfort.

PRONE SUPERMAN - BOSU

Lie face down over the Bosu. Slowly raise your arms and legs upward off the ground. Then lower slowly back to the ground.

_____ Reps _____ Sets _____X Day _____Hold

41   Notes:

Starting
Position

TRUNK EXTENSION - BOSU

Lie face down with your upper body on a Bosu and slowly raise your head and chest upwards as shown.
Your arms can be behind your back or alongside your body.

_____ Reps _____ Sets _____X Day _____Hold

42   Notes:

Starting
Position

TRUNK EXTENSION - HANDS BEHIND HEAD - BOSU

Lie face down with your upper body on a Bosu.
Touch the back of your head with both hands and slowly raise your head and chest upwards.

_____ Reps _____ Sets _____X Day _____Hold

43   Notes:

Starting
Position

TRUNK EXTENSION - HANDS CROSSED IN FRONT - BOSU

While lying face down with your upper body on a Bosu, slowly raise your head and chest upwards.
Keep your arms crossed on your chest as you perform.

_____ Reps _____ Sets _____X Day _____Hold

44   Notes:

SUPERMAN - ARMS BACK- EXERCISE BALL

Start in a kneeling position with an exercise ball in front of you. Roll forward so that you are face down on the ball with your feet on the ground and your stomach on the ball. Hold up your head and chest so that a straight line exists between your feet and head. Also bring your arms back along side of your body and hold this position.

_____ Reps	_____ Sets	_____ X Day	_____ Hold		_____ Reps	_____ Sets	_____ X Day _____ Hold

45	Notes:	46	Notes:

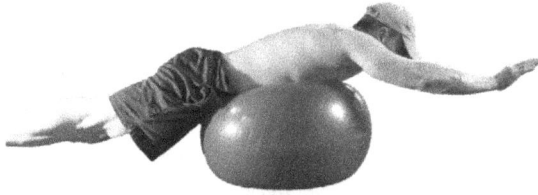

SUPERMAN – BOTH ARMS IN FRONT - EXERCISE BALL

Start in a kneeling position with an exercise ball in front of you. Next, roll forward so that you are face down on the ball with your feet on the ground and your stomach on the ball. Hold up your head and chest so that a straight line exists between your feet and head. Also bring your arms up and forward out in front of you and hold this position.

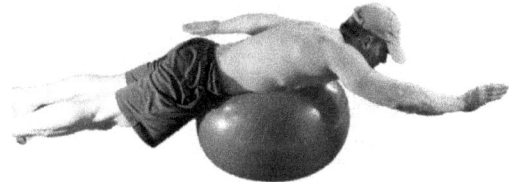

SUPERMAN – ONE ARM FORWARD / ONE ARM BACK - EXERCISE BALL

Start in a kneeling position with an exercise ball in front of you. Next, roll forward so that you are face down on the ball with your feet on the ground and your stomach on the ball. Hold up your head and chest so that a straight line exists between your feet and head. Raise one arm up and out in front of you as you bring the other arm back and along side your body as in a swimming motion.

Lateral Plank

_____ Reps _____ Sets _____ X Day _____ Hold	_____ Reps _____ Sets _____ X Day _____ Hold

47	Notes:	48	Notes:

Starting

Position

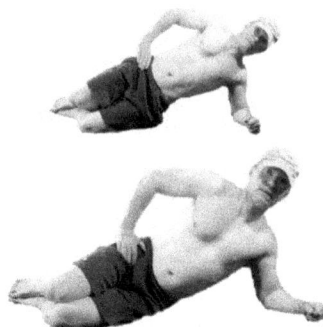

LATERAL PLANK MODIFIED

Lie on your side with your knees bent, lift your body up on your elbow and knees. Try and maintain a straight spine.

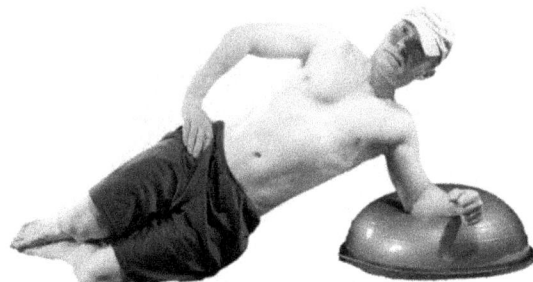

LATERAL PLANK MODIFIED- BOSU- can be anything unstable

Lie on your side with your knees bent and your elbow on the Bosu, lift your body up on your elbow and knees. Try and maintain a straight spine.

_____ Reps _____ Sets _____X Day _____Hold	_____ Reps _____ Sets _____X Day _____Hold

49   Notes: **50**   Notes:

LATERAL PLANK - 1 KNEE 1 FOOT

Lie on your side with bottom knee bent and top knee straight. Lift your body up on your elbow and knee on one side and foot on the other side. Try and maintain a straight spine.

LATERAL PLANK - 1 KNEE 1 FOOT – BOSU- Can be anything unstable

Lie on your side with elbow on Bosu with bottom knee bent and the top knee straight. Lift your body up on your elbow and knee on one side and foot on the other side. Try and maintain a straight spine.

_____ Reps _____ Sets _____X Day _____Hold	_____ Reps _____ Sets _____X Day _____Hold

51   Notes: **52**   Notes:

Starting Position

LATERAL PLANK

Lie on your side with both legs straight and lift your body up on your elbow and feet. Try and maintain a straight spine.

LATERAL PLANK - BOSU - Can be anything unstable

Lie on your side with your elbow on the Bosu and both legs straight. Lift your body up on your elbow and feet. Try and maintain a straight spine.

Backward Lean

	_____ Reps _____ Sets _____X Day _____Hold		_____ Reps _____ Sets _____X Day _____Hold
53	Notes:	**54**	Notes:

Starting
Position

LEAN BACK

Start in an upright seated position with knees bent. Hold onto thighs and lean back keeping spine as straight as possible.

Starting
Position

LEAN BACK - BOSU

Start in an upright seated position on Bosu with knees bent. Hold onto thighs or Bosu and lean back keeping spine as straight as possible.

	_____ Reps _____ Sets _____X Day _____Hold		_____ Reps _____ Sets _____X Day _____Hold
55	Notes:	**56**	Notes:

Starting
Position

LEAN BACK WITH ARMS OUT

Start in an upright seated position with knees bent. Hold arms straight out or overhead, brace core and lean back keeping spine as straight as possible

Starting
Position

LEAN BACK WITH ARMS OUT - BOSU

Start in an upright seated position on Bosu with knees bent. Hold arms straight out or overhead, brace core and lean back keeping spine as straight as possible.

	_____ Reps _____ Sets _____X Day _____Hold
57	Notes:

LEAN BACK WITH TWIST

Start in an upright seated position with knees bent. Hold arms straight out, brace core and lean back keeping spine as straight as possible. Rotate trunk/arms to one side and then repeat to the other side.

Starting Position

	_____ Reps _____ Sets _____X Day _____Hold
58	Notes:

LEAN BACK WITH TWIST – BOSU

Start in an upright seated position on Bosu with knees bent. Hold arms straight out, brace core and lean back keeping spine as straight as possible. Rotate trunk/arms to one side - repeat to the other side

Starting Position

	_____ Reps _____ Sets _____X Day _____Hold
59	Notes:

CRUNCHY FROG

Sit on floor or edge of couch/bench. Lean back and with arms wide apart and legs straight. Next, bring knees towards chest and arms forward and return to starting position.

	_____ Reps _____ Sets _____X Day _____Hold
60	Notes:

SEATED BIKE - FORWARD AND BACKWARDS

Sit on floor and lean back. With arms on floor or off ground, peddle feet forward for 15-30 repetitions, rest and then reverse. *Progress by moving hands forward near hips or remove arm support*

Abdominal Crunch Variations

_____ Reps _____ Sets _____X Day _____Hold

61 Notes:

Starting Position

CRUNCH – ARMS OUT

Lie on your back with your arms outstretched forward, brace core and curl up lifting your shoulder blades off the ground. Exhale as you come up and squeeze/tighten your abdominal muscles.

_____ Reps _____ Sets _____X Day _____Hold

62 Notes:

Starting Position

CRUNCH – ARMS OUT - BOSU

Lie on your back on Bosu with your arms out-stretched forward, brace core and curl up lifting your shoulder blades off the ground. Exhale as you come up and squeeze/tighten your abdominal muscles.

_____ Reps _____ Sets _____X Day _____Hold

63 Notes:

Starting Position

CRUNCH – ARMS IN BACK OF HEAD

Lie on your back with your arms behind your head, brace core and curl up lifting your shoulder blades off the ground. Exhale as you come up and squeeze/tighten your abdominal muscles. Do not pull on your neck/head.

_____ Reps _____ Sets _____X Day _____Hold

64 Notes:

CRUNCH – ARMS IN BACK OF HEAD - BOSU

Lie on your back on Bosu with your arms behind your head, brace core and curl up lifting your shoulder blades off the ground. Exhale as you come up and squeeze/tighten your abdominal muscles. Do not pull on your neck/head.

_____ Reps _____ Sets _____X Day _____Hold

65   Notes:

OBLIQUE CRUNCH

Lie on your back with one or both hands in back of head. Brace core and curl up targeting elbow to opposite knee as shown. Keep shoulders off floor. Exhale as you come up and squeeze/tighten your abdominal muscles. Do not pull on your neck/head.

_____ Reps _____ Sets _____X Day _____Hold

66   Notes:

OBLIQUE CRUNCH - BOSU

Lie back on Bosu with one or both hands in back of head. Brace core and curl up targeting elbow to opposite knee as shown. Keep shoulders off Bosu. Exhale as you come up and squeeze/tighten your abdominal muscles. Do not pull on your neck/head.

_____ Reps _____ Sets _____X Day _____Hold

67   Notes:

90 DEGREE CRUNCH

Lie on your back with legs straight in air. Reach your hands towards toes, crunching shoulders off ground. Exhale as you come up and squeeze/tighten your abdominal muscles.

_____ Reps _____ Sets _____X Day _____Hold

68   Notes:

BALL CRUNCH – Can put legs on seat of chair

Lie on back with legs up on ball so knees and hips are at ~ 90 degrees. Cross hands over chest or behind head. Brace core and curl up lifting your shoulder blades off the ground. Exhale as you come up and squeeze/tighten your abdominal muscles. Do not pull on your neck/head.

_____ Reps _____ Sets _____ X Day _____ Hold

69 | Notes:

Starting
Position

CURL UPS – ARMS ON LEGS - EXERCISE BALL

While sitting on an exercise ball, roll forward so that your back lies against the ball. Put hands on thighs/legs. Brace core and curl up lifting your shoulder blades off the ball. Exhale as you come up and squeeze/tighten your abdominal muscles.

_____ Reps _____ Sets _____ X Day _____ Hold

70 | Notes:

CURL UPS- ARMS CROSSED IN FRONT - EXERCISE BALL

While sitting on an exercise ball, roll forward so that your back lies against the ball. Cross hands over your chest. Brace core and curl up lifting your shoulder blades off the ball. Exhale as you come up and squeeze/tighten your abdominal muscles.

_____ Reps _____ Sets _____ X Day _____ Hold

71 | Notes:

CURL UPS – ARMS BEHIND HEAD - EXERCISE BALL

While sitting on an exercise ball, roll forward so that your back lies against the ball. Place your hands behind your head. Brace core and curl up lifting your shoulder blades off the ball. Exhale as you come up and squeeze/tighten your abdominal muscles. Do not pull on your neck/head.

_____ Reps _____ Sets _____ X Day _____ Hold

72 | Notes:

Starting   Position

SUPINE CRUNCH TOUCH - EXERCISE BALL

Lie on the floor with your knees bend and holding a ball over your head. Bring both your knees and ball towards each other above your chest and touch your knees to the ball. Slowly return both to original positions and repeat.

_____ Reps _____ Sets _____ X Day _____ Hold

73 Notes:

LOWER ABDOMINAL CRUNCH – WITH or WITHOUT BALL

Sit on a solid surface with or without a ball/pillow between your knees. Maintaining a straight spine, contract your lower abdominals. Lift both knees up. Hold and control movement back to starting position. Repeat. Can be done holding onto surface for added stability with or without ball (3rd picture)

_____ Reps _____ Sets _____ X Day _____ Hold

74 Notes:

HIGH MARCH CRUNCH

Lift knee towards chest keeping hips forward in a high march position. Continue to alternate sides while standing in place. Exhale as you come up and squeeze/tighten your abdominal muscles.

_____ Reps _____ Sets _____ X Day _____ Hold

75 Notes:

Starting Position

STANDING SIDE CRUNCH

Standing with hip rotated out bring knee up towards same side elbow squeezing your obliques. Continue alternating sides while standing in place. Exhale as you come up and squeeze/tighten muscles.

_____ Reps _____ Sets _____ X Day _____ Hold

76 Notes:

Starting Position

STANDING BIKE CRUNCH

Lift knee to chest and rotate pulling opposite elbow towards knee. Continue to alternate sides while standing in place. Exhale as you come up and squeeze/tighten muscles.

Strengthening

Anaerobic - without oxygen: Single repetition with maximum resistance
Lifting lighter weights with a high number of repetitions will result in 'toning', whereas lifting heavier weights with a lower number of repetitions will result in 'bulking up'.

Benefits of strengthening	<ul><li>Increases muscle fiber size and contractile strength</li><li>Increases tendon and ligament strength</li><li>Increases bone strength / bone mineral density</li><li>Improves hormonal balances-decreased cortisol</li><li>Increases Peripheral (PNS) and Central (CNS) Nervous System communication/proprioception</li><li>Improves function for ADL's (Activities of Daily Living)</li></ul>
Range of Motion (ROM)	Refers to the distance and direction a joint can move between the flexed position and the extended position (stretching from flexion to extension for physiological gain). It is important to be able to complete full ROM before adding resistance. ***Before strengthening (adding resistance), make sure you can go through full ROM*** unless being followed by an MD or physical/occupational therapist or other professional.
Forms of strengthening exercise	<ul><li>**Isometric** – Muscles contract with no motion at the joint or change in length of the muscle. The exercises usually consist of maximal effort against an object that does not move, like a wall.</li><li>**Isotonic** – Muscles contract with motion at the joint; muscles either lengthen or shorten (*see **concentric/eccentric** below*). Tension is not constant through the range of motion. (During a bicep curl, holding a 5 lb weight, the contraction is not constant during the entire movement). Most common form of isotonic exercises use free weights with either dumbbells or a barbell.</li><li>**Concentric** – Muscle shortens, positive phase of lift. Bending the elbow in a bicep curl</li><li>**Eccentric** – Muscle lengthens, negative phase of lift or lowering. Straightening the elbow in a bicep curl.</li><li>**Isokinetic** – Muscles contract with motion at the joint; muscles either lengthen or shorten. Machines or equipment control the speed of the movement, so tension is constant providing the maximum amount of resistance throughout the entire movement.</li></ul>
Repetition (Reps)	Single cycle of lifting and lowering a weight in a controlled manner, moving through the form of the exercise. Example: 12 Bicep curls per set.
Set	Several repetitions performed one after another with no break between. There can be a number of reps per set and sets per exercise depending on the goal of the individual. Example: 12 reps x3 sets
Rep Maximum (RM)	The number of repetitions one can perform at a certain weight is called the Rep Maximum (RM). For example, if one could perform 10 repetitions with a 75 lbs dumbbell, then their RM for that weight would be 10RM. 1RM is the maximum weight that someone can lift in a given exercise - i.e. a weight that they can only lift once. (*Wikipedia*) (*See Bulk Up or Tone Up Below*)
Bulk up or Tone up	Do you want to 'bulk up' or 'tone up'? Although much of this depends on genetics and your ratio of slow and fast twitch fibers, discussed in the *Endurance* section, it is good to know what your goals are before starting. The average person should be able to perform at about 75% of their maximum resistance for 10 repetitions. If you can do ONE bicep curl with a 20-pound dumbbell/weight, then you should be able to do 10 with a 15 lbs. weight. (See *Set*) 20 lbs. x 75% = 15 lbs. Once you get into a routine, it will be easy for you to know when to increase the weight.

General rule of thumb	<ul><li>Work from the Ground up</li><li>Order: Isometric > ROM > Eccentric > Concentric</li><li>Use assistance before resistance – Start without weight to complete range of motion and then add weight with proper form. *(See ROM above)*</li><li>Add weight: 8-12 reps x 2-3 sets of each exercise at 75% of one repetition maximum (one-rep max).</li><li>Once you reach 12 easily, you can then recheck your one-rep max. If it has increased, then increase your weight as above.</li><li>If you are looking to 'bulk up', perform low repetitions at a higher weight – up to 85-90% of the one-rep maximum. 5-8 reps x 2-3 sets. With increased weight, there is a higher risk of injury.</li><li>If you are looking to 'tone up', perform high repetitions with 65-75% of the one-rep max. 12-20 reps x 2-3 sets.</li><li>Do NOT exercise the same muscle group every day. The muscles need about 48-72 hours to repair. This includes the abdomen. **Muscle strengthening, if you are lifting weights, alternate upper and lower body with isolated abdomen exercises every other day as well. For those working out several days a week, find a schedule that works for you, but give each muscle group 48-72 hours to recover.</li><li>Cardiac/aerobic conditioning can be done daily.</li><li>Breathe!! Always exhale on the exertion. For example, when you are doing a crunch, exhale as you flexing the abs or 'curling'. Do not hold your breath.</li><li>Engage your core. Don't forget what you learned under core and balance.</li></ul>

Duration, Frequency, Intensity and Movement Patterns

Intensity: How *much* mental and physical *effort* it takes to sustain an activity.	This can be done using the target heart rate range THR (optimum exercise intensity levels through beats per minute, talk test or rate of perceived exertion.
Duration: How *long* the training lasts.	The higher the intensity, the shorter the duration. The American College of Sports Medicine guidelines recommend all healthy adults aged 18–65 yr should participate in moderate intensity aerobic physical activity for a minimum of 30 min on five days per week, or vigorous intensity aerobic activity for a minimum of 20 min on three days per week.
Frequency: How *often* the training occurs.	Strength training should be performed every other day or 2-3 days a week. It is important to give each muscle group 48-72 hours to recover. Alternate upper and lower body with isolated abdomen/core exercises every other day. For those working out several days a week, find a schedule that works for you as long as you give each muscle group 48 hours of recovery time.
Movement Patterns and Examples Basic movements that help to increase overall body strengthening	<ul><li>Bend and Lift: Squats, Dead Lifts and Leg presses<ul><li>Picking up item off floor</li></ul></li><li>Single Leg: Step ups, Single leg stance, Lunges<ul><li>Walking up steps</li></ul></li><li>Push: Shoulder press, Bench press, Push up<ul><li>Pushing Shopping cart or Lawn mower</li></ul></li><li>Pull: Lat pull downs, Seated rows<ul><li>Vacuuming, Raking</li></ul></li><li>Rotational<ul><li>Shoveling snow</li></ul></li></ul>

EXERCISE Lower Extremity - Lying & Seated Strengthening and Range of Motion	EXERCISE NUMBER	NOTES
INVERSION – SEATED - ELASTIC BAND	1	
INVERSION – SEATED - ELASTIC BAND - 2	2	
EVERSION – SEATED - ELASTIC BAND	3	
EVERSION – SEATED - ELASTIC BAND - 2	4	
ANKLE PUMPS - SEATED	5	
ANKLE PUMPS – SUPINE or FEET UP ON STOOL	6	
DORSIFLEXION – SEATED - ELASTIC BAND	7	
DORSIFLEXION – SEATED - ELASTIC BAND - 2	8	
PLANTARFLEXION - STRAP	9	
PLANTARFLEXION - SEATED – ELASTIC BAND	10	
HEEL SLIDES - SUPINE	11	
HEEL SLIDES - RESISTED EXTENSION – ELASTIC BAND	12	
QUAD SET –ISOMETRIC	13	
QUAD SET WITH TOWEL UNDER HEEL - ISOMETRIC	14	
SHORT ARC QUAD (SAQ) – SELF ASSISTED	15	
SHORT ARC QUAD - (SAQ)	16	
KNEE EXTENSION - SELF ASSISTED	17	
PARTIAL ARC QUAD - LOW SEAT	18	
LONG ARC QUAD (LAQ) – LOW SEAT (90 deg)	19	
LONG ARC QUAD (LAQ) – LOW SEAT - ANKLE WEIGHTS	20	
LONG ARC QUAD (LAQ) - HIGH SEAT	21	
LONG ARC QUAD (LAQ) - HIGH SEAT - ANKLE WEIGHTS	22	
LONG ARC QUAD - ELASTIC BAND – HAND HELD	23	
LONG ARC QUAD - ELASTIC BAND	24	

EXERCISE Lower Extremity - Lying & Seated Strengthening and Range of Motion	EXERCISE NUMBER	NOTES
HAMSTRING CURLS - PRONE - ASSISTED	25	
HAMSTRING CURLS - PRONE	26	
HAMSTRING CURLS - - PRONE - WEIGHTS	27	
HAMSTRING CURLS – PRONE - ELASTIC BAND	28	
HAMSTRING CURLS – ELASTIC BAND	29	
HAMSTRING CURLS – ELASTIC BAND - 2	30	
HAMSTRING CURLS ON BALL	31	
HAMSTRING CURLS - SINGLE LEG - EXERCISE BALL	32	
HIP FLEXION ISOMETRIC	33	
HIP FLEXION ISOMETRIC BILATERAL	34	
HIP FLEXION – ISOMETRIC	35	
STRAIGHT LEG RAISE (SLR)	36	
STRAIGHT LEG RAISE (SLR) – ANKLE WEIGHTS	37	
STRAIGHT LEG RAISE (SLR) - ELASTIC BAND	38	
SEATED MARCHING	39	
SEATED MARCHING - ELASTIC BAND	40	
HIP EXTENSION - PRONE	41	
HIP EXTENSION – PRONE – ANKLE WEIGHTS	42	
HIP EXTENSION – PRONE – ELASTIC BAND	43	
HIP EXTENSION – QUADRUPED	44	
HIP ABDUCTION - SUPINE	45	
HIP ABDUCTION - SUPINE – ANKLE WEIGHTS	46	
HIP ABDUCTION – SUPINE - ELASTIC BAND	47	
HIP ABDUCTION / CLAMS– SUPINE - ELASTIC BAND	48	
MODIFIED HIP ABDUCTION – SIDELYING	49	

EXERCISE Lower Extremity - Lying & Seated Strengthening and Range of Motion	EXERCISE NUMBER	NOTES
HIP ABDUCTION – SIDELYING	50	
HIP ABDUCTION – SIDELYING - WEIGHTS	51	
HIP ABDUCTION – SIDELYING - ELASTIC BAND	52	
CLAM SHELLS	53	
SIDELYING CLAM - ELASTIC BAND	54	
HIP ABDUCTION - FIRE HYDRANT - QUADRUPED	55	
HIP ABDUCTION - FIRE HYDRANT – QUADRUPED - ELASTIC BAND	56	
HIP ABDUCTION - SEATED - STRAIGHT LEG	57	
HIP ABDUCTION - SEATED - STRAIGHT LEG – ANKLE WEIGHT	58	
HIP ABDUCTION - SINGLE- SEATED	59	
HIP ABDUCTION - SINGLE- SEATED – ELASTIC BAND	60	
HIP ABDUCTION - BILATERAL- SEATED	61	
HIP ABDUCTION - BILATERAL- SEATED - ELASTIC BAND	62	
HIP ADDUCTION SQUEEZE – SUPINE – KNEES BENT	63	
HIP ADDUCTION SQUEEZE – SUPINE – LEGS STRAIGHT	64	
HIP ADDUCTION - SIDELYING	65	
INTERNAL ROTATION - HEEL SQUEEZE - ISOMETRIC	67	
HIP INTERNAL ROTATION - SUPINE	68	
REVERSE CLAMS - SIDELYING	69	
REVERSE CLAMS - SIDELYING - ELASTIC BAND	70	
HIP INTERNAL ROTATION - SEATED	71	
HIP INTERNAL ROTATION - ELASTIC BAND	72	
HIP EXTERNAL ROTATION - SUPINE	73	

EXERCISE Lower Extremity - Lying & Seated Strengthening and Range of Motion	EXERCISE NUMBER	NOTES
HIP EXTERNAL ROTATION - ELASTIC BAND	74	
HIP ROTATIONS – BILATERAL - SIDELYING	75	
HIP ROTATION - SEATED - BALL and ELASTIC BAND	76	
PRESS – BILATERAL – ELASTIC BAND	77	
PRESS – SINGLE LEG – ELASTIC BAND	78	
HIP HIKE - STANDING	79	
HIP HIKE – KNEELING	80	
GLUTE SETS - PRONE	81	
GLUTE SET - SUPINE	82	
GLUTE SQUEEZE - SITTING	83	
PT (MAX/MEDIUS)	84	

LOWER EXTREMITY - Range Of Motion > Isometric > Strength
Lying and Seated
Inversion (IV) / Eversion (EV)

_____ Reps _____ Sets _____X Day _____Hold		

1 **Notes:**
*Lymphedema: Do not wrap band around UE or LE

INVERSION – SEATED - ELASTIC BAND

In a seated position, cross your legs and using an elastic band attached to your foot, hook it under your opposite foot and up to your hand. Draw the resisted foot inward. Keep your heel in contact with the floor the entire time.

_____ Reps _____ Sets _____X Day _____Hold

2 **Notes:**
*Lymphedema: Do not wrap band around UE or LE

INVERSION – SEATED - ELASTIC BAND - 2

In a seated position, use an elastic band secured to a steady object and the other end attached to your foot. Draw the resisted foot inward. Keep your heel in contact with the floor the entire time.

_____ Reps _____ Sets _____X Day _____Hold

3 **Notes:**
*Lymphedema: Do not wrap band around UE or LE

EVERSION – SEATED - ELASTIC BAND

In a seated position, use an elastic band attached to your foot, hook it under your opposite foot and up to your hand. Draw the resisted foot outward. Keep your heel in contact with the floor the entire time.

_____ Reps _____ Sets _____X Day _____Hold

4 **Notes:**
*Lymphedema: Do not wrap band around UE or LE

EVERSION – SEATED - ELASTIC BAND - 2

In a seated position, use an elastic band secured to a steady object and the other end attached to your foot. Draw the resisted foot outward. Keep your heel in contact with the floor the entire time.

Dorsiflexion (DF) / Plantarflexion (PF)

	_____ Reps _____ Sets _____X Day _____Hold		_____ Reps _____ Sets _____X Day _____Hold
5	**Notes:**	**6**	**Notes:**

ANKLE PUMPS - SEATED

In a seated position keeping feet on the floor, first go up on toes (toes pointed towards the ground – PF). Then point toes up keeping heels on the ground (DF). Alternate back and forth in a pumping motion.

ANKLE PUMPS – SUPINE or FEET UP ON STOOL

Lying or with feet up on stool first point the toes forward (PF) and then back up with toes facing the ceiling. Alternate back and forth in a pumping motion.

	_____ Reps _____ Sets _____X Day _____Hold		_____ Reps _____ Sets _____X Day _____Hold
7	**Notes:** *Lymphedema: Do not wrap band around UE or LE	**8**	**Notes:** *Lymphedema: Do not wrap band around UE or LE

DORSIFLEXION – SEATED - ELASTIC BAND

In a seated position, use an elastic band attached to your target foot, hook it under your opposite foot and up to your hand. Draw the band upwards with the resisted foot as shown. Keep your heel in contact with the floor the entire time.

DORSIFLEXION – SEATED - ELASTIC BAND - 2

In a seated position, use an elastic band secured to a steady object and the other end attached to your foot. Draw the resisted foot upward. Keep your heel in contact with the floor the entire time.

_____ Reps _____ Sets _____X Day _____Hold		_____ Reps _____ Sets _____X Day _____Hold	
9	**Notes:** *Lymphedema: Do not wrap band around UE or LE	**10**	**Notes:** *Lymphedema: Do not wrap band around UE or LE

PLANTARFLEXION - STRAP

In a seated position, attach one loop of the strap to your foot and hold the other end. Move your foot forward and back at the ankle as shown. Keep your heel in contact with the floor the entire time.

PLANTARFLEXION - SEATED – ELASTIC BAND

In a seated position, hold an elastic band and attach the other end to your foot. Press your foot downward towards the floor. Keep your heel in contact with the floor the entire time.

Heel Slides

_____ Reps _____ Sets _____X Day _____Hold		_____ Reps _____ Sets _____X Day _____Hold	
11	**Notes:**	**12**	**Notes:** *Lymphedema: Do not wrap band around UE or LE

HEEL SLIDES - SUPINE

Lie on your back with knees straight and slide the target heel towards your buttock as you bend your knee. Hold a gentle stretch in this position and then return to original position.

Starting Position

HEEL SLIDES - RESISTED EXTENSION – ELASTIC BAND

Long sit with band around bottom of target foot. Slide the target heel towards your buttock as you bend your knee. Push your foot to straighten knee against resistance to the original position.

Quadriceps (QUAD) / Knee Extension

_____ Reps _____ Sets _____X Day _____Hold	_____ Reps _____ Sets _____X Day _____Hold

13 Notes:

14 Notes:

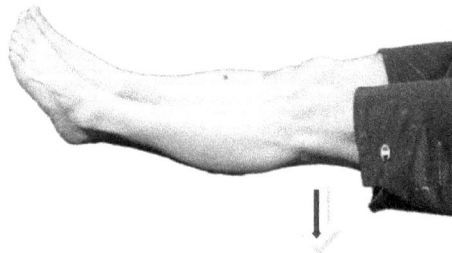

QUAD SET –ISOMETRIC

Tighten your top thigh muscle as you attempt to press the back of your knee downward towards the table. Hold 5-10 seconds. Repeat.

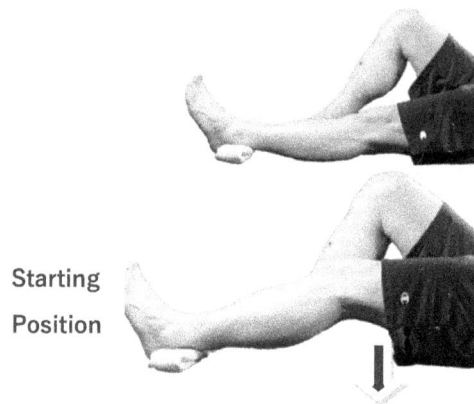

QUAD SET WITH TOWEL UNDER HEEL - ISOMETRIC

Lying or sitting with a small towel roll under your ankle, tighten your top thigh muscle to press the back of your knee downward towards the ground. Hold 5-10 seconds. Repeat.

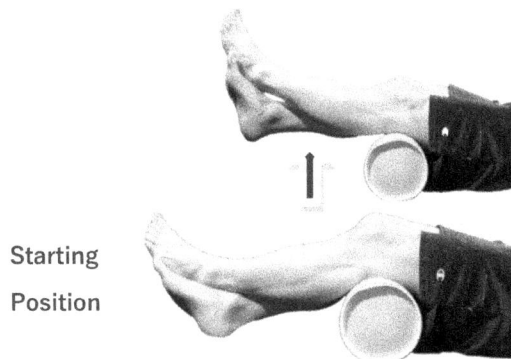

Starting Position

_____ Reps _____ Sets _____X Day _____Hold	_____ Reps _____ Sets _____X Day _____Hold

15 Notes:

16 Notes:

Starting

Position

SHORT ARC QUAD (SAQ) – SELF ASSISTED

Place a rolled-up towel or other rounded object under your knee. Hook one foot under the other to assist the affected leg. Slowly straighten your knee as your raise up your foot tightening the top thigh muscle.

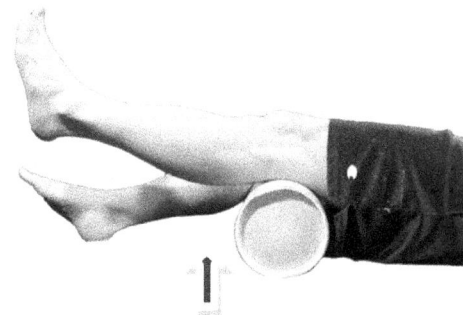

SHORT ARC QUAD - (SAQ) - Can add ankle weight

Place a rolled-up towel or object under your knee and slowly straighten your knee as your raise up your foot tightening the top thigh muscle. Flex your foot to increase the stretch.

	_____ Reps _____ Sets _____X Day _____Hold		_____ Reps _____ Sets _____X Day _____Hold
17	Notes:	**18**	Notes:

KNEE EXTENSION - SELF ASSISTED

In a seated position, place the unaffected leg under the target leg. Use the unaffected leg to assist the target leg up to a straightened knee position.

PARTIAL ARC QUAD - LOW SEAT - Can add ankle weight

Sit with your knee in a semi bent position and your heel touching the ground and then slowly straighten your knee as you raise your foot upwards as shown. Lower your foot back down slowly controling the muscle until your heel touches the ground and then repeat.

	_____ Reps _____ Sets _____X Day _____Hold		_____ Reps _____ Sets _____X Day _____Hold
19	Notes:	**20**	Notes:

LONG ARC QUAD (LAQ) – LOW SEAT (90 deg)

Sit with your knee in a bent position and then tighten the quadricep. Slowly straighten your knee as you raise your foot upwards as shown. Lower your foot back down to original bent knee position slowly controlling the muscle and then repeat.

LONG ARC QUAD (LAQ) – LOW SEAT - ANKLE WEIGHTS

Attach and ankle weight. Sit with your knee in a bent position and then tighten the quadricep. Slowly straighten your knee as you raise your foot upwards as shown. Lower your foot back down to original bent knee position slowly controlling the muscle - repeat.

	_____ Reps _____ Sets _____ X Day _____ Hold
21	Notes:

LONG ARC QUAD (LAQ) - HIGH SEAT

Sit with your knee in a bent position and then tighten the quadricep. Slowly straighten your knee as you raise your foot upwards as shown. Lower your foot back down to original bent knee position slowly controlling the muscle and then repeat.

	_____ Reps _____ Sets _____ X Day _____ Hold
22	Notes:

LONG ARC QUAD (LAQ) - HIGH SEAT - ANKLE WEIGHTS

Attach and ankle weight. Sit with your knee in a bent position and then tighten the quadricep. Slowly straighten your knee as you raise your foot upwards as shown. Lower your foot back down to original bent knee position slowly controlling the muscle and then repeat.

	_____ Reps _____ Sets _____ X Day _____ Hold
23	Notes: *Lymphedema: Do not wrap band around UE or LE

LONG ARC QUAD - ELASTIC BAND – HANDHELD

Attach a looped elastic band to your ankle and to the opposite foot or hold with your hand. Sit with your knee in a bent position and then tighten the quadricep. Draw your lower leg upwards to a straighten knee position while your other foot or hand secures the band. Lower your foot back down to original bent knee position slowly controlling the muscle and then repeat.

	_____ Reps _____ Sets _____ X Day _____ Hold
24	Notes: *Lymphedema: Do not wrap band around UE or LE

LONG ARC QUAD - ELASTIC BAND

Attach a looped elastic band to your ankle and to a steady object behind you. Sit with your knee in a bent position and then tighten the quadricep. Draw your lower leg upwards to a straightened knee position. Lower your foot back down to original bent knee position slowly controlling the muscle and then repeat.

Hamstrings	

_____ Reps _____ Sets _____ X Day _____ Hold	_____ Reps _____ Sets _____ X Day _____ Hold
25 Notes:	**26** Notes:

HAMSTRING CURLS - PRONE - ASSISTED

Lie face down and hook one foot under the other to assist the affected leg. Bend the target leg with the assistance of your unaffected leg.

HAMSTRING CURLS - PRONE

Lie face down and slowly bend your knee as you bring your foot towards your buttock.

_____ Reps _____ Sets _____ X Day _____ Hold	_____ Reps _____ Sets _____ X Day _____ Hold
27 Notes:	**28** Notes: *Lymphedema: Do not wrap band around UE or LE

HAMSTRING CURLS - - PRONE - WEIGHTS

Attach and ankle weight. Lie face down and slowly bend your knee as you bring your foot towards your buttock.

HAMSTRING CURLS – PRONE - ELASTIC BAND

Attach an elastic band around your foot and opposite ankle as shown. While lying face down, slowly bend your target knee as you bring your foot towards your buttock. Keep your other foot on the floor to fixate the band.

_____Reps _____Sets _____X Day _____Hold		_____Reps _____Sets _____X Day _____Hold

29

Notes:
*Lymphedema: Do not wrap band around UE or LE

30

Notes:
*Lymphedema: Do not wrap band around UE or LE

HAMSTRING CURLS – ELASTIC BAND

Sit and use an elastic band secured to a steady object and the other end attached to your ankle. Bend your knee and draw back your foot.

HAMSTRING CURLS – ELASTIC BAND - 2

Attach a looped elastic band to your ankle and to the opposite foot while one leg is propped on stool or another raised object. Draw your lower leg downwards to a bent knee position while your other ankle anchors the band on the chair.

_____Reps _____Sets _____X Day _____Hold		_____Reps _____Sets _____X Day _____Hold

31

Notes:

32

Notes: **Advanced**

HAMSTRING CURLS ON BALL – can add ankle weight.

Lie prone on an exercise ball as shown. Slowly bend your knee as you bring your foot towards your buttock.

Starting

Position

HAMSTRING CURLS - SINGLE LEG - EXERCISE BALL

Lie on the floor and place your heel on an exercise ball.
Lift your buttocks and then bend your knees to draw the ball towards your buttocks. Keep your buttocks elevated off the floor the entire time.

Hip Flexion

_____ Reps _____ Sets _____ X Day _____ Hold	_____ Reps _____ Sets _____ X Day _____ Hold
33 Notes:	**34** Notes:

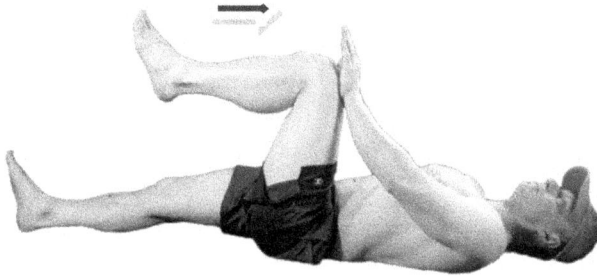

HIP FLEXION ISOMETRIC

Lie on your back, lift up your knee and press it into your hand. Hold. Return to the original position and repeat.

HIP FLEXION ISOMETRIC - ALTERNATING
Lie on your back, lift up your knee and press it into your hand. Hold. Return to the original position and repeat on the other side.

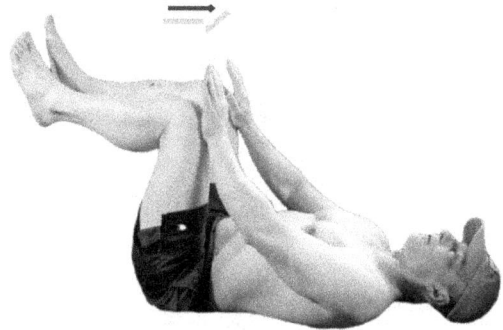

HIP FLEXION ISOMETRIC BILATERAL

Lie on your back, lift up your knees and press them into your hands. Hold. Return to the original position and repeat.

_____ Reps _____ Sets _____ X Day _____ Hold	_____ Reps _____ Sets _____ X Day _____ Hold
35 Notes:	**36** Notes:

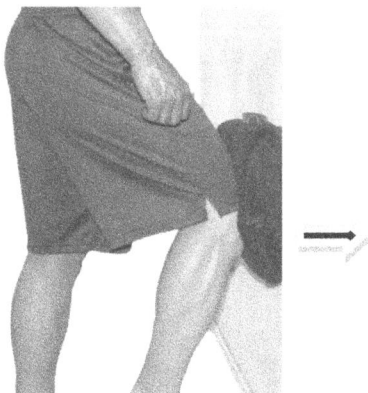

HIP FLEXION – ISOMETRIC - Can use towel roll for comfort

While standing in front of a wall, draw your knee forward and press it into the wall. Place a folded towel between your knee and the wall for comfort if needed.

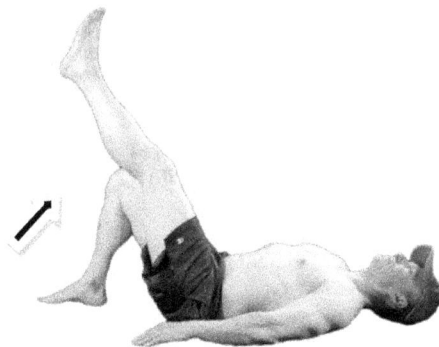

STRAIGHT LEG RAISE (SLR)

Lie on your back, tighten the quad of the target leg and lift up with a straight knee. Keep the opposite knee bent with the foot planted on the ground. (see #37 for starting position)

_____ Reps _____ Sets _____X Day _____Hold

37	Notes:

Starting
Position

STRAIGHT LEG RAISE (SLR) – ANKLE WEIGHTS

Attach ankle weights. Lie on your back and lift up your leg with a straight knee. Keep the opposite knee bent with the foot planted on the ground

_____ Reps _____ Sets _____X Day _____Hold

38	Notes: *Lymphedema: Do not wrap band around UE or LE

STRAIGHT LEG RAISE (SLR) - ELASTIC BAND

Lie on your back with an elastic band looped around your ankles, lift the target leg upwards.

_____ Reps _____ Sets _____X Day _____Hold

39	Notes:

SEATED MARCHING - can add ankle weights for resistance

Sit in a chair and move a knee upward, set it back down and then alternate to the other side

_____ Reps _____ Sets _____X Day _____Hold

40	Notes: *Lymphedema: Do not wrap band around UE or LE

SEATED MARCHING - ELASTIC BAND

Sit in a chair with an elastic band wrapped around your thighs. Move a knee upward, set it back down and then alternate to the other side.

Hip Extension

_____ Reps _____ Sets _____X Day _____Hold	_____ Reps _____ Sets _____X Day _____Hold

41   Notes: **42**   Notes:

HIP EXTENSION - PRONE

Lie face down with your knee straight and slowly lift up leg off the ground. Maintain a straight knee the entire time.

HIP EXTENSION – PRONE – ANKLE WEIGHTS

Attach ankle weights. Lie face down with your knee straight and slowly lift up leg off the ground. Maintain a straight knee the entire time.

_____ Reps _____ Sets _____X Day _____Hold	_____ Reps _____ Sets _____X Day _____Hold

43   Notes:
*Lymphedema: Do not wrap band around UE or LE

44   Notes:

HIP EXTENSION – PRONE – ELASTIC BAND

Lie on your stomach with an elastic band looped around your ankles and lift the targeted leg upwards. Maintain a straight knee the entire time.

HIP EXTENSION – QUADRUPED with or without ankle weights

Start in a crawl position and then raise your leg up behind you as shown. Keep your knee bent at 90 degrees the entire time.

Hip Abduction (ABD)

	_____ Reps _____ Sets _____X Day _____Hold		_____ Reps _____ Sets _____X Day _____Hold
45	Notes:	**46**	Notes:

HIP ABDUCTION - SUPINE

Lie on your back and slowly bring your leg out to the side. Return to original position and repeat. Keep your knee straight the entire time.

HIP ABDUCTION - SUPINE – ANKLE WEIGHTS

Attach and weights. Lie on your back and slowly bring your leg up slightly and then out to the side. Return to original position and repeat. Keep your knee straight the entire time.

	_____ Reps _____ Sets _____X Day _____Hold		_____ Reps _____ Sets _____X Day _____Hold
47	Notes: *Lymphedema: Do not wrap band around UE or LE	**48**	Notes: *Lymphedema: Do not wrap band around UE or LE

HIP ABDUCTION – SUPINE - ELASTIC BAND

Lie on your back and slowly bring your leg out to the side. Return to original position and repeat. Keep your knee straight the entire time.

HIP ABDUCTION / CLAMS– SUPINE - ELASTIC BAND

Lie down on your back with your knees bent. Place an elastic band around your knees and then draw your knees apart. Return to original position and repeat.

_____ Reps _____ Sets _____ X Day _____ Hold	_____ Reps _____ Sets _____ X Day _____ Hold

49	Notes:	50	Notes:

MODIFIED HIP ABDUCTION – SIDELYING can add weights

Lie on your side and slowly lift up your top leg to the side. The bottom leg can be bent to stabilize your body. Keep your knee straight and maintain your toes pointed forward the entire time. Keep your leg in-line with your body. Return to original position and repeat.

HIP ABDUCTION – SIDELYING

Lie on your side and slowly lift up your top leg to the side. Keep your knee straight and maintain your toes pointed forward the entire time. Keep your leg in-line with your body. Return to original position and repeat.

_____ Reps _____ Sets _____ X Day _____ Hold	_____ Reps _____ Sets _____ X Day _____ Hold

51	Notes:	52	Notes:
			*Lymphedema: Do not wrap band around UE or LE

HIP ABDUCTION – SIDELYING - WEIGHTS

Attach ankle weights. Lie on your side and slowly lift up your top leg to the side. Keep your knee straight and maintain your toes pointed forward the entire time. Keep your leg in-line with your body. Return to original position and repeat.

HIP ABDUCTION – SIDELYING - ELASTIC BAND

Lie on your side with an elastic band looped around your ankles. Lift the top leg upwards keeping your knee straight and maintaining your toes pointed forward the entire time. Keep your leg in-line with your body. Return to original position and repeat.

_____ Reps _____ Sets _____X Day _____Hold

53 | **Notes:**

Starting
Position

CLAM SHELLS

Lie on your side with your knees bent, draw up the top knee while keeping contact of your feet together.
Do not let your pelvis roll back during the lifting movement.

_____ Reps _____ Sets _____X Day _____Hold

54 | **Notes:**
*Lymphedema: Do not wrap band around UE or LE

Starting
Position

SIDELYING CLAM - ELASTIC BAND

Lie on your side with your knees bent and an elastic band wrapped around your knees, draw up the top knee while keeping contact of your feet together as shown. Do not let your pelvis roll back during the lifting movement.

_____ Reps _____ Sets _____X Day _____Hold

55 | **Notes:**

Starting
Position

HIP ABDUCTION - FIRE HYDRANT - QUADRUPED

Start in a crawl position and raise your leg out to the side as shown. Maintain a straight upper and mid back.

_____ Reps _____ Sets _____X Day _____Hold

56 | **Notes:**
*Lymphedema: Do not wrap band around UE or LE

Starting
Position

HIP ABDUCTION - FIRE HYDRANT – QUADRUPED - ELASTIC BAND

Start in a crawl position with an elastic band around your thighs. Raise your leg out to the side as shown. Maintain a straight upper and mid back.

_____ Reps _____ Sets _____ X Day _____ Hold		_____ Reps _____ Sets _____ X Day _____ Hold	
57	Notes:	**58**	Notes:

HIP ABDUCTION - SEATED - STRAIGHT LEG

Sit close to the edge of a chair with your target leg straight at the knee. Move your target leg to the side lifting slightly off the ground and then return to straight ahead.. You can slide your heel across the floor as you move and then return to straight ahead if unable to lift. Maintain your toes pointed up the entire time.

HIP ABDUCTION - SEATED - STRAIGHT LEG – ANKLE WEIGHT

Attach an ankle weight. Sit close to the edge of a chair with your target leg straight at the knee. Move your target leg to the side lifting slightly off the ground and then return to straight ahead. Maintain your toes pointed up the entire time.

_____ Reps _____ Sets _____ X Day _____ Hold		_____ Reps _____ Sets _____ X Day _____ Hold	
59	Notes:	**60**	Notes: *Lymphedema: Do not wrap band around UE or LE

HIP ABDUCTION - SINGLE- SEATED

Sit close to the edge of a chair with knees bent and both feet on the floor. Move your target knee out to the side as shown and then return to straight ahead. Maintain contact of your feet on the floor the entire time.

HIP ABDUCTION - SINGLE- SEATED – ELASTIC BAND

With band tied around the thighs, sit close to the edge of a chair with knees bent and both feet on the floor. Move your target knee out to the side as shown and then return to straight ahead. Maintain contact of your feet on the floor the entire time.tact of your feet on the floor the entire time.

	_____ Reps _____ Sets _____ X Day _____ Hold

61   Notes:

HIP ABDUCTION - BILATERAL- SEATED

Sit close to the edge of a chair with knees bent and both feet on the floor. Move your knees out to the side as shown and then return to straight ahead. Maintain contact of your feet on the floor the entire time.

	_____ Reps _____ Sets _____ X Day _____ Hold

62   Notes:
*Lymphedema: Do not wrap band around UE or LE

HIP ABDUCTION - BILATERAL- SEATED - ELASTIC BAND

Sit close to the edge of a chair with an elastic band wrapped around your knees. Move both knees to the sides to separate your legs. Keep contact of your feet on the floor the entire time.

Hip Adduction (ADD)

	_____ Reps _____ Sets _____ X Day _____ Hold

63   Notes:

HIP ADDUCTION SQUEEZE – SUPINE – KNEES BENT

Lie on your back with legs bent and place a rolled up towel, ball or pillow between your knees. Press your knees together so that you squeeze the object firmly. Hold, release and repeat.

	_____ Reps _____ Sets _____ X Day _____ Hold

64   Notes:

HIP ADDUCTION SQUEEZE – SUPINE – LEGS STRAIGHT

Lie on your back and place a rolled up towel, ball or pillow between your knees. Squeeze the object with your knees. Hold, release and repeat.

	_____ Reps _____ Sets _____ X Day _____ Hold		_____ Reps _____ Sets _____ X Day _____ Hold
65	Notes:	66	Notes:

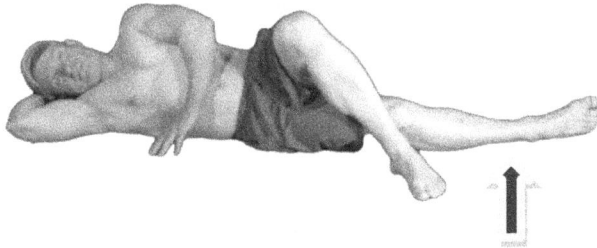

HIP ADDUCTION - SIDELYING

Lie on your side, slowly lift up your bottom leg towards the ceiling. Keep your knee straight the entire time. Your top leg should be bent at the knee and your foot planted on the ground supporting your body.

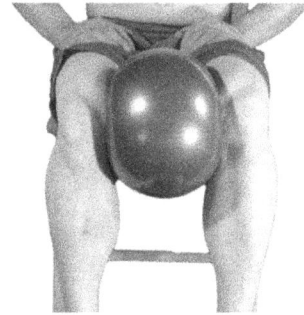

BALL SQUEEZE - SEATED

Sit and place a rolled-up towel, ball or pillow between your knees and squeeze the object firmly. Hold, release and repeat.

Hip Internal Rotation (IR)

	_____ Reps _____ Sets _____ X Day _____ Hold		_____ Reps _____ Sets _____ X Day _____ Hold
67	Notes:	68	Notes:

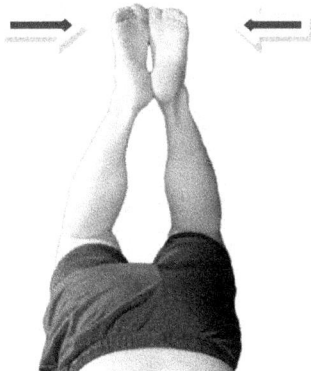

INTERNAL ROTATION - HEEL SQUEEZE - ISOMETRIC

Lie face down, spead your knees apart and press your heels together. Hold, release and repeat.

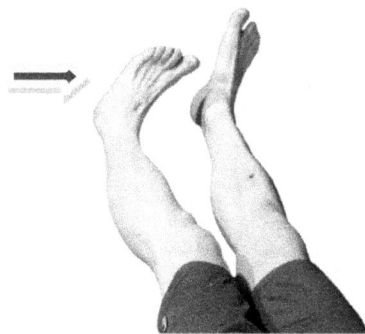

HIP INTERNAL ROTATION - SUPINE

Lie on your back with your knees straight, roll your hip in so that your toes point inward. Be sure that your knee cap faces inward as well.

_____ Reps _____ Sets _____X Day _____Hold

69	Notes:

REVERSE CLAMS - SIDELYING

Starting Position

Lie on your side with your knees bent and raise your top foot towards the ceiling while keeping contact of your knees together. Lower back down to original position. Do not let your pelvis roll forward during the lifting movement.

_____ Reps _____ Sets _____X Day _____Hold

70	Notes: *Lymphedema: Do not wrap band around UE or LE

REVERSE CLAMS - SIDELYING - ELASTIC BAND

Starting Position

Lie on your side with your knees bent and an elastic band around your ankles. Raise your top foot towards the ceiling while keeping contact of your knees together. Lower back down to original position. Do not let your pelvis roll forward during the lifting movement.

_____ Reps _____ Sets _____X Day _____Hold

71	Notes:

HIP INTERNAL ROTATION - SEATED

Sit on a chair with your legs spread apart and feet planted on the ground. Use your hand on the inside of your knee to resist the movement inward.

_____ Reps _____ Sets _____X Day _____Hold

72	Notes: *Lymphedema: Do not wrap band around UE or LE

HIP INTERNAL ROTATION - ELASTIC BAND - High chair

Attach one end of an elastic band at your ankle and the other to a sturdy object. Pull away from your other leg while keeping your thigh from moving.

Hip External Rotation (ER)

	_____ Reps _____ Sets _____X Day _____Hold		_____ Reps _____ Sets _____X Day _____Hold
73	**Notes:**	**74**	**Notes:** *Lymphedema: Do not wrap band around UE or LE

HIP EXTERNAL ROTATION - SUPINE

Lie on your back with your knees straight and roll your hip out so that your toes point outward. Be sure that your knee cap faces outward as well.

HIP EXTERNAL ROTATION - ELASTIC BAND

Sit and use an elastic band secured to a steady object and the other end attached to your ankle from the side.
Pull towards your other leg while keeping your thigh from moving across the table.

Bilateral Hip Rotation

	_____ Reps _____ Sets _____X Day _____Hold		_____ Reps _____ Sets _____X Day _____Hold
75	**Notes:**	**76**	**Notes:** *Lymphedema: Do not wrap band around UE or LE

HIP ROTATIONS – BILATERAL - SIDELYING

Lie on your side in fetal position with knees and hips bent.
Slowly raise up both lower legs and feet as shown.
Your feet and knees should be touching the entire time.

HIP ROTATION - SEATED - BALL and ELASTIC BAND – High chair

Sit and place a rolled-up towel, ball or pillow between your knees and an elastic band around your ankles. Squeeze the ball, sustain and hold. Next, pull the band as you move your feet apart from each other.

Leg Press

_____ Reps _____ Sets _____ X Day _____ Hold	_____ Reps _____ Sets _____ X Day _____ Hold
77 **Notes:** *Lymphedema: Do not wrap band around UE or LE	**78** **Notes:** *Lymphedema: Do not wrap band around UE or LE

Starting Position

PRESS – BILATERAL – ELASTIC BAND

Lie on back put elastic band on bottom of both feet. Start with knees bent and push with feet to straighten both legs.

PRESS – SINGLE LEG – ELASTIC BAND

Lie on back put elastic band on bottom of one foot. Start with knees bent and push with foot to straighten leg.

Hip Hikes (Gluteus Medius)

_____ Reps _____ Sets _____ X Day _____ Hold	_____ Reps _____ Sets _____ X Day _____ Hold
79 **Notes:**	**80** **Notes:**

HIP HIKE - STANDING on Step or Pad

Stand with one foot on a step or pad and the other hanging off as shown. Raise and lower the side of your pelvis that is hanging off the edge.

HIP HIKE – KNEELING on towel or pad

Kneel on both knees with one knee on a folded towel or pad. Raise and lower the side of your pelvis that is not on the towel/pad.

Glutes (Glute Max)

_____ Reps _____ Sets _____ X Day _____ Hold	_____ Reps _____ Sets _____ X Day _____ Hold
81 Notes:	**82** Notes:

GLUTE SETS - PRONE

Lie face down, squeeze your buttocks and hold. Repeat.

GLUTE SET - SUPINE

Lie on your back, squeeze your buttocks and hold. Repeat.

_____ Reps _____ Sets _____ X Day _____ Hold	_____ Reps _____ Sets _____ X Day _____ Hold
83 Notes:	**84** Notes:

GLUTE SQUEEZE - SITTING

While sitting, squeeze your buttocks and hold. Repeat.

GLUTE SCULPT (MAX/MEDIUS)

Lie on your side leaning towards your stomach. Bend leg on target side, raise up and hold.

EXERCISE Upper Extremity Strengthening and Range of Motion	EXERCISE NUMBER	NOTES
ELBOW FLEXION EXTENSION - SUPINE	1	
ELBOW FLEXION / EXTENSION - GRAVITY ELIMINATED	2	
BICEPS CURLS – ALTERNATING	3	
BICEPS CURL - SELF FIXATION – ELASTIC BAND	4	
SEATED BICEPS CURLS - ALTERNATING	5	
SEATED BICEPS CURLS - BILATERAL	6	
CONCENTRATION CURLS – SITTING	7	
PREACHER CURL ON BALL	8	
BICEPS CURLS	9	
BICEPS CURLS - RADIOBRACHIALIS - HAMMER CURL	10	
BICEPS CURLS - BRACHIALIS	11	
BICEPS CURLS – ROTATE OUTWARD	12	
BICEPS CURLS – ONE ARM - ELASTIC BAND	13	
BICEPS CURLS – BILATERAL - ELASTIC BAND	14	
BICEPS CURLS - RADIOBRACHIALIS - HAMMER CURL – ONE ARM - ELASTIC BAND	15	
BICEPS CURLS - RADIOBRACHIALIS - HAMMER CURL – BILATERAL - ELASTIC BAND	16	
BICEPS CURLS – BRACHIALIS - ONE ARM - ELASTIC BAND	17	
BICEPS CURL – BRACHIALIS – BILATERAL - ELASTIC BAND	18	
TRICEPS - SELF FIXATION - ELASTIC BAND	19	
OVERHEAD TRICEPS - SELF FIXATION –SEATED OR STANDING - ELASTIC BAND	20	
TRICEP EXTENSION – SITTING OR STANDING - WEIGHT	21	
TRICEP EXTENSION – SITTING OR STANDING – BILATERAL - WEIGHT	22	
ELBOW EXTENSION - BALL	23	

EXERCISE Upper Extremity Strengthening and Range of Motion	EXERCISE NUMBER	NOTES
ELBOW EXTENSION - SKULL CRUSHER - BALL	24	
TRICEPS - ELASTIC BAND	25	
TRICEPS - BENT OVER	26	
CHAIR DIPS / PUSH UPS	27	
DIPS OFF CHAIR	28	
PENDULUM SHOULDER FORWARD/BACK	29	
PENDULUM SHOULDER – SIDE TO SIDE	30	
PENDULUM SHOULDER CIRCLES	31	
PENDULUMS - SUPINE	32	
ISOMETRIC FLEXION	33	
SHOULDER FLEXION – SIDELYING	34	
FLEXION – SUPINE - SINGLE OR BILATERAL	35	
FLEXION – SUPINE – SINGLE OR BILATERAL - WEIGHT	36	
FLEXION – SUPINE - DOWEL	37	
FLEXION – SUPINE - DOWEL - Weight	38	
FLEXION - SELF FIXATION – ELASTIC BAND	39	
FLEXION – ELASTIC BAND	40	
FLEXION - STANDING - PALMS DOWN / OVERHAND DOWEL	41	
FLEXION - STANDING - PALMS UP / UNDERHAND DOWEL	42	
FLEXION – PALMS FACING INWARD	43	
FLEXION – PALMS DOWN	44	
V RAISE	45	
V RAISE – WEIGHTS	46	
MILITARY PRESS – DOWEL	47	
MILITARY PRESS - FREE WEIGHTS	48	

EXERCISE Upper Extremity Strengthening and Range of Motion	EXERCISE NUMBER	NOTES
ISOMETRIC EXTENSION	49	
PRONE EXTENSION - EXERCISE BALL	50	
SHOULDER EXTENSION - STANDING	51	
SHOULDER EXTENSION - STANDING - WEIGHTS	52	
EXTENSION – STANDING – DOWEL	53	
EXTENSION - SELF FIXATION - ELASTIC BAND	54	
EXTENSION - ELASTIC BAND	55	
EXTENSION - BILATERAL - ELASTIC BAND	56	
INTERNAL ROTATION – ISOMETRIC	57	
INTERNAL ROTATION - ISOMETRIC- ELEVATED	58	
INTERNAL ROTATION - SIDELYING	59	
INTERNAL ROTATION - ELASTIC BAND	60	
INTERNAL / EXTERNAL ROTATION - STANDING – DOWEL	61	
INTERNAL ROTATION – DOWEL	62	
EXTERNAL ROTATION - ISOMETRIC	63	
EXTERNAL ROTATION - ISOMETRIC – ELEVATED	64	
EXTERNAL ROTATION WITH TOWEL - SIDELYING	65	
EXTERNAL ROTATION – 90/90 - WEIGHTS	66	
EXTERNAL ROTATION - BILATERAL - ELASTIC BAND	67	
EXTERNAL ROTATION - ELASTIC BAND	68	
ADDUCTION – ISOMETRIC	69	
ADDUCTION - ELASTIC BAND	70	
ABDUCTION – ISOMETRIC	71	
HORIZONTAL ABDUCTION - DOWEL	72	

EXERCISE Upper Extremity Strengthening and Range of Motion	EXERCISE NUMBER	NOTES
HORIZONTAL ABDUCTION/ADDUCTTION - SUPINE	73	
HORIZONTAL ABDUCTION/ADDUCTTION - SUPINE -WEIGHT	74	
ABDUCTION - SIDELYING	75	
HORIZONTAL ABDUCTION - SIDELYING	76	
ABDUCTION – WEIGHT	77	
ABDUCTION – ELASTIC BAND	78	
HORIZONTAL ABDUCTION – BILATERAL - ELASTIC BAND	79	
90/90 ABDUCTION - WEIGHT	80	
LATERAL RAISES	81	
LATERAL RAISES – LEAN FORWARD	82	
LATERAL RAISES – LEAN FORWARD - ARM ROTATION	83	
FRONTAL RAISE – WEIGHTS	84	
UPRIGHT ROW – WEIGHTS	85	
UPRIGHT ROW – ELASTIC BAND	86	
SHRUGS	87	
SHRUGS - WEIGHTS	88	
SHOULDER ROLLS	89	
SHOULDER ROLLS - WEIGHTS	90	
SCAPULAR RETRACTIONS - BILATERAL	91	
SCAPULAR RETRACTION – SINGLE ARM	92	
ELASTIC BAND SCAPULAR RETRACTIONS WITH MINI SHOULDER EXTENSIONS	93	
PRONE RETRACTION	94	
SCAPULAR PROTRACTION - SUPINE - BILATERAL	95	
SCAPULAR PROTRACTION - SUPINE - WEIGHT	96	

EXERCISE Upper Extremity Strengthening and Range of Motion	EXERCISE NUMBER	NOTES
SCAPULAR PROTRACTION - SUPINE - ELASTIC BAND	97	
SCAPULAR PROTRACTION / TABLE PLANK	98	
CHEST PRESS – SEATED or STANDING - ELASTIC BAND	99	
CHEST PRESS – BALL, FLOOR or BENCH- WEIGHTS	100	
DOWEL PRESS – STANDING	101	
CHEST PRESS – STANDING or SEATED	102	
BENT OVER ROWS	103	
ROWS – PRONE	104	
ROWS - ELASTIC BAND	105	
WIDE ROWS - ELASTIC BAND	106	
LOW ROW – ELASTIC BAND	107	
HIGH ROW – ELASTIC BAND	108	
FLY'S – FLOOR - WEIGHT	109	
FLY'S – BALL or BENCH – WEIGHT	110	
WALL PUSH UPS	111	
WALL PUSH UP - BALL	112	
WALL PUSH UP - Triceps uneven	113	
WALL PUSH UP - Hands inverted	114	
WALL PUSH UP - Narrow	115	
WALL PUSH UP – Wide	116	
PUSH UPS - BALL	117	
PUSH UP - MODIFIED	118	
PUSH UP	119	
PUSH UP -DIAMOND	120	
PUSH UP – MODIFIED - BOSU - UNSTABLE	121	

EXERCISE Upper Extremity Strengthening and Range of Motion	EXERCISE NUMBER	NOTES
PUSH UP – BOSU - UNSTABLE	122	
PUSH UP – MODIFIED – INVERTED BOSU - UNSTABLE	123	
PUSH UP – INVERTED BOSU - UNSTABLE	124	

UPPER EXTREMITY - Range Of Motion > Isometric > Strength

Elbow Flexion/Extension

	_____ Reps _____ Sets _____X Day _____Hold		_____ Reps _____ Sets _____X Day _____Hold
1	Notes:	**2**	Notes:

Extension

Flexion

ELBOW FLEXION EXTENSION - SUPINE

Lie on your back and rest your elbow on a small rolled up towel. Bend at your elbow and then lower back down.

Flexion   Extension

ELBOW FLEXION / EXTENSION - GRAVITY ELIMINATED

Sit and hold your arm up with the help of your other arm. Bend and straighten your elbow.

Elbow Flexion (Biceps)

	_____ Reps _____ Sets _____X Day _____Hold		_____ Reps _____ Sets _____X Day _____Hold
3	Notes:	**4**	Notes: *Lymphedema: Do not wrap band around UE or LE

BICEPS CURLS – ALTERNATING

Bend your elbow and move your forearm upwards. As you lower back down, begin bending the opposite elbow upwards.

BICEPS CURL - SELF FIXATION – ELASTIC BAND

Sit and hold an elastic band with one hand. Hold the other end of elastic band with the opposite hand and fixate hand on your knee. Slowly draw up your hand by bending at the elbow. Return to starting position and repeat.

*Can increase resistance by doubling band as shown.

	_____ Reps _____ Sets _____X Day _____Hold		_____ Reps _____ Sets _____X Day _____Hold
5	**Notes:** *Neuropathy/Hands – Precaution holding weights	**6**	**Notes:** *Neuropathy/Hands – Precaution holding weights

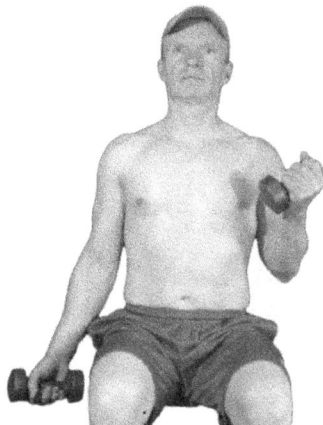

SEATED BICEPS CURLS - ALTERNATING

Sit in a chair and hold free weights on each thigh. Lift one side while bending at the elbow and squeezing bicep muscle. Perform on one side and then alternate to the other side.

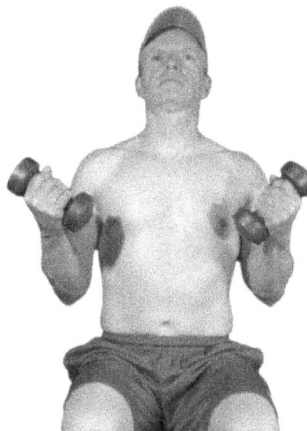

SEATED BICEPS CURLS - BILATERAL

Sit in a chair and hold free weights on each thigh. Lift both sides while bending at the elbows and squeezing bicep muscles. Lower back down and repeat.

	_____ Reps _____ Sets _____X Day _____Hold		_____ Reps _____ Sets _____X Day _____Hold
7	**Notes:** *Neuropathy/Hands – Precaution holding weights	**8**	**Notes:** *Neuropathy/Hands – Precaution holding weights

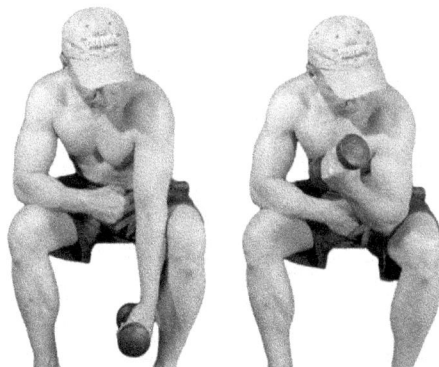

CONCENTRATION CURLS – SITTING

Sit in a chair, lean slightly forward and hold a free weight with arm straight with elbow on inside of thigh. Bend elbow squeezing bicep muscle. Lower back down - repeat.

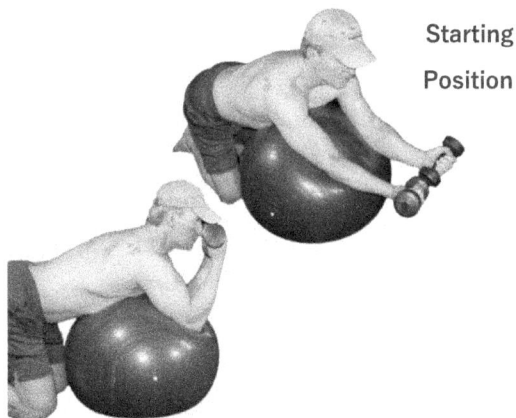

Starting Position

PREACHER CURL ON BALL

Lie on stomach over ball in crawling position. Hold weights in both hands with back of arms against ball. Lift both sides while bending at the elbows and squeezing bicep muscles. Lower back down - repeat.

_____ Reps _____ Sets _____X Day _____Hold	_____ Reps _____ Sets _____X Day _____Hold

9	Notes: *Neuropathy/Hands – Precaution holding weights	10	Notes: *Neuropathy/Hands – Precaution holding weights

BICEPS CURLS

Holding weights and keeping your arm at your side, draw up your hand by bending at the elbow squeezing bicep muscle. Keep your palm face up the entire time. Can perform set on one side and then other or alternate arms.

BICEPS CURLS - RADIOBRACHIALIS - HAMMER CURL

Holding weights and keeping your arm at your side, draw up your hand by bending at the elbow squeezing bicep muscle. Keep your wrist in a neutral position as shown above the entire time. Can perform set on one side and then other or alternate arms.

_____ Reps _____ Sets _____X Day _____Hold	_____ Reps _____ Sets _____X Day _____Hold

11	Notes: *Neuropathy/Hands – Precaution holding weights	12	Notes: *Neuropathy/Hands – Precaution holding weights

BICEPS CURLS - BRACHIALIS

Holding weights and keeping your arm at your side, draw up your hand by bending at the elbow squeezing bicep muscle. Keep your palm face down the entire time. Can perform set on one side and then other or alternate arms.

BICEPS CURLS – ROTATE OUTWARD

Holding weights and keeping your arm at your side, draw up your hand by bending at the elbow squeezing bicep muscle. Keep your palm face up the entire time. You can do this one arm at a time or bilateral.

	_____ Reps _____ Sets _____X Day _____Hold
13	**Notes:** *Lymphedema: Do not wrap band around UE or LE

BICEPS CURLS – ONE ARM - ELASTIC BAND

In a standing position, step on the band with one leg. Keep your arm at your side holding an elastic band and draw up your hand by bending at the elbow squeezing bicep muscle. Keep your palm face up the entire time.

	_____ Reps _____ Sets _____X Day _____Hold
14	**Notes:** *Lymphedema: Do not wrap band around UE or LE

BICEPS CURLS – BILATERAL - ELASTIC BAND

In a standing position, step on the band with both feet, shoulder width apart. Keep your arms at your side holding an elastic band and draw up your hands by bending at the elbows squeezing bicep muscles. Keep your palms facing upward the entire time.

	_____ Reps _____ Sets _____X Day _____Hold
15	**Notes:** *Lymphedema: Do not wrap band around UE or LE

BICEPS CURLS - RADIOBRACHIALIS - HAMMER CURL – ONE ARM - ELASTIC BAND

In a standing position, step on the band with one leg. Keep your arm at your side holding an elastic band and draw up your hand by bending at the elbow squeezing bicep muscle. Keep your palm facing inward the entire time.

	_____ Reps _____ Sets _____X Day _____Hold
16	**Notes:** *Lymphedema: Do not wrap band around UE or LE

BICEPS CURLS - RADIOBRACHIALIS - HAMMER CURL – BILATERAL - ELASTIC BAND

In a standing position, step on the band with both feet, shoulder width apart. Keep your arms at your side holding an elastic band and draw up your hands by bending at the elbows squeezing bicep muscles. Keep your palms facing inward the entire time.

_____ Reps _____ Sets _____X Day _____Hold		_____ Reps _____ Sets _____X Day _____Hold
17	Notes: *Lymphedema: Do not wrap band around UE or LE	**18**	Notes: *Lymphedema: Do not wrap band around UE or LE

BICEPS CURLS – BRACHIALIS - ONE ARM - ELASTIC BAND

In a standing position, step on the band with one leg. Keep your arm at your side holding an elastic band and draw up your hand by bending at the elbow squeezing bicep muscle. Keep your palm face down the entire time.

BICEPS CURL – BRACHIALIS – BILATERAL - ELASTIC BAND

In a standing position, step on the band with both feet, shoulder width apart. Keep your arms at your side holding an elastic band and draw up your hands by bending at the elbows squeezing bicep muscles. Keep your palms facing downward the entire time.

Elbow Extension (Triceps)

_____ Reps _____ Sets _____X Day _____Hold		_____ Reps _____ Sets _____X Day _____Hold
19	Notes: *Lymphedema: Do not wrap band around UE or LE	**20**	Notes: *Lymphedema: Do not wrap band around UE or LE

TRICEPS - SELF FIXATION - ELASTIC BAND

Hold an elastic band across your chest with the unaffected arm. Pull the band downward with the other arm so that the elbow goes from a bent position to a straightened position as shown.

OVERHEAD TRICEPS - SELF FIXATION –SEATED OR STANDING - ELASTIC BAND

Hold an elastic band with one arm fixated behind back as shown and other hand behind head. Extend elbow with arm overhead and return to starting position.

	_____ Reps _____ Sets _____X Day _____Hold		_____ Reps _____ Sets _____X Day _____Hold
21	**Notes:** *Neuropathy/Hands – Precaution holding weights	22	**Notes:** *Neuropathy/Hands – Precaution holding weights

Starting

Position

TRICEP EXTENSION – SITTING OR STANDING - WEIGHT

Start with hand behind head holding free weight. Extend your elbow as shown. Maintain your upper arm in an upward direction and only bend and straighten at your elbow.
*Can hold the triceps area with opposite arm to stabilize.

Starting

Position

TRICEP EXTENSION – SITTING OR STANDING – BILATERAL - WEIGHT

Start with hands behind head holding free weight Extend your elbows while holding a free weight in both hands. Maintain your upper arms in an upward direction and only bend and straighten at your elbows.

	_____ Reps _____ Sets _____X Day _____Hold		_____ Reps _____ Sets _____X Day _____Hold
23	**Notes:** *Neuropathy/Hands – Precaution holding weights	24	**Notes:** *Neuropathy/Hands – Precaution holding weights

Starting

Position

ELBOW EXTENSION - BALL

Lie on your back on ball. Extend your elbow as shown while holding a free weight in each hand. Maintain your upper arms in an upward direction and only bend and straighten at your elbows.

ELBOW EXTENSION - SKULL CRUSHER - BALL

Lie on your back on ball with a free weight in each hand. Bend your elbows to lower the weight towards the side of your head and then extend arms straight up towards the ceiling.

	_____ Reps _____ Sets _____X Day _____Hold		_____ Reps _____ Sets _____X Day _____Hold
25	**Notes:** *Lymphedema: Do not wrap band around UE or LE	**26**	**Notes:** *Neuropathy/Hands – Precaution holding weights

TRICEPS - ELASTIC BAND

Fixate the band at top of door. Start with your elbow bent and holding an elastic band as shown. Pull the elastic band downward as you extend your elbow. Keep your elbow by your side the entire time.

TRICEPS - BENT OVER

Stand and bend over with either support or placing your unaffected arm on thigh for support. With your targeted arm and elbow at your side, extend your elbow as you straighten your arm as shown. Keep your elbow at your side and back flat the entire time.

	_____ Reps _____ Sets _____X Day _____Hold		_____ Reps _____ Sets _____X Day _____Hold
27	**Notes:**	**28**	**Notes:**

CHAIR DIPS / PUSH UPS

While sitting in a chair with arm rests, push yourself upawards so that you lift your buttocks of the chair and then lower down controlled back to normal seated position.   *If you are unable to lift yourself up, you can perform "pressure releases" so that you simply push to take some weight off your buttocks.

DIPS OFF CHAIR

Push yourself up to a straight elbow position as shown. Then lower your buttocks down towards the floor by bending your elbows.

Shoulder PENDULUMS

	_____Reps _____Sets _____X Day _____Hold		_____Reps _____Sets _____X Day _____Hold
29	Notes:	**30**	Notes:

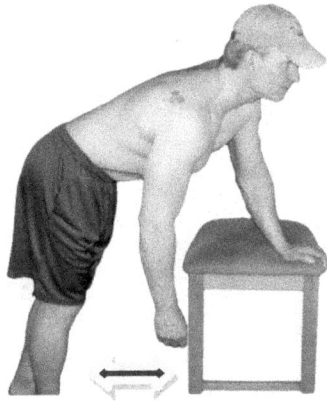

PENDULUM SHOULDER FORWARD/BACK

Shift your body weight forward then back to allow your injured arm to swing forward and back freely. Your affected arm should be fully relaxed.

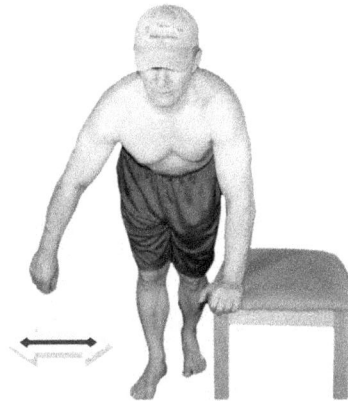

PENDULUM SHOULDER – SIDE TO SIDE

Shift your body weight side to side to allow your injured arm to swing side to side freely. Your affected arm should be fully relaxed.

	_____Reps _____Sets _____X Day _____Hold		_____Reps _____Sets _____X Day _____Hold
31	Notes:	**32**	Notes: *Neuropathy/Hands – Precaution holding weights

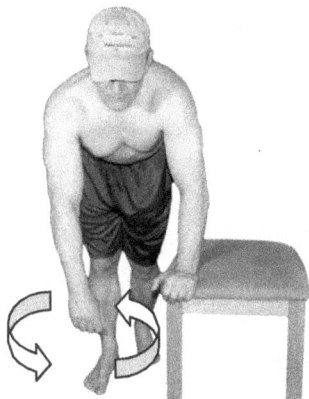

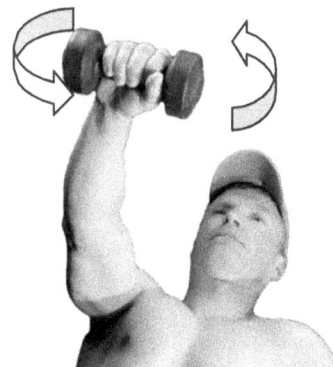

PENDULUM SHOULDER CIRCLES
Shift your body weight in circles to allow your injured arm to swing in circles freely. Your injured arm should be fully relaxed.
REVERSE PENDULUM SHOULDER CIRCLES
Shift your body weight into reverse circles to allow your injured arm to swing in circles freely. Your injured arm should be fully relaxed.

PENDULUMS - SUPINE

Lie on your back and straighten your arm towards the ceiling. Move your arm in small circles in a clockwise motion. After a few seconds, reverse the direction to a counterclockwise motion. Change directions every few seconds.

Shoulder Flexion

_____ Reps _____ Sets _____X Day _____Hold	_____ Reps _____ Sets _____X Day _____Hold
33 Notes:	**34** Notes:

ISOMETRIC FLEXION - Can use towel roll for comfort

Gently push your fist forward into a wall with your elbow bent. Hold for 5-10 seconds. Repeat.

Starting Position

SHOULDER FLEXION – SIDELYING - Can add weight

Lie on your side with arm at your side. Slowly raise the arm forward towards overhead and in front of your body.

_____ Reps _____ Sets _____X Day _____Hold	_____ Reps _____ Sets _____X Day _____Hold
35 Notes:	**36** Notes: *Neuropathy/Hands – Precaution holding weights

Starting Position

FLEXION – SUPINE - SINGLE OR BILATERAL

Lie on your back with your arm at your side. Slowly raise arm up and forward towards overhead.

Starting Position

FLEXION – SUPINE – SINGLE OR BILATERAL - WEIGHT

Lie on your back with your arm at your side. Holding a weight, slowly raise arm up and forward towards overhead.

	_____ Reps _____ Sets _____X Day _____Hold
37	Notes:

FLEXION – SUPINE - DOWEL

Lie on your back holding dowel with both hands. Slowly raise up and forward towards overhead. Return to starting position. Repeat.
*If you have an injury/weakness, allow your unaffected arm to perform most of the effort. Your affected arm should be partially relaxed.

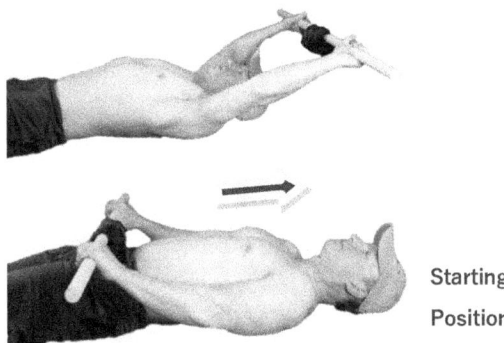

	_____ Reps _____ Sets _____X Day _____Hold
38	Notes:

FLEXION – SUPINE - DOWEL – Add weight only if equal strength

Attach ankle weight to dowel. Lie on your back holding dowel with both hands. Slowly raise up and forward towards overhead. Return to starting position. Repeat.

	_____ Reps _____ Sets _____X Day _____Hold
39	Notes: *Lymphedema: Do not wrap band around UE or LE

FLEXION - SELF FIXATION – ELASTIC BAND

Hold an elastic band in front and fixate unaffected arm straight by your side or on your leg. Pull the band upward towards the ceiling with your target arm.

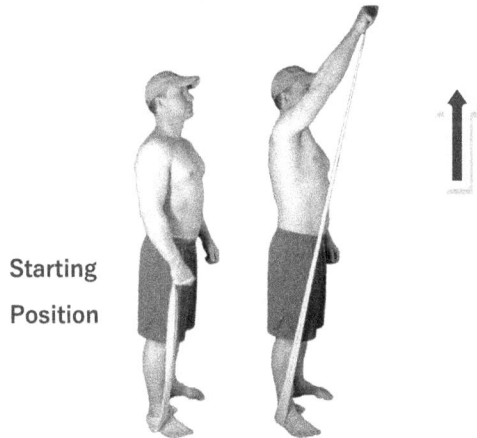

	_____ Reps _____ Sets _____X Day _____Hold
40	Notes: *Lymphedema: Do not wrap band around UE or LE

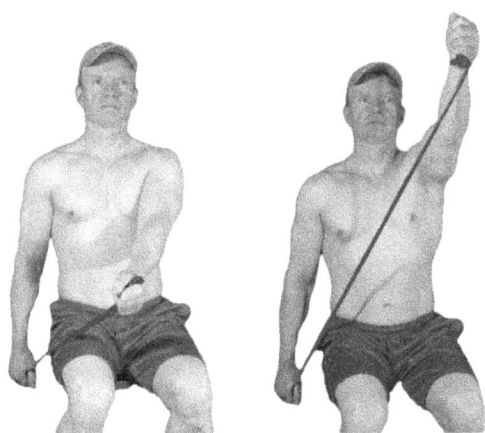

FLEXION – ELASTIC BAND

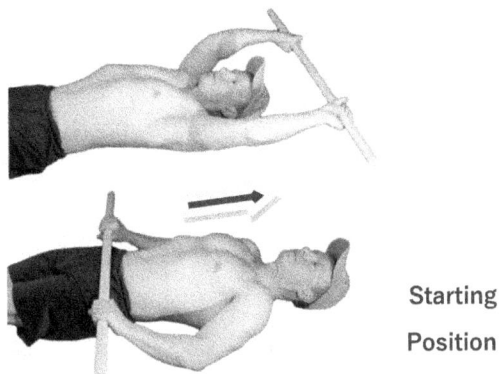

In a standing position, step on the band with one leg. Keep your arm at your side holding an elastic band and draw up your arm up in front of you keeping your elbow straight.

_____ Reps _____ Sets _____ X Day _____ Hold

41 Notes:

FLEXION - STANDING - PALMS DOWN / OVERHAND DOWEL - Add weight only if equal strength

Hold a dowel/cane with both arms, palm down on both sides. Raise the dowel forward and up. (see #39/40)
*Do not use weight if you have an injury/weakness. Allow your unaffected arm to perform most of the work. Your affected arm should be partially relaxed.

_____ Reps _____ Sets _____ X Day _____ Hold

42 Notes:

FLEXION - STANDING - PALMS UP /UNDERHAND DOWEL - Add weight only if equal strength

Hold a dowel/cane with both arms and palms up on both sides. Raise the dowel forward and up.
*Do not use weight if you have an injury/weakness. Allow your unaffected arm to perform most of the work. Your affected arm should be partially relaxed.

_____ Reps _____ Sets _____ X Day _____ Hold

43 Notes:
*Neuropathy/Hands – Precaution holding weights

FLEXION – PALMS FACING INWARD - Can remove weight BILATERAL or ALTERNATE ARMS.

Sit or stand with your arm at your side. Hold a free weight with your palm facing your side and your elbows straight. Raise up your arm forward as shown then return to starting position. Do not let your shoulder shrug upwards unless instructed to go over shoulder level height.

_____ Reps _____ Sets _____ X Day _____ Hold

44 Notes:
*Neuropathy/Hands – Precaution holding weights

FLEXION – PALMS DOWN - Can remove weight BILATERAL or ALTERNATE ARMS.

Sit or stand with your arm at your side. Hold a weight with your palm facing down and your elbows straight. Raise up your arm forward as shown then return to starting position. Do not let your shoulder shrug upwards unless instructed to go over shoulder height.

V Raises

	_____ Reps _____ Sets _____X Day _____Hold		_____ Reps _____ Sets _____X Day _____Hold
45	Notes:	**46**	Notes: *Neuropathy/Hands – Precaution holding weights

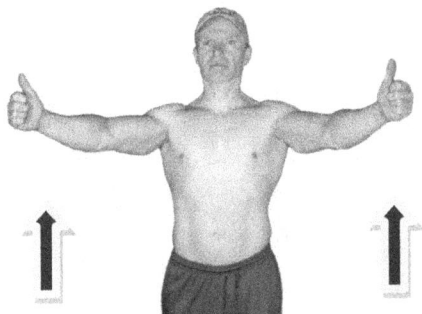

V RAISE

Start with your arms down by your side, palms facing inward, thumbs up and your elbows straight. Raise up your arms in the form of a V to shoulder height as shown keeping elbows straight then return to starting position.

Starting Position

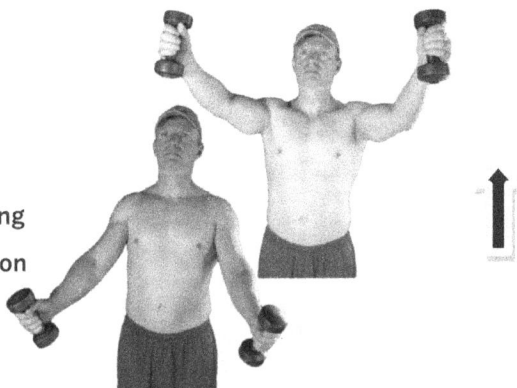

V RAISE – WEIGHTS

Holding free weights, start with your arms down by your side, palms facing inward and your elbows straight. Raise up your arms in the form of a V to shoulder height keeping elbows straight – return.

Shoulder Press

	_____ Reps _____ Sets _____X Day _____Hold		_____ Reps _____ Sets _____X Day _____Hold
47	Notes:	**48**	Notes: *Neuropathy/Hands – Precaution holding weights

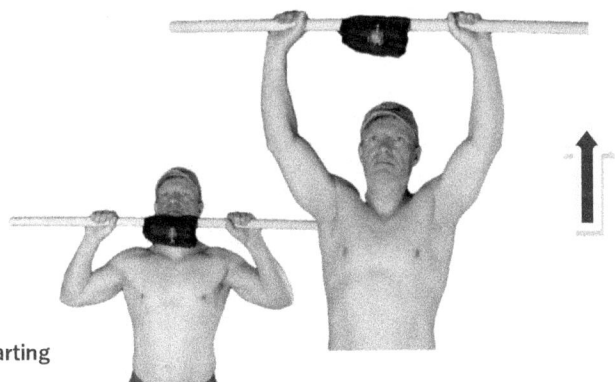

Starting Position

MILITARY PRESS – DOWEL- Add weight only if equal strength

Hold a dowel or cane at chest height. Slowly push the wand upwards towards the ceiling until your elbows become fully straightened. Return to the original position.

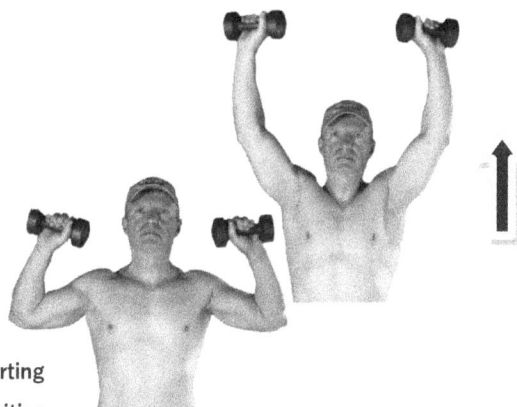

Starting Position

MILITARY PRESS - FREE WEIGHTS

Hold free weights at 90-degree angle as shown above.
Slowly push your arms upwards towards the ceiling until your elbows become fully straightened. Return to the original position.

Shoulder Extension

	_____ Reps _____ Sets _____ X Day _____ Hold
49	**Notes:**

ISOMETRIC EXTENSION - Can use towel roll for comfort

Gently push your bent elbow back into a wall. Hold for 5-10 seconds. Relax and repeat.

	_____ Reps _____ Sets _____ X Day _____ Hold
50	**Notes:**

PRONE EXTENSION - EXERCISE BALL – Can add weights.

Lie face down over an exercise ball with your elbows straight and along the side of your body. Slowly raise your arms upward along your side and then return to original position.

	_____ Reps _____ Sets _____ X Day _____ Hold
51	**Notes:**

SHOULDER EXTENSION - STANDING

Start with arms by your side. Draw your arm back behind your waist. Keep your elbows straight.

	_____ Reps _____ Sets _____ X Day _____ Hold
52	**Notes:** *Neuropathy/Hands – Precaution holding weights

SHOULDER EXTENSION - STANDING - WEIGHTS

Hold a weight by your side and draw your arm back. Keep your elbows straight.

	_____ Reps _____ Sets _____X Day _____Hold
53	**Notes:**

EXTENSION – STANDING – DOWEL - Add weight only if equal strength

Hold a dowel or cane behind your back with both arms. Draw your arms back.

	_____ Reps _____ Sets _____X Day _____Hold
54	**Notes:** *Lymphedema: Do not wrap band around UE or LE

EXTENSION - SELF FIXATION - ELASTIC BAND

Hold an elastic band out in front of you with your fixated arm. Pull the band downward towards the ground and backwards with your target arm.

	_____ Reps _____ Sets _____X Day _____Hold
55	**Notes:** *Lymphedema: Do not wrap band around UE or LE

EXTENSION - ELASTIC BAND

Fixate the end of an elastic band at top of door. Hold the elastic band in front of you with your elbows straight. Slowly pull the band down and back towards your side.

	_____ Reps _____ Sets _____X Day _____Hold
56	**Notes:** *Lymphedema: Do not wrap band around UE or LE

EXTENSION - BILATERAL - ELASTIC BAND

Fixate the middle of an elastic band at top of door. Hold the elastic band with both arms in front of you with your elbows straight. Slowly pull the band downwards and back towards your side.

Shoulder Internal Rotation (IR)

_____ Reps _____ Sets _____ X Day _____ Hold		_____ Reps _____ Sets _____ X Day _____ Hold	
57	Notes:	**58**	Notes:

INTERNAL ROTATION – ISOMETRIC - Can use towel roll for comfort

Press your hand into a wall using the palm side of your hand and hold. Maintain a bent elbow the entire time.

INTERNAL ROTATION - ISOMETRIC- ELEVATED - Can use towel roll for comfort

Push the front of your hand into a wall with your elbow bent and arm elevated and hold.

_____ Reps _____ Sets _____ X Day _____ Hold		_____ Reps _____ Sets _____ X Day _____ Hold	
59	Notes:	**60**	Notes: *Lymphedema: Do not wrap band around UE or LE

INTERNAL ROTATION - SIDELYING

Lie on your side with your shoulder flexed to 90 degrees and elbow bent and rested on the table/bed/matt. Your forearm should be pointing up towards the ceiling. Allow your forearm to lower toward the table as shown. Place a rolled-up towel under your elbow if needed.

INTERNAL ROTATION - ELASTIC BAND

Hold an elastic band at your side with your elbow bent. Start with your hand away from your stomach and then pull the band towards your stomach. Keep your elbow near your side the entire time.

	_____ Reps _____ Sets _____ X Day _____ Hold		_____ Reps _____ Sets _____ X Day _____ Hold
61	Notes:	**62**	Notes:

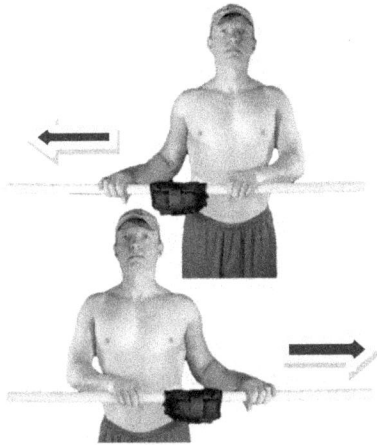

INTERNAL / EXTERNAL ROTATION - STANDING – DOWEL
Add weight only if equal strength

Stand and hold a dowel/cane with both hands keeping your elbows bent. Move your arms and dowel/cane side-to-side. _If you have an injury/weakness, the affected arm should be partially relaxed while your unaffected arm performs most of the effort._

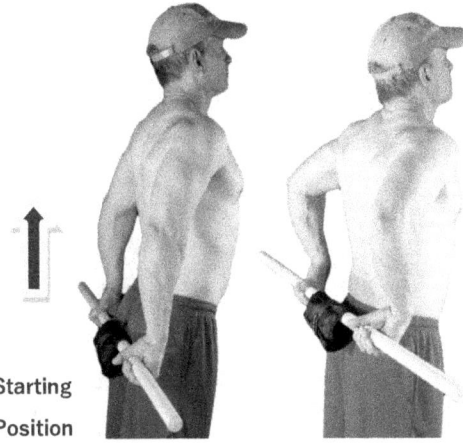

Starting

Position

INTERNAL ROTATION – DOWEL - Add weight only if equal strength

While holding a dowel/cane behind your back, slowly pull the wand up.

Shoulder External Rotation (ER)

	_____ Reps _____ Sets _____ X Day _____ Hold		_____ Reps _____ Sets _____ X Day _____ Hold
63	Notes:	**64**	Notes:

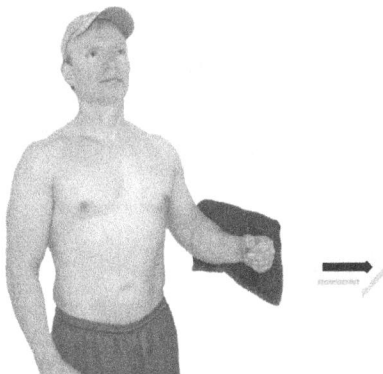

EXTERNAL ROTATION - ISOMETRIC – Can use towel roll for comfort

Gently press your hand into a wall using the back side of your hand. Maintain a bent elbow the entire time.

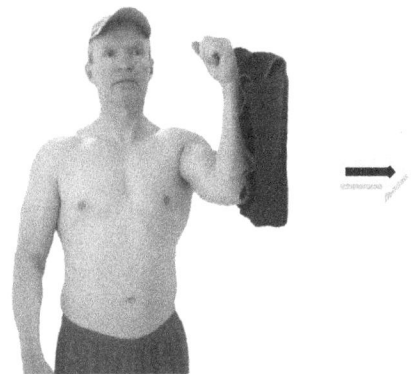

EXTERNAL ROTATION - ISOMETRIC – ELEVATED - Can use towel roll for comfort

Gently push the back of your hand/arm into a wall with your arm elevated.

_____ Reps _____ Sets _____X Day _____Hold		_____ Reps _____ Sets _____X Day _____Hold	
65	Notes:	**66**	Notes: *Neuropathy/Hands – Precaution holding weights

Starting
Position

EXTERNAL ROTATION WITH TOWEL - SIDELYING

Lie on your side with your elbow bent to 90 degrees. Place a rolled-up towel between your arm and the side your body as shown. Squeeze your shoulder blade back and rotate arm up and hold this position. Slowly rotate back to original position and repeat.

Starting
Position

EXTERNAL ROTATION – 90/90 - WEIGHTS

Hold weights with elbows bent to 90 degrees and away from your side. Rotate your shoulders back so that the palms of your hands face forward and then return as shown.

_____ Reps _____ Sets _____X Day _____Hold		_____ Reps _____ Sets _____X Day _____Hold	
67	Notes: *Lymphedema: Do not wrap band around UE or LE	**68**	Notes: *Lymphedema: Do not wrap band around UE or LE

EXTERNAL ROTATION - BILATERAL - ELASTIC BAND
Can put a towel between side and elbow (see #68)

Hold an elastic band with your elbows bent, pull your hands away from your stomach area. Keep your elbows near the side of your body.

EXTERNAL ROTATION - ELASTIC BAND – Can add roll between side and arm

Fixate an elastic band to the door at elbow height. Hold the other end of the band at your side with your elbow bent. Start with your hand near your stomach and then pull the band away. Keep your elbow at your side the entire time.

Shoulder Adduction (ADD)

	_____ Reps _____ Sets _____ X Day _____ Hold	_____ Reps _____ Sets _____ X Day _____ Hold
69	Notes:	**70** Notes: *Lymphedema: Do not wrap band around UE or LE

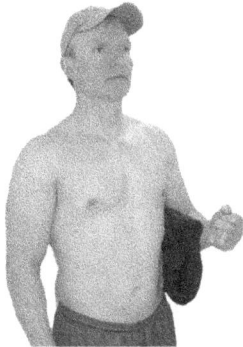

ADDUCTION – ISOMETRIC - Can use towel roll for comfort

Place a towel roll between your bent elbow and body. Gently push your elbow into the side of your body.

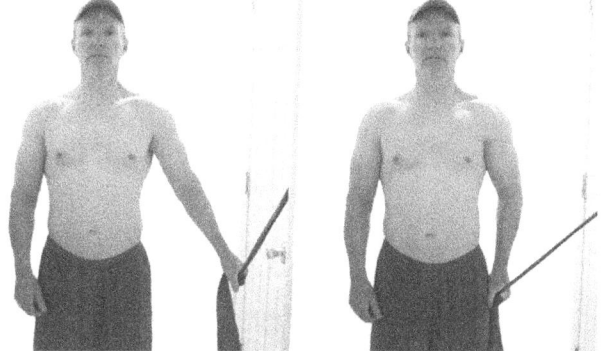

ADDUCTION - ELASTIC BAND

Fixate an elastic band to the door and hold the other end of the band away from your side. Pull the band towards your side keeping your elbow straight.

Shoulder Abduction (ABD)

	_____ Reps _____ Sets _____ X Day _____ Hold	_____ Reps _____ Sets _____ X Day _____ Hold
71	Notes:	**72** Notes:

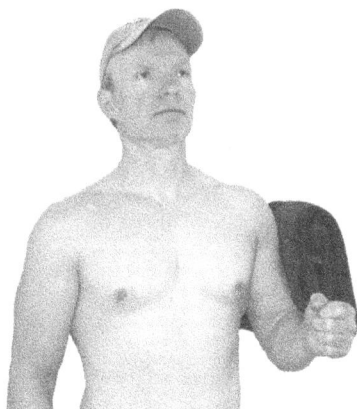

ABDUCTION – ISOMETRIC - Can use towel roll for comfort

Gently push your elbow out to the side into a wall with your elbow bent.

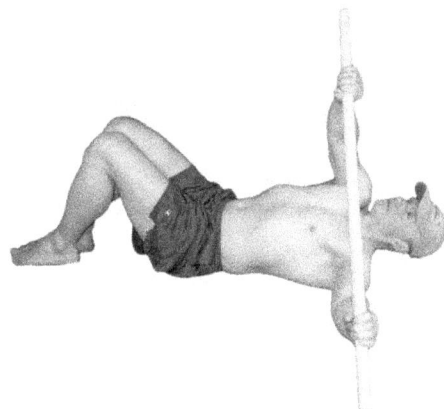

HORIZONTAL ABDUCTION - DOWEL

Lie on your back holding a dowel/cane straight up towards the ceiling with your elbows straight. Bring your arms and wand to the side and then towards the other.

_____ Reps _____ Sets _____ X Day _____ Hold

73	**Notes:**

HORIZONTAL ABDUCTION/ADDUCTTION - SUPINE
Lie on your back with arm straight up in front of your body. Slowly lower your arm out towards the side. Return to original position.

_____ Reps _____ Sets _____ X Day _____ Hold

74	**Notes:** *Neuropathy/Hands – Precaution holding weights

HORIZONTAL ABDUCTION/ADDUCTTION - SUPINE - WEIGHT

Hold a weight. Lie on your back with arm straight up in front of your body. Slowly lower your arm out towards the side. Return to original position

_____ Reps _____ Sets _____ X Day _____ Hold

75	**Notes:**

ABDUCTION - SIDELYING - Can add weight

Lie on your side with arm at your side. Slowly raise the target arm up towards head and away from your side.

_____ Reps _____ Sets _____ X Day _____ Hold

76	**Notes:**

HORIZONTAL ABDUCTION - SIDELYING - Can add weight

Lie on your side with arm out in front of your body. Slowly raise up the arm overhead towards the ceiling.

	_____ Reps _____ Sets _____ X Day _____ Hold
77	**Notes:** *Neuropathy/Hands – Precaution holding weights

ABDUCTION – WEIGHT – Can do without a weight

Hold a weight with your affected arm at your side.
Keeping your elbow straight, raise up your arm to the side.

	_____ Reps _____ Sets _____ X Day _____ Hold
78	**Notes:** *Lymphedema: Do not wrap band around UE or LE

ABDUCTION – ELASTIC BAND

Fixate an elastic band under a door and hold band
with hand farthest away from door at your side.
Keeping your elbow straight, raise up your arm to
the side.

	_____ Reps _____ Sets _____ X Day _____ Hold
79	**Notes:** *Lymphedema: Do not wrap band around UE or LE

HORIZONTAL ABDUCTION – BILATERAL - ELASTIC BAND

Hold an elastic band in both hands with your elbows
straight in front of your body. Slowly pull your arms apart
towards the sides.

	_____ Reps _____ Sets _____ X Day _____ Hold
80	**Notes:** *Neuropathy/Hands – Precaution holding weights

90/90 ABDUCTION - WEIGHT

Hold weights at your side with elbows bent to 90
degrees. Raise up your elbows away from your side
while maintaining your elbows bent at 90 degrees.

Lateral/Frontal Raise

_____ Reps _____ Sets _____ X Day _____ Hold	_____ Reps _____ Sets _____ X Day _____ Hold
81 Notes: *Neuropathy/Hands – Precaution holding weights	**82** Notes: *Neuropathy/Hands – Precaution holding weights

Starting Position

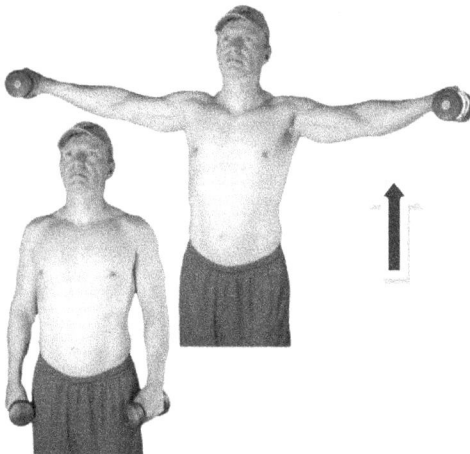

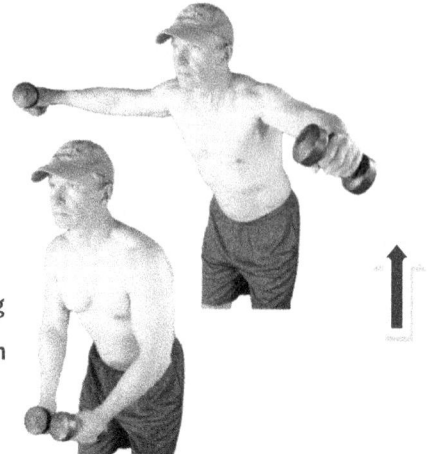

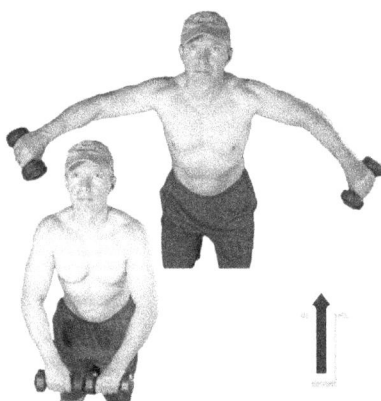

LATERAL RAISES

Hold weights at your side with arms straight. Raise up your elbows away from your side while keeping your elbow straight the entire time.

Starting Position

LATERAL RAISES – LEAN FORWARD

Bend slightly at the waist holding weights slightly in front. Raise up your elbows away from your side squeezing shoulder blades together.

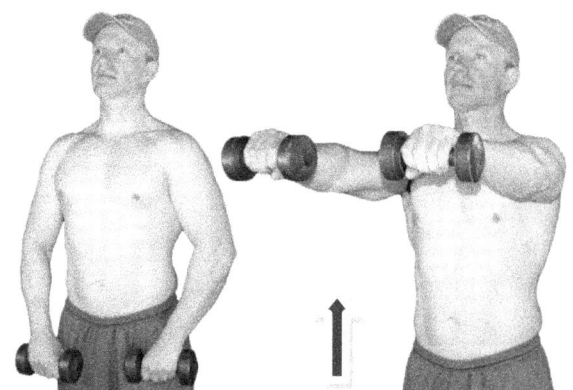

_____ Reps _____ Sets _____ X Day _____ Hold	_____ Reps _____ Sets _____ X Day _____ Hold
83 Notes: *Neuropathy/Hands – Precaution holding weights	**84** Notes: *Neuropathy/Hands – Precaution holding weights

Starting Position

LATERAL RAISES – LEAN FORWARD - ARM ROTATION

Bend slightly at the waist holding weights slightly in front as shown palms facing your body. Raise up your elbows away from your side squeezing shoulder blades together.

FRONTAL RAISE – WEIGHTS – Can do without weights

Hold weights at your side with arms straight. Slowly raise your arms in front of of your body.

Upright Rows

	_____ Reps _____ Sets _____X Day _____Hold
85	**Notes:** *Neuropathy/Hands – Precaution holding weights

	_____ Reps _____ Sets _____X Day _____Hold
86	**Notes:** *Lymphedema: Do not wrap band around UE or LE

UPRIGHT ROW – WEIGHTS - Can use kettle bell

Hold weights or kettlebell with both hands at waist height. Lift the weights to chest height as you bend at your elbows.

UPRIGHT ROW – ELASTIC BAND

Stand on an elastic band with either one or both feet. Hold band at waist height and raise it up to chest height as you bend at your elbows.

Shoulder Shrugs & Rolls

	_____ Reps _____ Sets _____X Day _____Hold
87	**Notes:**

	_____ Reps _____ Sets _____X Day _____Hold
88	**Notes:** *Neuropathy/Hands – Precaution holding weights

SHRUGS

Raise your shoulders upward towards your ears as shown. Shrug both shoulders at the same time.

SHRUGS - WEIGHTS

Hold weights in both hands with arms straight. Raise your shoulders upward towards your ears. Shrug both shoulders at the same time.

_____ Reps _____ Sets _____ X Day _____ Hold

89	Notes:

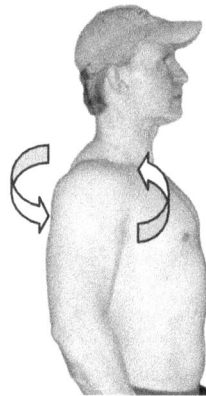

SHOULDER ROLLS

Move your shoulders in a circular pattern so that your are moving in an up, back and down direction. Perform small circles if needed for comfort.
Complete one set and then reverse direction

_____ Reps _____ Sets _____ X Day _____ Hold

90	Notes:

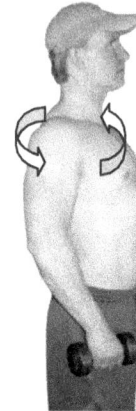

SHOULDER ROLLS - WEIGHTS

Hold weights in both or one hand. Move your shoulders in a circular pattern so that your are moving in an up, back and down direction.
Complete one set and then reverse direction

Scapular Retraction

_____ Reps _____ Sets _____ X Day _____ Hold

91	Notes:

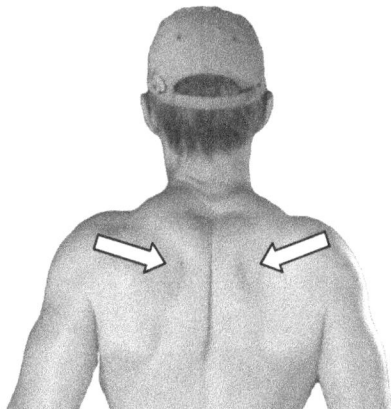

SCAPULAR RETRACTIONS - BILATERAL

Draw your shoulder blades back and down.

_____ Reps _____ Sets _____ X Day _____ Hold

92	Notes:

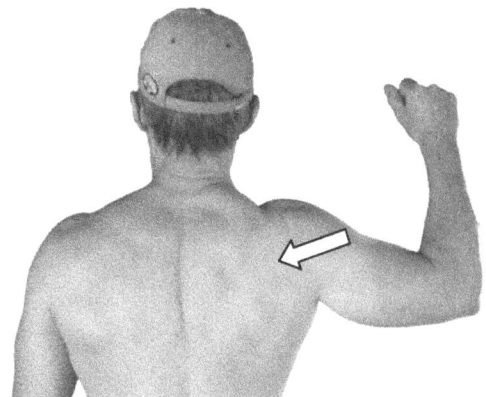

SCAPULAR RETRACTION – SINGLE ARM

With your arm raised up and elbow bent, draw your shoulder blade back and down.

_____ Reps _____ Sets _____X Day _____Hold	_____ Reps _____ Sets _____X Day _____Hold

93	Notes: *Lymphedema: Do not wrap band around UE or LE	94	Notes: *Neuropathy/Hands – Precaution holding weights

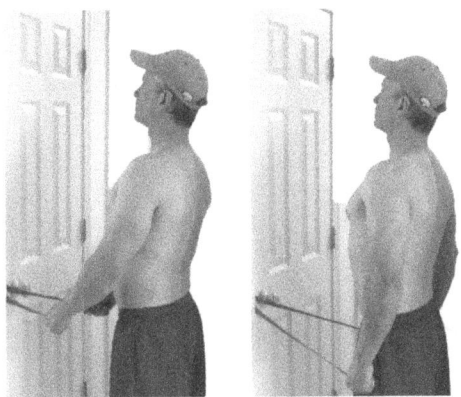

ELASTIC BAND SCAPULAR RETRACTIONS WITH MINI SHOULDER EXTENSIONS

Fixate an elastic band to the door and hold with both arms in front of you with your elbows straight. Slowly squeeze your shoulder blades together as you pull the band back. Be sure your shoulders do not rise up.

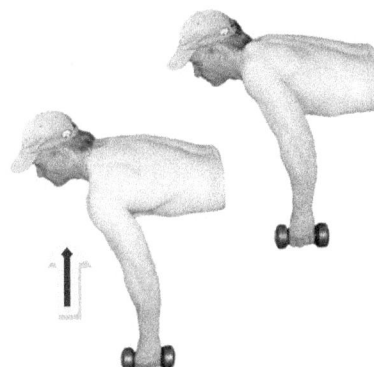

PRONE RETRACTION – Can do without weight

Lie face down with your elbows straight. Slowly draw your shoulder blade back towards your spine. Your whole arm should rise including your shoulder blade upward as shown. Your elbow should be straight the entire time.

Scapular Protraction

_____ Reps _____ Sets _____X Day _____Hold	_____ Reps _____ Sets _____X Day _____Hold

95	Notes:	96	Notes: *Neuropathy/Hands – Precaution holding weights

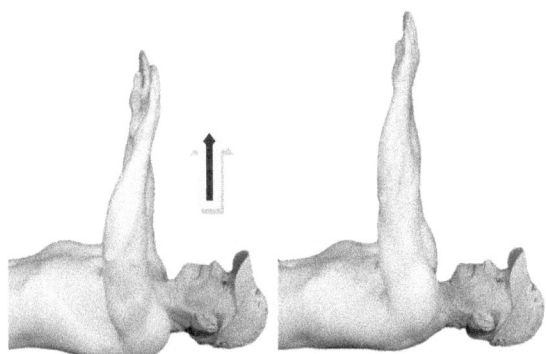

SCAPULAR PROTRACTION - SUPINE - BILATERAL

Lie on your back with your arms extended out in front of your body and towards the ceiling. While keeping your elbows straight, protract your shoulders reaching forward towards the ceiling. Keep your elbows straight the entire time.

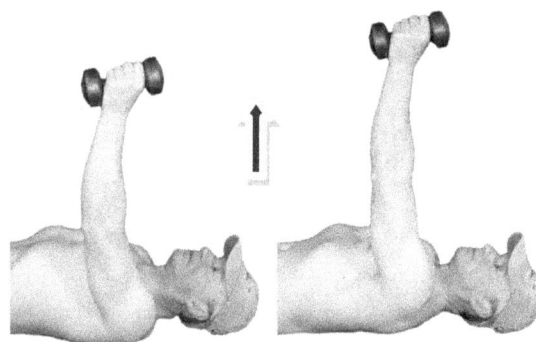

SCAPULAR PROTRACTION - SUPINE - WEIGHT

Lie on your back holding a weight with your arm extended out in front of your body and towards the ceiling. While keeping your elbows straight, protract your shoulders reaching forward towards the ceiling. Keep your elbows straight the entire time.

	_____ Reps _____ Sets _____X Day _____Hold		_____ Reps _____ Sets _____X Day _____Hold
97	Notes: *Lymphedema: Do not wrap band around UE or LE	**98**	Notes:

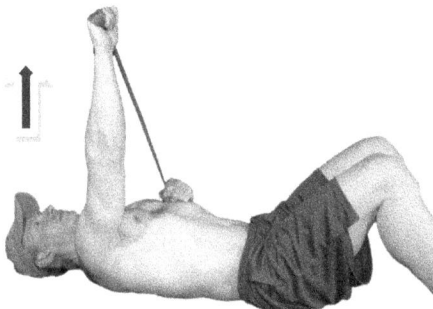

SCAPULAR PROTRACTION - SUPINE - ELASTIC BAND

Lie on your back and hold elastic band in both hands. Bend the unaffected arm to fixate the band. Extend the target arm out in front of your body and straight up towards the ceiling. While keeping your elbows straight, protract your shoulder blade forward towards the ceiling. Keep your elbows straight the entire time.

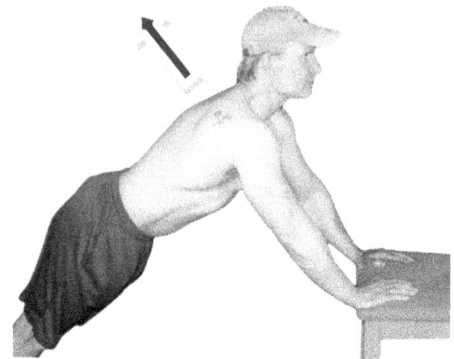

SCAPULAR PROTRACTION / TABLE PLANK

Start in a push up position on your hands and leaning up against a table or countertop as shown. Maintain this position as you protract your shoulder blades forward to raise your body upward a few inches. Return to original position.
*Progress by standing further away from the table.

Chest Press

	_____ Reps _____ Sets _____X Day _____Hold		_____ Reps _____ Sets _____X Day _____Hold
99	Notes: *Lymphedema: Do not wrap band around UE or LE	**100**	Notes: *Neuropathy/Hands – Precaution holding weights

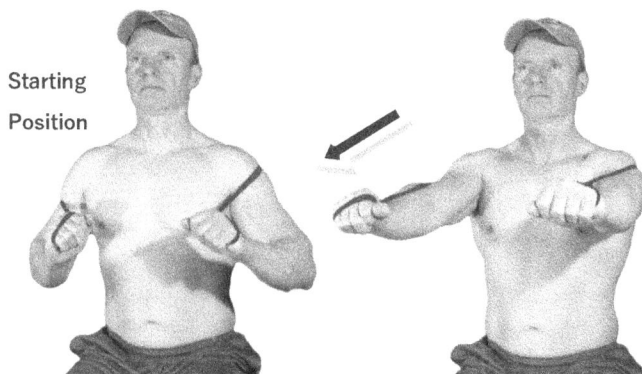

CHEST PRESS – SEATED or STANDING - ELASTIC BAND

Hold elastic band with both hands at your side and elbows bent with band wrapped around body or chair. Push the band out in front of your body as you straighten your elbows.

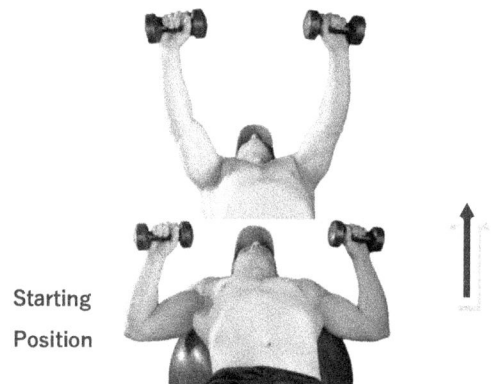

CHEST PRESS – BALL, FLOOR or BENCH- WEIGHTS

Lie on your back with your elbows bent. Slowly raise up your arms towards the ceiling while extending your elbows straight up above your head.

_____ Reps _____ Sets _____X Day _____Hold

101 | Notes:

102 | Notes:
*Neuropathy/Hands – Precaution holding weights

Starting
Position

DOWEL PRESS – STANDING – Add weight only if equal strength

Hold a dowel/cane at chest height. Slowly push the dowel outwards in front of your body so that your elbows become fully straightened. Return to the original position.

Starting
Position

CHEST PRESS – STANDING or SEATED

Hold weights in both hands with your arms at your side and elbows bent. Push your arms out in front of your body as you straighten your elbows.

Rows

_____ Reps _____ Sets _____X Day _____Hold

103 | Notes:
*Neuropathy/Hands – Precaution holding weights

104 | Notes:
*Neuropathy/Hands – Precaution holding weights

BENT OVER ROWS

Stand, bend over and support yourself with the unaffected arm. Slowly draw up your target arm as you bend your elbow. Keep your back flat the entire time.

ROWS – PRONE – On bed or table

Lie face down with your elbows straight, slowly raise your arms upward while bending your elbows.

	_____ Reps _____ Sets _____X Day _____Hold

105	**Notes:** *Lymphedema: Do not wrap band around UE or LE

ROWS - ELASTIC BAND

Fixate the elastic band in the door at elbow level. Hold the elastic band with both hands, draw back the band as you bend your elbows. Keep your elbows near the side of your body.

	_____ Reps _____ Sets _____X Day _____Hold

106	**Notes:** *Lymphedema: Do not wrap band around UE or LE

WIDE ROWS - ELASTIC BAND

Fixate the elastic band in the door and hold the band with both hands. Draw back the band as you bend your elbows squeezing shoulder blades together. Keep your arms about 90 degrees away from the side of your body.

	_____ Reps _____ Sets _____X Day _____Hold

107	**Notes:** *Lymphedema: Do not wrap band around UE or LE

LOW ROW – ELASTIC BAND

Fixate the elastic band in the door below elbow level. Hold the elastic band with both hands, draw back the band as you bend your elbows. Keep your elbows near the side of your body.

	_____ Reps _____ Sets _____X Day _____Hold

108	**Notes:** *Lymphedema: Do not wrap band around UE or LE

HIGH ROW – ELASTIC BAND

Fixate the elastic band at the top of the door. Hold the elastic band with both hands, draw back the band as you bend your elbows. Keep your elbows near the side of your body.

Flys

_____ Reps _____ Sets _____ X Day _____ Hold	_____ Reps _____ Sets _____ X Day _____ Hold
109 Notes: *Neuropathy/Hands – Precaution holding weights	**110** Notes: *Neuropathy/Hands – Precaution holding weights

Starting

Position

FLY'S – FLOOR - WEIGHT

Holding weights, lie on your back with your arms horizontally out to the side. Bring your arms up and forward towards the ceiling. Lower your arms back down to the original position. Your elbows should be partially bent the entire time.

FLY'S – BALL or BENCH – WEIGHT

Holding weights, lie on your back on a ball with your arms horizontally out to the side. Bring your arms up and forward towards the ceiling. Lower your arms back down to the original position with elbows partially bent the entire time.

Wall pushups – To progress, move feet further away from wall

_____ Reps _____ Sets _____ X Day _____ Hold	_____ Reps _____ Sets _____ X Day _____ Hold
111 Notes:	**112** Notes:

WALL PUSH UPS

Place your arms out in front of you with your elbows straight so that your hands just reach the wall. Bend your elbows slowly to bring your chest closer to the wall. Straighten your arms pushing your body away from wall. Maintain your feet planted on the ground the entire time.

WALL PUSH UP - BALL

Place a ball on a wall while holding the ball with both hands as shown. Bend your elbows slowly to bring your chest closer to the wall and then straighten your arms pushing your body away from wall. Maintain your feet planted on the ground the entire time.

	_____ Reps _____ Sets _____X Day _____Hold
113	Notes:

WALL PUSH UP - Triceps uneven

Place your arms out in front of you with your elbows straight in an uneven position so that your hands just reach the wall. Bend your elbows slowly to bring your chest closer to the wall and then straighten your arms pushing your body away from wall. Maintain your feet planted on the ground the entire time.

	_____ Reps _____ Sets _____X Day _____Hold
114	Notes:

WALL PUSH UP – Hands inverted

Place your arms out in front of you with your elbows straight and hands inverted just reaching the wall. Bend your elbows slowly to bring your chest closer to the wall and then straighten your arms pushing your body away from wall. Maintain your feet planted on the ground the entire time.

	_____ Reps _____ Sets _____X Day _____Hold
115	Notes:

WALL PUSH UP - Narrow

Place your arms out in front of you with your elbows straight and hands close togther just reaching the wall. Bend your elbows slowly to bring your chest closer to the wall and then straighten your arms pushing your body away from wall. Maintain your feet planted on the ground the entire time.

	_____ Reps _____ Sets _____X Day _____Hold
116	Notes:

WALL PUSH UP – Wide

Place your arms out in front of you with your elbows straight and your arms and hands far apart just reaching the wall. Bend your elbows slowly to bring your chest closer to the wall and then straighten your arms pushing your body away from wall. Maintain your feet planted on the ground the entire time.

Push ups

_____ Reps _____ Sets _____X Day _____Hold		_____ Reps _____ Sets _____X Day _____Hold

117	Notes:	**118**	Notes:

PUSH UPS - BALL

Start in a kneeling position with an exercise ball in front of you. Slowly walk yourself out with your arms so that the ball is positioned under your legs. Then perform push ups. *Progress by moving ball back towards thighs

Starting Position

PUSH UP - MODIFIED

Lie face down and use your arms and push yourself up. Keep your knees in contact with the floor and maintain a straight back the entire time.

_____ Reps _____ Sets _____X Day _____Hold		_____ Reps _____ Sets _____X Day _____Hold

119	Notes:	**120**	Notes:

Starting Position

PUSH UP

Lie face down, use your arms and push yourself. Keep your toes in contact with the floor and maintain a straight back the entire time.

PUSH UP -DIAMOND

Lie face down and place your hands on the floor in the shape of a diamond with your thumbs and index fingers.
Use your arms and push yourself up.. Keep your toes in contact with the floor and maintain a straight back the entire time.

_____ Reps _____ Sets _____ X Day _____ Hold		_____ Reps _____ Sets _____ X Day _____ Hold
121	Notes:	**122**	Notes:

PUSH UP – MODIFIED - BOSU - UNSTABLE

Perform push-ups with your hands on a Bosu. Keep your knees in contact with the floor and maintain a straight back the entire time.

PUSH UP – BOSU - UNSTABLE

Perform push-ups with your hands on top of a Bosu. Keep your toes in contact with the floor and maintain a straight back the entire time.

_____ Reps _____ Sets _____ X Day _____ Hold		_____ Reps _____ Sets _____ X Day _____ Hold
123	Notes:	**124**	Notes:

PUSH UP – MODIFIED – INVERTED BOSU - UNSTABLE

Perform push-ups while holding an inverted Bosu. Try and maintain the Bosu platform as level as you can. Keep your knees in contact with the floor and maintain a straight back the entire time.

PUSH UP – INVERTED BOSU - UNSTABLE

Perform push-ups while holding an inverted Bosu. Try and maintain the Bosu platform as level as you can. Keep your toes in contact with the floor and maintain a straight back the entire time.

BALANCE – CORE – STANDING LE STRENGTH

Basics
- Requires LE strengthening for progression
- Perform exercises 2-3x a week
- Should be performed at beginning of exercise routine or can be the main exercise routine for endurance with increased repetitions or strength with resistance.

Duration, Frequency, Intensity, Sets and Reps
- Balance – 1 set, 2-4 repetitions for hold of 5-60 seconds
- Endurance – Less than 30 second rests in between sets
  - Static - 1 set, 5-10 repetitions as tolerated
  - Dynamic – 1 set, 3-10 reps for 10-30+ second hold as tolerated
- Strengthening – Add resistance with bands or weights (*see Strengthening for more information*)
  - Static – 2-3 sets, 3-12 reps – slow controlled movements
  - Dynamic – 1-3 sets, 2-4 reps

Static Balance Progression:
1. Bilateral – Both feet on the ground
2. Unilateral – One foot on the ground
3. Arm Movement – Overhead, can do arm exercises (*See Arm Strengthening for exercises*)
4. Trunk rotation – Rotate with or without arm movement
5. Eyes Shut (lack of visual cues – sensory removal)
6. Head Turns, hand/eye tracking, shifting focal point (vestibular – sensory alteration)
7. Reading (coordination)
8. Unstable – progression
   Repeat above on unstable surface such as balance pad, pillow, balance disc or Bosu.

Decrease Base of Support (BOS) Progression:
- Wide BOS
- Narrow Bos
- Staggered/Split Stance/Semi-tandem
- Tandem Stance
- Single Leg Stance

SOLID GROUND:
1. Support: Hold onto chair, counter, sink or another stationary object.
2. No Support: Stand next to stable surface if needed for security.
   - Can start with 1-2 hands and as you become more stable, decrease the number of fingers used for support. For example, take away the thumb and hold with 4 fingers, 3 fingers, 2 fingers, 1 finger and then without support.
3. Resistance: Add ankle weights on use elastic band for resistance

UNSTABLE SURFACE: Balance pad, Bosu, Half foam roll, Pillow or Other unstable surface
1. Support: Hold onto chair, counter or another stationary object.
2. No Support: Stand next to stable surface if needed for security.
   - Can start with 1-2 hands and as you become more stable, decrease the number of fingers used for support. For example, take away the thumb and hold with 4 fingers, 3 fingers, 2 fingers, 1 finger and then without support.
3. Resistance: Add ankle weights on use elastic band for resistance

Peripheral Neuropathy **Caution Balancing on Uneven Surface**	<ul><li>Peripheral neuropathy can be a side effect of diabetes or may be as a result of damage to the peripheral nerves. These nerves carry information from the brain to other parts of the body.</li><li>Feet or lower extremity – Caution standing on uneven surface, such as a Bosu ball or balance pads due to decreased sensation in feet. Increased risk of falling.</li><li>Hands – Caution with holding dumbbells or grasping resistance bands.</li></ul>

EXERCISE Balance	EXERCISE NUMBER	NOTES
WIDE BOS DECREASING TO NARROW BOS	1	
NARROW BOS	2	
ARM MOVEMENT	3	
TRUNK ROTATION	4	
EYES SHUTS	5	
HEAD TURNS	6	
READING ALOUD	7	
BALANCE PAD	8	
SPLIT STANCE – SEMI TANDEM	9	
SPLIT STANCE - *Progression*	10	
TANDEM- SHARPENED ROMBERG STANCE	11	
TANDEM STANCE - Progression	12	
SINGLE LEG STANCE (SLS)	13	
SINGLE LEG STANCE (SLS) - *Progression*	14	
SLS – LEG FORWARD	15	
SLS – LEG BACKWARDS	16	
SLS – LEG FORWARD / OPPOSITE ARM UP	17	
SLS – LEG BACKWARDS / OPPOSITE ARM UP	18	
SLS - REACH FORWARD	19	
SLS - REACH TWIST	20	
SINGLE LEG TOE TAP	21	
SINGLE LEG STANCE - CLOCKS	22	
BALL ROLLS - HEEL TOE	23	
BALL ROLLS - LATERAL	24	
SQUAT	25	
SIT TO STAND	26	

EXERCISE Balance	EXERCISE NUMBER	NOTES
SQUATS – WALL WITH BALL	27	
SQUATS WITH WEIGHTS	28	
MINI SQUAT - UNSTABLE SUPPORT - FOAM PAD	29	
SQUATS - SINGLE LEG	30	
SIDE TO SIDE WEIGHT SHIFT	31	
FORWARD AND BACKWARDS WEIGHT SHIFTS	32	
SPLIT STANCE WEIGHT SHIFT SIDE TO SIDE	33	
SPLIT STANCE WEIGHT SHIFT FORWARD AND BACKWARDS	34	
WALL FALLS - FORWARD - BALANCE DRILL	35	
WALL FALLS - LATERAL - BALANCE DRILL	36	
WALL FALLS - BACKWARDS - BALANCE DRILL	37	
WALL FALLS - SINGLE LEG - FORWARD - BALANCE DRILL	38	
WALL FALLS - SINGLE LEG - LATERAL - BALANCE DRILL	39	
WALL FALLS - SINGLE LEG - MEDIAL - BALANCE DRILL	40	
WALL FALLS - SINGLE LEG - BACKWARDS - BALANCE DRILL	41	
FALL LATERAL - STEP RECOVERY	42	
FALL FORWARD - STEP RECOVERY	43	
FALL BACKWARD - STEP RECOVERY	44	
TOE TAP ABDUCTION	45	
HIP ABDUCTION - STANDING	46	
HIP EXTENSION – STANDING	47	
HIP FLEXION - STANDING – STRAIGHT LEG RAISE	48	
HIP / KNEE FLEXION - SINGLE LEG	49	
STANDING MARCHING	50	

EXERCISE	EXERCISE	NOTES
Balance	NUMBER	
HAMSTRING CURL	51	
TOE RAISES	52	
TOE RAISES IR AND ER	53	
ONE LEGGED TOE RAISE	54	
SINGLE LEG BALANCE FORWARD	55	
SINGLE LEG BALANCE LATERAL	56	
SINGLE LEG BALANCE RETRO	57	
SINGLE LEG STANCE RETROLATERAL	58	
SQUAT	59	
SINGLE LEG SQUAT	60	
LUNGE – STATIC	61	
LUNGE FORWARD/BACKWARD	62	
FOUR CORNER MARCHING IN PLACE	63	
FOUR CORNER MARCHING IN PLACE WITH HEAD TURNS	64	
WALKING ON HEELS FORWARD AND BACKWARDS	65	
WALKING ON TOES FORWARD AND BACKWARDS	66	
TANDEM STANCE AND WALK – FORWARD AND BACKWARDS	67	
RUNNING MAN	68	
HOP STICK - FORWARD	69	
HOP STICK - BACKWARDS	70	
MINI LATERAL LUNGE	71	
SIDE STEPPING	72	
HOP STICK - LATERAL	73	
SINGLE LEG DEAD LIFT	74	

EXERCISE	EXERCISE NUMBER	NOTES
Balance		
CONE TAPS - SINGLE LEG STANCE	75	
CONE TAPS - SINGLE LEG STANCE - UNSTABLE	76	
FIGURE 8 AROUND CONES	77	
FIGURE 8 AROUND CONES – FOOT OR HAND TAP	78	
BALANCE DOUBLE LEG STANCE - WIDE	79	
BALANCE DOUBLE LEG STANCE - NARROW	80	
TANDEM STANCE	81	
TANDEM WALK	82	
SINGLE LEG STANCE - ABDUCTION	83	
SINGLE LEG STANCE - ABDUCTION	84	
SINGLE LEG STANCE – FORWARD KICK	85	
SINGLE LEG STANCE – HAMSTRING CURL	86	
SINGLE LEG SQUAT – LEG FORWARD	87	
SINGLE LEG SQUAT – LEG BACKWARDS	88	
TOE TAP OR HEEL PLACEMENT	89	
PULL UP FOOT TOUCHES ON STEP	90	
ALTERNATING SUSTAINED FOOT TOUCHES ON STEP	91	
STEP UP AND OVER	92	
FORWARD SWING THROUGH STEP	93	
SIDE STEPPING - *REPEAT STEPS 89-93 from a side approach.*	94	

BALANCE PROGRESSION- STATIC – See WARNING above Re: Peripheral Neuropathy

Hip Width/Narrow Stance >>>>> Staggered Stance >>>>> Tandem Stance   >>>>> Single-Leg Stance

1. Hold onto a chair, counter or other steady object.
2. Continue steps 2-8 holding on to a sturdy object.
3. Can start with 1-2 hands and as you become more stable, decrease the number of fingers used for support. For example, take away the thumb and hold with 4 fingers, 3 fingers, 2 fingers, 1 finger and then without support.
4. When feeling comfortable, take away support staying close to object for security
5. When able to complete with decreased support, add balance pad or unstable surface completing 2-8 as above.

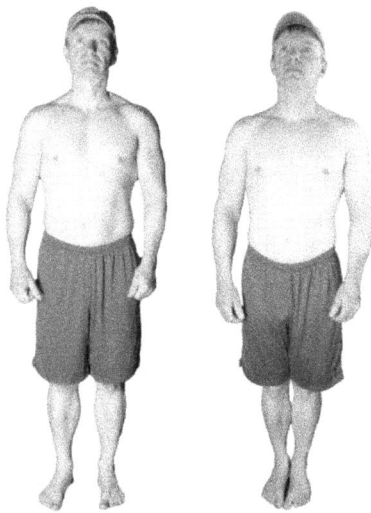

HIP WIDTH OR WIDE BASE OF SUPPORT (BOS) > NARROW BASE OF SUPPORT (BOS)

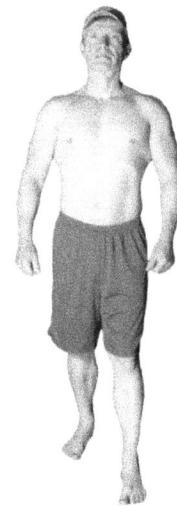

STAGGERED STANCE – SPLIT STANCE

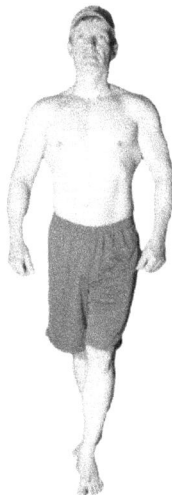

TANDEM STANCE

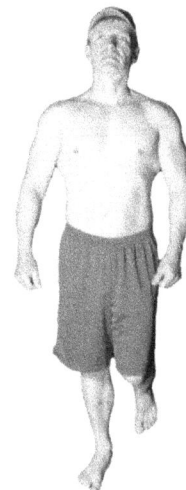

SINGLE LEG STANCE

	_____ Reps _____ Sets _____ X Day _____ Hold		_____ Reps _____ Sets _____ X Day _____ Hold
1	Notes:	**2**	Notes:

WIDE BOS DECREASING TO NARROW BOS

Continue steps 2-8 holding on to a sturdy object and then progress with decreased support as outlined above.

NARROW BOS

Stand with your feet together Count to 10. Increase time up to 60 seconds as tolerated maintaining your balance in this position.

	_____ Reps _____ Sets _____ X Day _____ Hold		_____ Reps _____ Sets _____ X Day _____ Hold
3	Notes:	**4**	Notes:

ARM MOVEMENT

Examples:
- Throw ball up in arm and catch
- Play catch with partner
- Reach hands above head and then down by side
- Do standing arm exercises (_See Arm Strengthening for examples)_

TRUNK ROTATION – reach side to side

Examples:
- Reach side to side within BOS
- Reach side to side and forward out of BOS

_____ Reps _____ Sets _____ X Day _____ Hold		_____ Reps _____ Sets _____ X Day _____ Hold	
5	Notes:	**6**	Notes:

EYES SHUTS - Lack of visual cues – *Sensory Removal*

Stand with eyes shut and count to 10. Increase time up to 60 seconds as tolerated.

HEAD TURNS - Vestibular – *Sensory Alteration*

Examples:
- Turn head slowly from side to side
- Move head up and down slowly
- Put one finger out in front of face at arm's length moving in outward/inward direction and move head to follow with eyes. Slow hand tracking.
- Shift focal point to different objects in the room
- *Can add head turns with eyes closed*

_____ Reps _____ Sets _____ X Day _____ Hold		_____ Reps _____ Sets _____ X Day _____ Hold	
7	Notes:	**8**	Notes:

READING ALOUD - *Coordination / Cognitive Task*

Hold reading material, such as a book, paper, tablet, or magazine in one or both hands.   Read out loud and progress to moving your head and the object on occasion to the side or up/down.

BALANCE PAD or another unstable surface

Place balance pad, Bosu, pillow or other unstable surface by a chair or counter for support. Stand on the pad.

****REPEAT STEPS 2-8 on unstable surface****

	_____ Reps _____ Sets _____X Day _____Hold
9	**Notes:**

SPLIT STANCE – SEMI TANDEM

Place one foot forward and the opposite foot to the back and slightly out to the side. Count to 10. Increase time up to 60 seconds as tolerated maintaining your balance in this position.

	_____ Reps _____ Sets _____X Day _____Hold
10	**Notes:**

SPLIT STANCE

FOLLOW STEPS 2-8 AS SEEN WITH NARROW BOS AS OUTLINED IN BALANCE PROGRESSION

1. HOLD STEADY OBJECT PROGRESSING TO NO SUPPORT
2. STAND FOR 10-60 SECONDS
3. ARM MOVEMENT
4. TRUNK ROTATION
5. EYES SHUT
6. HEAD TURNS
7. READING
8. **UNSTABLE**

REPEAT ABOVE ON UNSTABLE SURFACE SUCH AS BALANCE PAD, PILLOW, BALANCE DISC, HALF FOARM ROLL OR BOSU.

	_____ Reps _____ Sets _____X Day _____Hold
11	**Notes:**

TANDEM- SHARPENED ROMBERG STANCE

Place the heel of one foot so that it touches the toes of the other foot. Count to 10. Increase time up to 60 seconds as tolerated maintaining your balance in this position.

	_____ Reps _____ Sets _____X Day _____Hold
12	**Notes:**

TANDEM STANCE

FOLLOW STEPS 2-8 AS SEEN WITH NARROW BOS AS OUTLINED IN BALANCE PROGRESSION

1. HOLD STEADY OBJECT PROGRESSING TO NO SUPPORT
2. STAND FOR 10-60 SECONDS
3. ARM MOVEMENT
4. TRUNK ROTATION
5. EYES SHUT
6. HEAD TURNS
7. READING
8. **UNSTABLE**

REPEAT ABOVE ON UNSTABLE SURFACE SUCH AS BALANCE PAD, PILLOW, BALANCE DISC, HALF FOARM ROLL OR BOSU.

_____ Reps _____ Sets _____ X Day _____ Hold	_____ Reps _____ Sets _____ X Day _____ Hold

13 Notes:

14 Notes:

SINGLE LEG STANCE (SLS)

Stand on one foot. Count to 10 > 60 seconds as tolerated maintaining your balance in this position. Maintain a slightly bent knee on the stance side.

SINGLE LEG STANCE

FOLLOW STEPS 2-8 AS SEEN WITH NARROW BOS AS OUTLINED IN BALANCE PROGRESSION

1. HOLD STEADY OBJECT PROGRESSING TO NO SUPPORT
2. STAND FOR 10-60 SECONDS
3. ARM MOVEMENT
4. TRUNK ROTATION
5. EYES SHUT
6. HEAD TURNS
7. READING
8. **UNSTABLE**

REPEAT ABOVE ON UNSTABLE SURFACE SUCH AS BALANCE PAD, PILLOW, BALANCE DISC, HALF FOARM ROLL OR BOSU.

Single Leg Stance (SLS) with Arm and/or Leg Movements- *Progress to Balance Pad*

_____ Reps _____ Sets _____ X Day _____ Hold	_____ Reps _____ Sets _____ X Day _____ Hold

15 Notes:

16 Notes:

SLS – LEG FORWARD

Stand on one leg and maintain your balance. Hold your leg out in front of your body and then return to the original position. Repeat on opposite side. Maintain a slightly bent knee on the stance side.

SLS – LEG BACKWARDS

Stand on one leg and maintain your balance. Hold your leg in the back of your body and then return to original position. Repeat on opposite side. Maintain a slightly bent knee on the stance side.

_____ Reps _____ Sets _____X Day _____Hold

17 | Notes:

SLS – LEG FORWARD / OPPOSITE ARM UP

Stand on one leg and maintain your balance. Hold your leg out in front of your body and opposite arm up over your head. Return to the original position. Repeat on opposite side. Maintain a slightly bent knee on the stance side.

_____ Reps _____ Sets _____X Day _____Hold

18 | Notes:

SLS – LEG BACKWARDS / OPPOSITE ARM UP

Stand on one leg and maintain your balance. Hold your leg out in front of your body and opposite arm up over your head. Return to the original position. Repeat on opposite side. Maintain a slightly bent knee on the stance side.

_____ Reps _____ Sets _____X Day _____Hold

19 | Notes:

SLS - REACH FORWARD

Stand on one leg and maintain your balance. Reach forward with your opposite arm as far as you can without losing your balance and then return to original position. Repeat on opposite side. Maintain a slightly bent knee on the stance side.

_____ Reps _____ Sets _____X Day _____Hold

20 | Notes:

SLS - REACH TWIST

Stand on one leg and maintain your balance. Reach forward and across your body with your opposite arm as far as you can without losing your balance and then return to original position. Repeat on opposite side. Maintain a slightly bent knee on the stance side.

	_____ Reps _____ Sets _____X Day _____Hold		_____ Reps _____ Sets _____X Day _____Hold
21	Notes:	**22**	Notes:

SINGLE LEG TOE TAP

Start by standing on one leg and maintain your balance. Tap the opposite foot on a slightly raised object, such as a box or balance pad. To progress, increase the height of object, such as a stair step or cone. Can alternate feet or repeat on same side for several repetitions and then repeat on opposite side.

SINGLE LEG STANCE - CLOCKS

Start by standing on one leg and maintain your balance. Image a clock on the floor where your stance leg is in the center. Lightly touch position 1 as illustrated with the opposite foot. Then return that leg to the starting position. Next, touch position 2 and return. Maintain a slightly bent knee on the stance side.

	_____ Reps _____ Sets _____X Day _____Hold		_____ Reps _____ Sets _____X Day _____Hold
23	Notes:	**24**	Notes:

BALL ROLLS - HEEL TOE

In a standing position, place one foot on a ball and roll it forward and back in a controlled motion from heel to toe while maintaining your balance.

BALL ROLLS - LATERAL

In a standing position, place one foot on a ball and roll it side to side in a controlled motion from the inner side of your foot to the outer side of your foot while maintaining your balance.

Squats

_____ Reps _____ Sets _____ X Day _____ Hold	_____ Reps _____ Sets _____ X Day _____ Hold
25 Notes:	**26** Notes:

SQUAT – Can use chair or counter for support and chair behind if needed.

Stand with feet shoulder width apart (in front of a stable support for balance if needed.) Bend your knees and lower your body towards the floor. Your body weight should mostly be directed through the heels of your feet. Return to a standing position. Knees should bend in line with toes and not pass the front of the foot.

SIT TO STAND - Can use armchair to push off if needed

Start by scooting close to the front of the chair. Lean forward at your trunk and reach forward with your arms and rise to standing. (You may use a chair with arms to push off if needed and progress as tolerated).

Use your arms as a counterbalance by reaching forward when in sitting and lower them as you approach standing.

_____ Reps _____ Sets _____ X Day _____ Hold	_____ Reps _____ Sets _____ X Day _____ Hold
27 Notes:	**28** Notes:

SQUATS – WALL WITH BALL

Place either a small ball or therapy ball between you and the wall. Bend your knees and lower your body towards the floor. Return to a standing position. Knees should bend in line with toes and not pass the front of the foot.

SQUATS WITH WEIGHTS

Hold dumbbells or other weights in both hands by your side. Bend your knees and lower your body towards the floor. Return to a standing position. Knees should bend in line with toes and not pass the front of the foot

_____ Reps _____ Sets _____ X Day _____ Hold		_____ Reps _____ Sets _____ X Day _____ Hold	
29	Notes:	**30**	Notes:

MINI SQUAT - UNSTABLE SUPPORT - FOAM PAD

Start with your feet shoulder-width apart, toes pointed straight ahead and standing on a balance pad. Next, bend your knees to approximately 30 degrees of flexion to perform a mini squat as shown. Then, return to original position. Knees should not pass the front of the foot.

SQUATS - SINGLE LEG

While standing on one leg in front of a stable support for assisted balance, bend your knee and lower your body towards the floor. Return to a standing position.
Knees should not pass the front of the foot.

Weight Shifts, Wall Falls, Balance Recovery (Balance Drills)

_____ Reps _____ Sets _____ X Day _____ Hold		_____ Reps _____ Sets _____ X Day _____ Hold	
31	Notes:	**32**	Notes:

SIDE TO SIDE WEIGHT SHIFT
Stand next to stable surface if needed for support.

Keep feet shoulder width apart. Lean from side to side maintaining balance. *May stand in hallway with walls on both sides.*
*Advance to using balance pad

FORWARD AND BACKWARDS WEIGHT SHIFTS
Stand next to stable surface if needed for support.

Keep feet shoulder width apart. Lean from body forward and then backwards maintaining balance. *May stand in hallway with wall in front and in back.*
 *Advance to using balance pad

_____ Reps _____ Sets _____X Day _____Hold	_____ Reps _____ Sets _____X Day _____Hold
33 Notes:	**34** Notes:

SPLIT STANCE WEIGHT SHIFT SIDE TO SIDE
Stand next to stable surface if needed for support.

Stand in a split stance position. Lean side to side
maintaining balance. *May stand in hallway with wall on
both sides.*

SPLIT STANCE WEIGHT SHIFT FORWARD AND
BACKWARDS Stand next to stable surface if needed
for support.

Stand in a split stance position. Lean forward and
backwards maintaining balance. *May stand in
hallway with wall in front and in back.*

_____ Reps _____ Sets _____X Day _____Hold	_____ Reps _____ Sets _____X Day _____Hold
35 Notes:	**36** Notes:

WALL FALLS - FORWARD - BALANCE DRILL

Stand facing wall, a couple feet away from the wall.
Slowly and controlled, lean forward towards the wall. Try
to control your balance to prevent falling forward. Keep
leaning forward gradually until eventually you do lose
your balance and fall. Use your arms to catch yourself.
Push yourself back upright.

WALL FALLS - LATERAL - BALANCE DRILL

Stand to the side next to a wall, a couple feet away
from the wall. Slowly and controlled, lean to the
side towards the wall. Try to control your balance to
prevent falling sideways. Keep leaning to the side
gradually until eventually you do lose your balance
and fall. Use your arm to catch yourself. Push
yourself back upright.

	_____ Reps _____ Sets _____ X Day _____ Hold
37	Notes:

WALL FALLS - BACKWARDS - BALANCE DRILL

Stand facing away from a wall. Slowly and controlled, lean backward towards the wall. Try to control your balance to prevent falling backwards. Keep leaning backwards gradually until eventually you do lose your balance and fall. Use your upper back to catch the fall. Push yourself back upright.

	_____ Reps _____ Sets _____ X Day _____ Hold
38	Notes:

WALL FALLS - SINGLE LEG - FORWARD - BALANCE DRILL

Stand on one leg facing a wall, a couple feet away from the wall. Slowly and controlled, lean forward towards the wall. Try to control your balance to prevent falling forward. Keep leaning forward gradually until eventually you do lose your balance and fall. Use your arms to catch yourself. Push yourself back upright.

	_____ Reps _____ Sets _____ X Day _____ Hold
39	Notes:

WALL FALLS - SINGLE LEG - LATERAL - BALANCE DRILL

Stand on one leg with a wall a couple feet off to the side of that leg. Slowly and controlled, lean to the side towards the wall. Try to control your balance to prevent falling to the side. Keep leaning gradually towards the wall until eventually you lose your balance and fall. Use your arms to catch yourself. Push yourself back upright.

	_____ Reps _____ Sets _____ X Day _____ Hold
40	Notes:

WALL FALLS - SINGLE LEG - MEDIAL - BALANCE DRILL

Stand on one leg with a wall a couple feet off to the opposite side of that leg as shown. Slowly and controlled, lean sideways towards the wall. Try to control your balance to prevent falling to the side. Keep leaning gradually towards the wall until eventually you lose your balance and fall. Use your arms to catch yourself. Push yourself back upright.

	_____ Reps _____ Sets _____X Day _____Hold

41 | Notes:

WALL FALLS - SINGLE LEG - BACKWARDS - BALANCE DRILL

Stand on one leg facing away from a wall. Slowly and controlled, lean backward towards the wall. Try and control your balance to prevent falling backwards. Keep leaning backwards gradually until eventually you do lose your balance and fall. Use your upper back to catch the fall. Push yourself back upright.

	_____ Reps _____ Sets _____X Day _____Hold

42 | Notes:

FALL LATERAL - STEP RECOVERY
Stand next to stable surface if needed for support.

Start in a standing position with feet apart. Slowly lean to the side and try and prevent losing your balance. Continue to lean to the side until eventually you lose your balance and need to take a step to prevent falling.

	_____ Reps _____ Sets _____X Day _____Hold

43 | Notes:

FALL FORWARD - STEP RECOVERY
Stand next to stable surface if needed for support.

Start in a standing position with feet apart. Slowly lean forward and try and prevent losing your balance. Continue to lean forward until eventually you lose your balance and need to take a step to prevent falling.

	_____ Reps _____ Sets _____X Day _____Hold

44 | Notes:

FALL BACKWARD - STEP RECOVERY
Stand next to stable surface if needed for support.

Start in a standing position with feet apart. Slowly lean back and try and prevent losing your balance. Continue to lean backwards until eventually you lose your balance and need to take a step to prevent falling.

LEG EXERCISES > BALANCE > RESISTANCE

SOLID GROUND:
1. **Support:** Hold onto chair, counter, sink or another stationary object
2. **No Support:** Stand next to stable surface if needed for support
3. **Resistance:** Add ankle weights on use elastic band for resistance

UNSTABLE SURFACE: Balance pad, Bosu, Half foam roll, Pillow or Other unstable surface
1. **Support:** Hold onto chair, counter or another stationary object.
2. **No Support:** Stand next to stable surface if needed for support.
3. **Resistance:** Add ankle weights on use elastic band for resistance

Peripheral Neuropathy – See beginning of section for Caution on Unstable Surface

	_____ Reps _____ Sets _____ X Day _____ Hold		_____ Reps _____ Sets _____ X Day _____ Hold
45	Notes:	**46**	Notes:

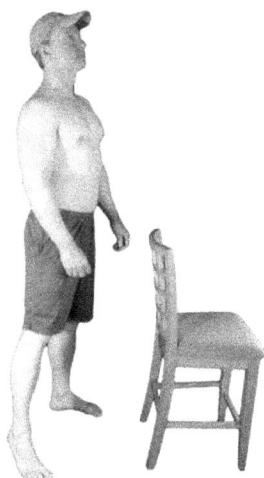

TOE TAP ABDUCTION

Standing upright and move your leg out to the side and tap your toe on the ground. Return to starting position and repeat.

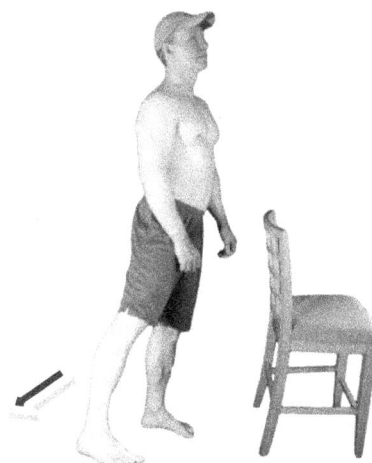

HIP ABDUCTION - STANDING – Can add ankle weights or elastic band.

Standing upright, raise your leg out to the side. Keep your knee straight and maintain your toes pointed forward the entire time. Return to starting position and repeat. Maintain a slow, controlled movement throughout.

_____ Reps _____ Sets _____ X Day _____ Hold

47 | Notes:

HIP EXTENSION – STANDING - Can add ankle weights or band.

Standing upright, balance on one leg and move your other leg in a backward direction. Do not swing the leg and tighten the buttock at end range. Keep your trunk stable and without arching or bending forward during the movement. Return to starting position and repeat. Maintain a slow, controlled movement throughout.

_____ Reps _____ Sets _____ X Day _____ Hold

48 | Notes:

HIP FLEXION - STANDING – STRAIGHT LEG RAISE - Can add ankle weights or band.

Standing upright, balance on one leg and lift your other leg forward with a straight knee as shown. Return to starting position and repeat. Maintain a slow, controlled movement throughout.

_____ Reps _____ Sets _____ X Day _____ Hold

49 | Notes:

HIP / KNEE FLEXION - SINGLE LEG - Can add ankle weights

Standing upright, lift your foot and knee up, set it down. Repeat. Maintain a slow, controlled movement throughout.

_____ Reps _____ Sets _____ X Day _____ Hold

50 | Notes:

STANDING MARCHING- Can add ankle weights

Standing upright, draw up your knee, set it down and then alternate to your other side. Maintain a slow, controlled movement throughout.

_____ Reps _____ Sets _____ X Day _____ Hold

51 | Notes:

HAMSTRING CURL - Can add ankle weights.

Standing upright, balance on one leg while bending the knee of the opposite leg towards the buttocks. Return to starting position and repeat. Maintain a slow, controlled movement throughout.

_____ Reps _____ Sets _____ X Day _____ Hold

52 | Notes:

TOE RAISES - Can add hand weights.

Standing upright, go up on your toes slowly towards the ceiling and then return to the starting position. Maintain a slow, controlled movement throughout.

_____ Reps _____ Sets _____ X Day _____ Hold

53 | Notes:

TOE RAISES IR AND ER - Can add hand weights.

IR (Internal Rotation)
Standing upright, rotate feet/legs inward and go up on your toes slowly towards the ceiling and then return to the starting position. Maintain a slow, controlled movement throughout.
ER (External Rotation)
Standing upright, rotate feet/legs outward and go up on your toes slowly towards the ceiling and then return to the starting position.

_____ Reps _____ Sets _____ X Day _____ Hold

54 | Notes:

ONE LEGGED TOE RAISE - Can add hand weights.

Standing upright and balance on one leg. Go up on your toes on the opposite leg towards the ceiling and then return to the starting position. Maintain a slow, controlled movement throughout.

BOSU – Can use chair for stability

_____ Reps _____ Sets _____X Day _____Hold		_____ Reps _____ Sets _____X Day _____Hold

55 Notes:

56 Notes:

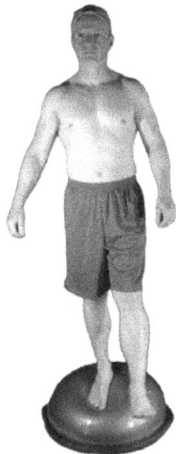

SINGLE LEG BALANCE FORWARD

Stand on a Bosu with one leg and maintain your balance. Hold your opposite leg out in front of your body and then return to original position. Maintain a slightly bent knee on the stance side.

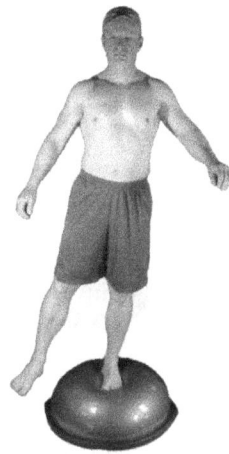

SINGLE LEG BALANCE LATERAL

Stand on a Bosu with one leg and maintain your balance. Hold your opposite leg out to the side of your body and then return to original position. Maintain a slightly bent knee on the stance side.

_____ Reps _____ Sets _____X Day _____Hold		_____ Reps _____ Sets _____X Day _____Hold

57 Notes:

58 Notes:

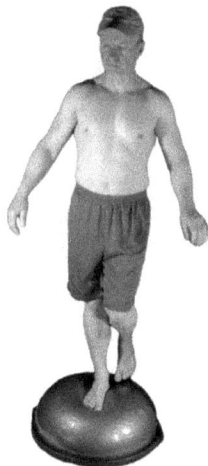

SINGLE LEG BALANCE RETRO

Stand on a Bosu Ball with one leg and maintain your balance. Hold your opposite leg back behind your body and then return to original position. Maintain a slightly bent knee on the stance side.

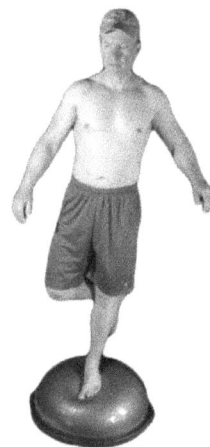

SINGLE LEG STANCE RETROLATERAL

Stand on a Bosu Ball with one leg and maintain your balance. Hold your opposite leg back behind and across your body and then return to original position. Maintain a slightly bent knee on the stance side.

_____ Reps _____ Sets _____ X Day _____ Hold	_____ Reps _____ Sets _____ X Day _____ Hold
59 Notes:	**60** Notes:

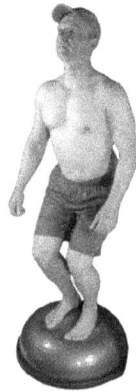

SQUAT

While standing and maintaining your balance on a Bosu, squat and return to a standing position. Knees should bend in line with the 2nd toe and not pass the front of the foot.

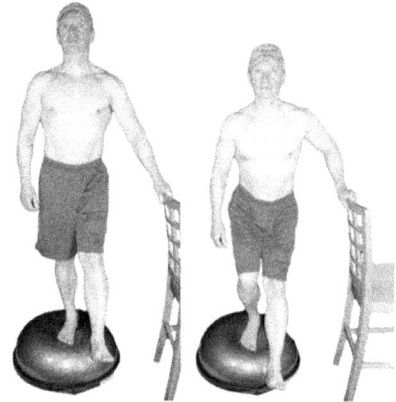

SINGLE LEG SQUAT

While standing and balancing on a Bosu with one leg, bend your knee and lower your body towards the ground. Return to a standing position. Your stance knee should bend in line with the 2nd toe and not pass the front of the foot.

Lunges

_____ Reps _____ Sets _____ X Day _____ Hold	_____ Reps _____ Sets _____ X Day _____ Hold
61 Notes:	**62** Notes:

Starting Position

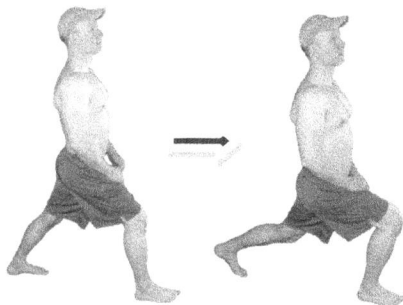

LUNGE – STATIC

Start in standing position with back leg straight and front leg with flexed/bent knee. Lean forward on front knee keeping knee in line with foot and back leg remaining straight. Return to starting position and repeat for several repetitions and then repeat on opposite side.
*Make sure front knee does not go past the foot.

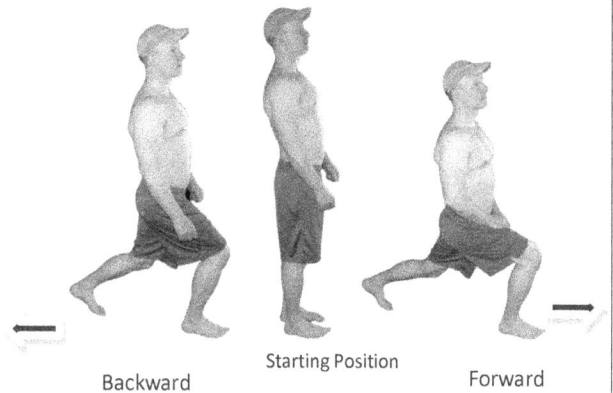

Backward   Starting Position   Forward

LUNGE FORWARD/BACKWARD

Start in standing (*middle picture*).
Backward: Keep one foot planted and step back with the opposite foot. Return to original position - repeat. *Forward:* Keep one foot planted and step forward with the opposite foot. Return to original position - repeat.

DYNAMIC MOVEMENTS

_____ Reps _____ Sets _____X Day _____Hold		_____ Reps _____ Sets _____X Day _____Hold

63 | Notes: | **64** | Notes:

FOUR CORNER MARCHING IN PLACE

Marching in place, move your body clockwise stopping at each corner for several seconds and move to the next corner. After completing the square, march counterclockwise.

FOUR CORNER MARCHING IN PLACE WITH HEAD TURNS

With Head and Body Moving Simultaneously
March in place to four corners, as previous exercise (#63). Move your head and body moving simultaneously as you complete the square.
With Head Turn And Then Body Turn.
March in place to four corners, as previous exercise (#63). Turn head and then body as you complete the square.

_____ Reps _____ Sets _____X Day _____Hold		_____ Reps _____ Sets _____X Day _____Hold

65 | Notes: | **66** | Notes:

WALKING ON HEELS FORWARD AND BACKWARDS – May walk along kitchen counter or wall until feeling steady.

Standing up tall, walk forward on heels. After feeling secure with a forward motion, try walking backwards on heels.

WALKING ON TOES FORWARD AND BACKWARDS – May walk along kitchen counter or wall until feeling steady.

Standing up tall, walk forward on up on toes. After feeling secure with a forward motion, try walking backwards up on toes.

	_____ Reps _____ Sets _____ X Day _____ Hold
67	Notes:

TANDEM STANCE AND WALK – FORWARD AND BACKWARDS

Maintaining your balance, stand with one foot directly in front of the other so that the toes of one foot touches the heel of the other. Progress by taking steps with your heel touching your toes with each step.

**Progress by walking backwards with your toe touching your heel with each step. Can also add head turns.

	_____ Reps _____ Sets _____ X Day _____ Hold
68	Notes:

RUNNING MAN

Stand and balance on one leg. Lean forward as you bring your other leg back behind you to tap the floor. Bring the same side arm forward as shown during the movement. Return to starting position and repeat.

	_____ Reps _____ Sets _____ X Day _____ Hold
69	Notes:

HOP STICK - FORWARD

Stand on one leg and then hop forward onto the other leg. Maintain your balance the entire time. Increase the difficulty by hoping forward further or higher.

	_____ Reps _____ Sets _____ X Day _____ Hold
70	Notes:

HOP STICK - BACKWARDS

Stand on one leg and then hop backward onto the other leg. Maintain your balance the entire time. Increase the difficulty by hoping back further or higher.

	_____ Reps _____ Sets _____ X Day _____ Hold
71	Notes:

MINI LATERAL LUNGE

Step to the side and balance on the leg. Next return to the original position. Repeat in the opposite direction. Your knees should be bent about 30 degrees.

	_____ Reps _____ Sets _____ X Day _____ Hold
72	Notes:

SIDE STEPPING – May step along kitchen counter or in hallway for support.

Step to the side continuing for length of room or counter – repeat in opposite direction.

	_____ Reps _____ Sets _____ X Day _____ Hold
73	Notes:

HOP STICK - LATERAL

Stand on one leg and then hop to the side onto the other leg. Maintain your balance the entire time. Increase the difficulty by hoping to the side further and higher.

	_____ Reps _____ Sets _____ X Day _____ Hold
74	Notes:

SINGLE LEG DEAD LIFT

While standing on one leg, bend forward with arms in front towards the ground as you extend your leg behind you and then return to the original position. Keep your legs straight and maintain your balance the entire time.

_____ Reps _____ Sets _____ X Day _____ Hold

75 Notes:

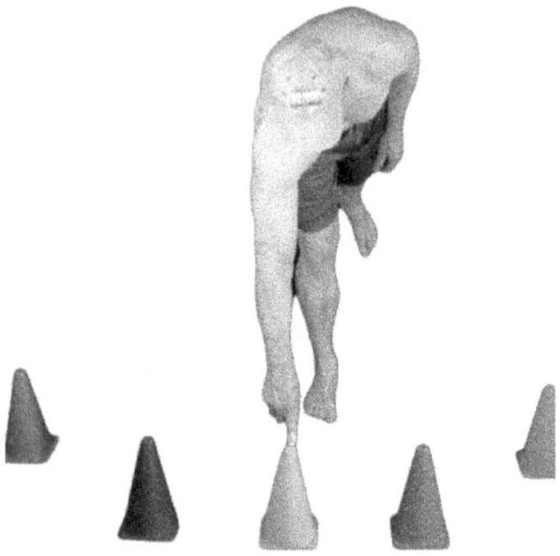

CONE TAPS - SINGLE LEG STANCE

Place 3-5 cones or cups around you as shown. Balance on a slightly bent knee. Lower yourself down to tap the top of a cone with your finger. Return to original position and repeat touching a different cone. Advance exercise with smaller cones/cups and or faster speed.

_____ Reps _____ Sets _____ X Day _____ Hold

76 Notes:

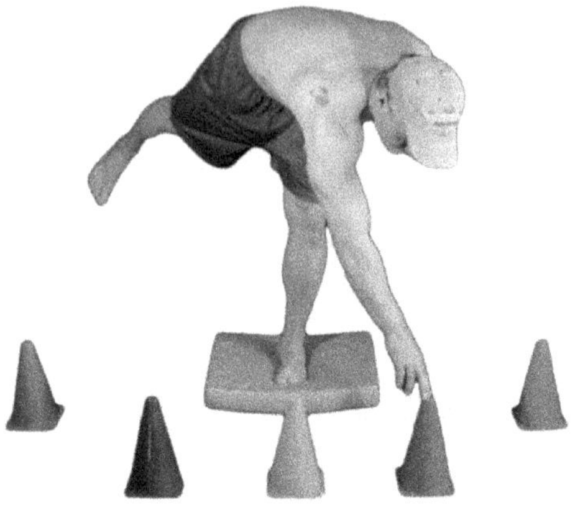

CONE TAPS - SINGLE LEG STANCE - UNSTABLE

Place 3-5 cones or cups around you. Balance on an unstable surface such as a foam pad with a slightly bent knee. Lower yourself down to tap the top of a cone. Return to original position and repeat touching a different cone. Advance exercise with smaller cones/cups and or faster speed.

_____ Reps _____ Sets _____ X Day _____ Hold

77 Notes:

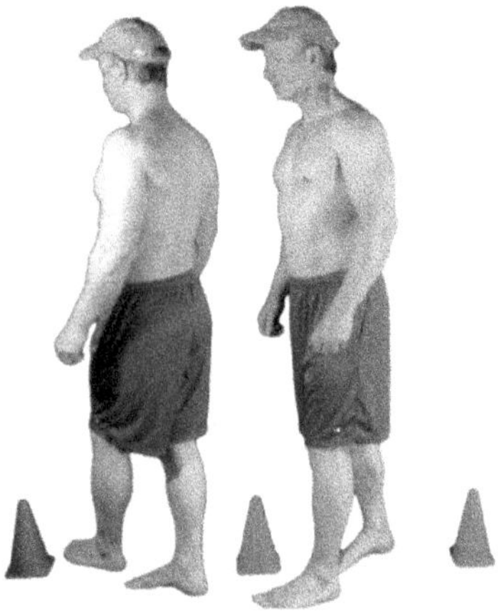

FIGURE 8 AROUND CONES

Set up 4-8 cones on the floor about 12 inches apart, although can vary to increase or decrease difficulty. Weave in and out of cones and then turn and repeat.

_____ Reps _____ Sets _____ X Day _____ Hold

78 Notes:

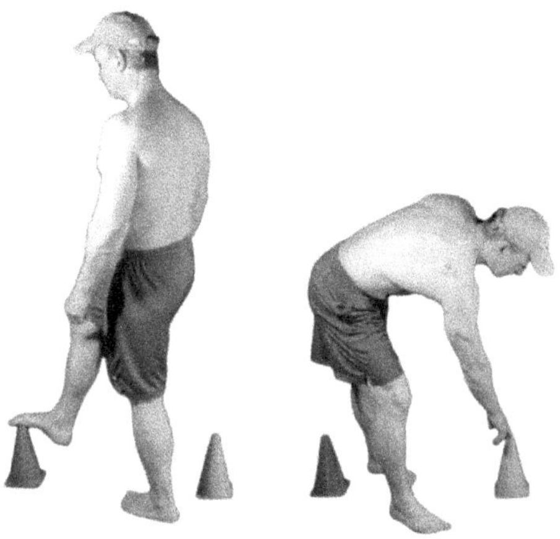

FIGURE 8 AROUND CONES – FOOT OR HAND TAP

Follow #75 figure around 4- 8 cones. To increase difficulty, you can tap each cone with your foot or lean over and tap with your hand.

HALF ROLLER (static and dynamic) – FLAT SIDE UP OR DOWN

	_____ Reps _____ Sets _____X Day _____Hold		_____ Reps _____ Sets _____X Day _____Hold
79	Notes:	**80**	Notes:

BALANCE DOUBLE LEG STANCE - WIDE

Place a half foam roll on the ground in a side-to-side direction. Stand on the foam roll with your feet spread apart and maintain your balance.

BALANCE DOUBLE LEG STANCE - NARROW

Place a half foam roll on the ground in a side-to-side direction. Stand on the foam roll with your feet together and maintain your balance.

	_____ Reps _____ Sets _____X Day _____Hold		_____ Reps _____ Sets _____X Day _____Hold
81	Notes:	**82**	Notes:

TANDEM STANCE

Place a half foam roll on the ground in a forward-back direction. Stand on the foam roll in tandem stance (with your heel and toe touching as shown) and maintain your balance.

TANDEM WALK

Place a half foam roll on the ground in a forward-back direction. Stand on the foam roll and begin tandem walking (heel-toe pattern walking as shown). Once you get to the end of the roll, either turn around or tandem walk backward.

_____ Reps _____ Sets _____ X Day _____ Hold	_____ Reps _____ Sets _____ X Day _____ Hold

83 Notes:

84 Notes:

SINGLE LEG STANCE - ABDUCTION

Place a half foam roll on the ground in a side-to-side direction. Balance on one leg and move the opposite leg to the side.

SINGLE LEG STANCE - ABDUCTION

Place a half foam roll on the ground in a forward-back direction. Balance on one leg with the opposite leg to the side.

_____ Reps _____ Sets _____ X Day _____ Hold	_____ Reps _____ Sets _____ X Day _____ Hold

85 Notes:

86 Notes:

SINGLE LEG STANCE – FORWARD KICK

Place a half foam roll on the ground in a forward-back direction. Balance on one leg and move the opposite leg forward.

SINGLE LEG STANCE – HAMSTRING CURL

Place a half foam roll on the ground in a forward-back direction. Balance on one leg and with the opposite leg, bend the knee backwards as shown.

_____ Reps _____ Sets _____ X Day _____ Hold		_____ Reps _____ Sets _____ X Day _____ Hold	
87	Notes:	**88**	Notes:

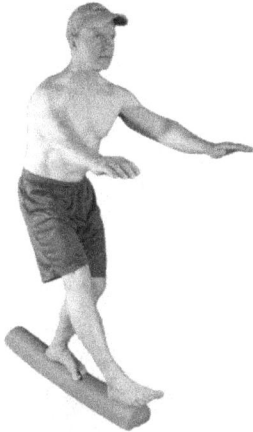

SINGLE LEG SQUAT – LEG FORWARD

Place a half foam roll on the ground in a forward-back direction. Balance on one leg with a slight bend in the supporting knee and move the opposite leg forward. Straighten supporting knee and repeat.

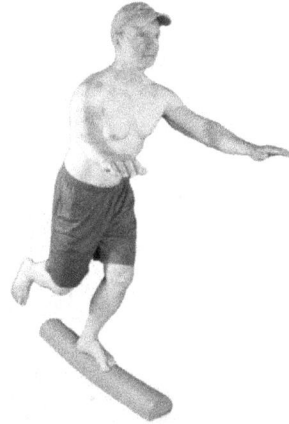

SINGLE LEG SQUAT – LEG BACKWARDS

Place a half foam roll on the ground in a forward-back direction. Balance on one leg with a slight bend in the supporting knee and with the opposite leg, move the leg backwards as shown with bent knee. Straighten supporting knee and repeat.

STAIR STEP – *To progress, increase step height*

_____ Reps _____ Sets _____ X Day _____ Hold		_____ Reps _____ Sets _____ X Day _____ Hold	
89	Notes:	**90**	Notes:

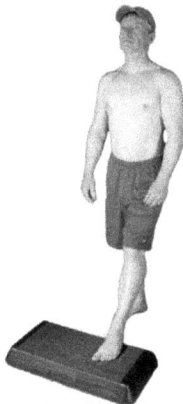

TOE TAP OR HEEL PLACEMENT

While standing with both feet on the floor, place one foot on the top of the step. Next, return the foot back to the floor and then repeat with the other leg.
You can either put your foot up for several repetitions or alternate.

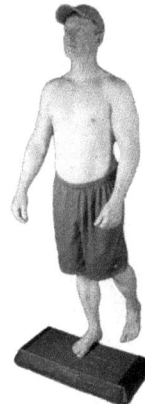

PULL UP FOOT TOUCHES ON STEP

Whie standing with both feet on the ground, put one foot on the step. Push through the foot straightening the knee until the opposite foot is off the ground. Lower the foot back to the starting position. Repeat with the opposite foot for several repetitions.

	_____ Reps _____ Sets _____X Day _____Hold
91	Notes:

ALTERNATING SUSTAINED FOOT TOUCHES ON STEP

Whie standing with both feet on the ground, put one foot on the step. Push through the foot straightening the knee until the opposite foot is also on the step. Step off backwards to the starting position. Repeat with the opposite foot for several repetitions.

	_____ Reps _____ Sets _____X Day _____Hold
92	Notes:

STEP UP AND OVER

Step up onto the step and then onto the ground on the other side. Turn around and repeat.
Repeat several repetitions on one side and then the other or alternate legs.

	_____ Reps _____ Sets _____X Day _____Hold
93	Notes:

FORWARD SWING THROUGH STEP

Step up onto the step without stopping on the top, swing opposite leg through and onto the floor on the other side.

	_____ Reps _____ Sets _____X Day _____Hold
94	Notes:

SIDE STEPPING

****REPEAT STEPS 89-93 from a side approach****

EXERCISE Agility/Reactivity/Speed	EXERCISE NUMBER	NOTES
Four Square Drills	1	
Dots	2	
Ladder Drills	3	
Box Drills	4	
Cones	5	
Hurdles	6	

Agility/Reactivity/Speed

According to the Twist Conditioning workbook, "Agility is the ability to link several fundamental movement skills into a multidirectional pattern. Reaction skills are the 'whole body' responsiveness to external stimuli, as well as muscle and joint internal reactivity. Quickness is the ability to explosively initiate movement from a stationary position, as well as shifting the gears of speed". (*Twist, Peter, Twist Agility, Quickness and & Reactivity Workbook, 2009, pg 16*)

Agility is a combination of acceleration, deceleration, coordination, power, strength and dynamic balance. With agility training, always keep your head in a neutral position looking straight ahead no matter which way you turn. "Powerful arm movement during transitional and directional changes is essential in order to reacquire a high rate of speed". (*Brown & Ferrigno, 2005, pp 73-74*)

Agility exercises can be done with cones, hurdles, dots or squares on the floor, box drills, Bosu or ladders. Agility can also be high impact or explosive movements. If you are not comfortable with this in the beginning or have any contraindications, stick with low impact movements. In other words, if you are jumping over hurdles, keep them low to the ground and jump over with one leg leading for low impact and jump with both legs for high impact.

If you are doing box drills or Bosu, please do NOT JUMP off backwards.

AGILITY / SPEED / REACTIVITY

4 Square Drills

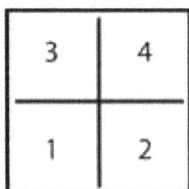 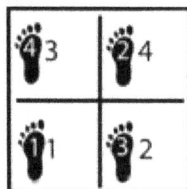 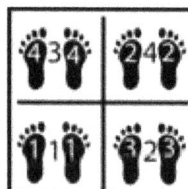 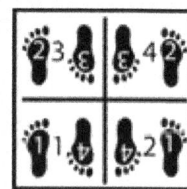

Dots

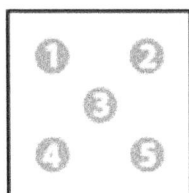 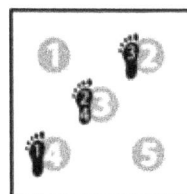 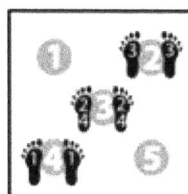 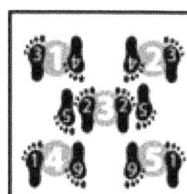

Ladder

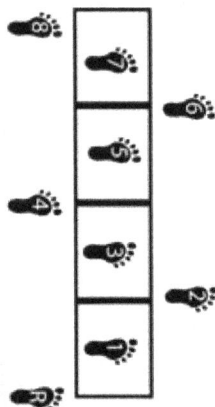 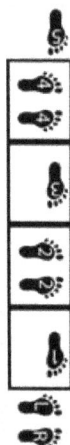 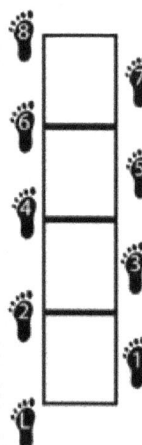 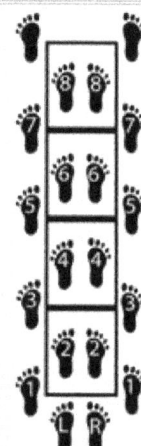

Box Drills – Box should be no higher than the middle of your shin. This can be done on Bosu for balance.

Alt Tap Box With Foot

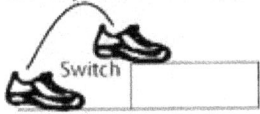

Switch

Down Up Both
Feet Together

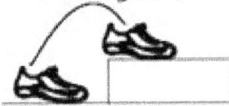

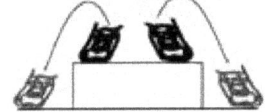

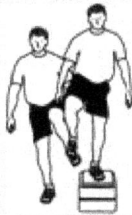

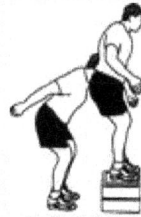

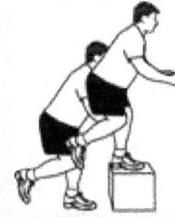

Quickly Move
Side to Side

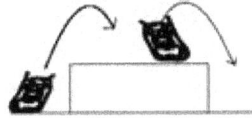

Down Up Both
Feet Together

Cones

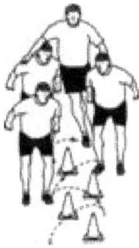

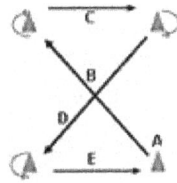

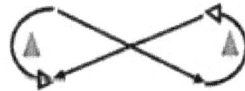

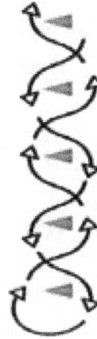

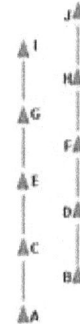

Hurdles – can run or
jump over hurdles

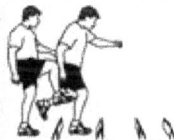

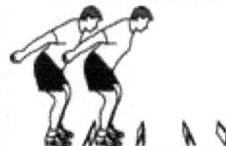

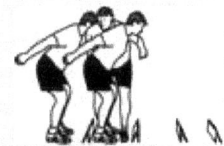

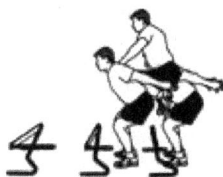

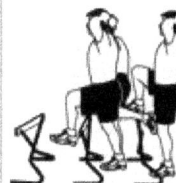

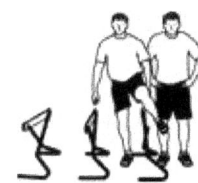

Endurance / Aerobic Capacity

Aerobic - with oxygen: Muscular and Cardiovascular

Many repetitions with sub-maximal weight (weight that is less than the maximum you can lift).

Muscular endurance is the ability of the muscle or group of muscles to sustain repeated contractions against resistance for an extended period of time. This is needed to build muscle. (See *Strengthening*). Cardiovascular endurance is the ability of the heart, lungs and blood vessels to deliver oxygen to working muscles and tissues, as well as the ability of those muscles and tissues to utilize that oxygen. This is needed to help endure long runs or sustained activity, as with biking or running. In short, endurance or aerobic exercises increase the heart rate and respiratory rate.

As far as long-term performance goes, there are two types of muscle fibers that can determine the likelihood of success: slow and fast twitch, which may determine whether you are more likely to be a powerlifter or sprinter (*fast twitch*), or a marathon runner (*slow twitch*). Your ability depends on the distribution of these fibers in the body. In other words, you could have a certain percentage of slow twitch in your biceps, but a different percentage in your quadriceps. There is some controversy over whether you can change the percentage or distribution of these fibers with endurance training or training for a specific event, although you may be able to change the glycolytic capacity.

Type of Fibers	***Slow twitch fibers:*** Have a high aerobic capacity and are resistant to fatigue. People that have a higher percentage of slow twitch fibers tend to have better endurance abilities.
	Fast twitch fibers: Contract faster than slow twitch, and thus fatigue faster. People that have a higher percentage of fast twitch fibers tend to have better sprinting or muscle building abilities.

The following research is from the: **MAYO CLINIC**

Mayo Clinic - *https://www.mayoclinic.org/healthy-lifestyle/fitness/in-depth/aerobic-exercise/art-20045541*
Regular aerobic activity, such as walking, bicycling or swimming, can help you live longer and healthier. Need motivation? See how aerobic exercise affects your heart, lungs and blood flow.

How your body responds to aerobic exercise
- During aerobic activity, you repeatedly move large muscles in your arms, legs and hips. You'll notice your body's responses quickly.
- You'll breathe faster and more deeply. This maximizes the amount of oxygen in your blood. Your heart will beat faster, which increases blood flow to your muscles and back to your lungs.
- Your small blood vessels (capillaries) will widen to deliver more oxygen to your muscles and carry away waste products, such as carbon dioxide and lactic acid.
- Your body will even release endorphins, natural painkillers that promote an increased sense of well-being.

What aerobic exercise does for your health
Regardless of age, weight or athletic ability, aerobic activity is good for you. As your body adapts to regular aerobic exercise, you'll get stronger and fitter.
Consider the following 10 ways that aerobic activity can help you feel better and enjoy life to the fullest.

Aerobic activity can help you:

1. **Keep excess pounds at bay**
   Combined with a healthy diet, aerobic exercise helps you lose weight and keep it off.

2. **Increase your stamina**
   You may feel tired when you first start regular aerobic exercise. But over the long term, you'll enjoy increased stamina and reduced fatigue.

3. **Ward off viral illnesses**

Aerobic exercise activates your immune system in a good way. This may leave you less susceptible to minor viral illnesses, such as colds and flu.

4. **Reduce your health risks**
Aerobic exercise reduces the risk of many conditions, including obesity, heart disease, high blood pressure, type 2 diabetes, metabolic syndrome, stroke and certain types of cancer.
Weight-bearing aerobic exercises, such as walking, help decrease the risk of osteoporosis.

5. **Manage chronic conditions**
Aerobic exercise may help lower blood pressure and control blood sugar. If you have coronary artery disease, aerobic exercise may help you manage your condition.

6. **Strengthen your heart**
A stronger heart doesn't need to beat as fast. A stronger heart also pumps blood more efficiently, which improves blood flow to all parts of your body.

7. **Keep your arteries clear**
Aerobic exercise boosts your high-density lipoprotein (HDL), the "good," cholesterol, and lowers your low-density lipoprotein (LDL), the "bad," cholesterol. This may result in less buildup of plaques in your arteries.

8. **Boost your mood**
Aerobic exercise may ease the gloominess of depression, reduce the tension associated with anxiety and promote relaxation.

9. **Stay active and independent as you age**
Aerobic exercise keeps your muscles strong, which can help you maintain mobility as you get older. Studies have found that regular physical activity may help protect memory, reasoning, judgment and thinking skills (cognitive function) in older adults, and may improve cognitive function in young adults.

10. **Live longer**
Studies show that people who participate in regular aerobic exercise live longer than those who don't exercise regularly.

Take the first step

Ready to get more active? Great. Just remember to start with small steps. If you've been inactive for a long time or if you have a chronic health condition, get your doctor's OK before you start. When you're ready to begin exercising, start slowly. You might walk five minutes in the morning and five minutes in the evening.
The next day, add a few minutes to each walking session. Pick up the pace a bit, too. Soon, you could be walking briskly for at least 30 minutes a day and reaping all the benefits of regular aerobic activity.
Other options for aerobic exercise could include cross-country skiing, aerobic dancing, swimming, stair climbing, bicycling, jogging, elliptical training or rowing.
Mayo Clinic - *https://www.mayoclinic.org/healthy-lifestyle/fitness/in-depth/aerobic-exercise/art-20045541*

Calories

Calorie: A unit of food energy. The word calorie is ordinarily used instead of the more precise, scientific term kilocalorie. A kilocalorie represents the amount of energy required to raise the temperature of a liter of water 1' centigrade at sea level. Technically, a kilocalorie represents 1,000 true calories of energy. *(MedicineNet.com)*

Calories are a measurement tool, like inches or cups. Calories measure the energy a food or beverage provides from the carbohydrate, fat, protein, and alcohol* it contains. Calories give you the fuel or energy you need to work and play – even to rest and sleep! When choosing what to eat and drink, it's important to get the right mix – enough nutrients without too many calories. Paying attention to calories is an important part of managing your weight. The amount of calories you need are different if you want to gain, lose, or maintain your weight. Tracking what and how much you eat, and drink can help you better understand your calorie intake over time. Each person's body may have different needs for calories and exercise. A healthy lifestyle requires balance in the foods you eat, the beverages you drink, the way you do daily activities, adequate sleep, stress management, and in the amount of activity in your daily routine. (*ChooseMyPlate.gov & CDC*)

Example of Activities and Calories Burned (*ChooseMyPlate.gov*)
A 154-pound man who is 5' 10" will use up (burn) about the number of calories listed doing each activity below. Those who weigh more will use more calories; those who weigh less will use fewer calories. The calorie values listed include both calories used by the activity and the calories used for normal body functioning during the activity time.

EXAMPLE	Approximate calories used (burned) by a 154-pound man	
MODERATE physical activities:	In 1 hour	In 30 minutes
Hiking	370	185
Light gardening/ yard work	330	165
Dancing	330	165
Golf (walking and carrying clubs)	330	165
Bicycling (less than 10 mph)	290	145
Walking (3.5 mph)	280	140
Weight training (general light workout)	220	110
Stretching	180	90
VIGOROUS physical activities:	In 1 hour	In 30 minutes
Running/ jogging (5 mph)	590	295
Bicycling (more than 10 mph)	590	295
Swimming (slow freestyle laps)	510	255
Aerobics	480	240
Walking (4.5 mph)	460	230
Heavy yard work (chopping wood)	440	220
Weightlifting (vigorous effort)	440	220
Basketball (vigorous)	440	220

References

Also, Some Good Books, Websites & DVD'

ACE Idea Fitness Journal: *Martina M. Cartwright, PhD, RD http://www.ideafit.com/fitness-library/protein-today-are-consumers-getting-too-much-of-a-good-thing?ACE_ACCESS=ebec6bcf61abff08f7b1d8b27c555758*

ACE Senior Fitness Manual, *American Council on Exercise* (2014)

American Physical Therapy Association, (APTA), 2007. *Basic Science for Animal Physical Therapy: Canine, 2nd edition*

Arleigh J Reynolds, DVM, PhD - *www.absasleddogracing.org.uk/newgang/src/gangline/role.htm*

Australian Institute of Sports - *http://www.ausport.gov.au*

BodyBuilder.com

Brown & Ferrigno, (2005). *Training for Speed, Agility and Quickness*, Champaign, IL: Human Kinetics.

Bryant, C & Green, D, editors (2003), *Ace Personal Trainer Manual, 3rd ed.*, San Diego, CA: American Council on Exercise (ACE)

ChooseMyPlate.gov

Examine.com

ExRx.net

Feher & Szunyoghy (1996). *Cyclopedia Anatomicae,* Tess Press

Gillette, R (2002). Temperature Regulation of the Dog. Retrieved June 2011 from *http://www.sportsvet.com/11Nwsltr.PDF*

Gillette, R (2008). *Feeding the Canine Athlete for Optimal Performance.* Retrieved September 25, 2008 from *www.sports vet.com/Art3.html.*

Glucose (Wikipedia) - *http://en.wikipedia.org/wiki/Glucose*

Glycemic Index (Wikipedia) - *http://en.wikipedia.org/wiki/Glycemic_index*

LiveStrong.com

Mayo Clinic - *https://www.mayoclinic.org/healthy-lifestyle/fitness/in-depth/aerobic-exercise/art-20045541*

MedicineNet.com

Myofascial Release: (Wikipedia) - https://en.wikipedia.org/wiki/Myofascial_release

Rikli, Roberta and Jones, Jessie (2013) *Senior Fitness Test Manual, 2nd Ed.,*

Strength Training: (Wikipedia) *http://en.wikipedia.org/wiki/Strength_training*

Twist, Peter (2009). *Twist Agility, Quickness and & Reactivity Workbook.* British Columbia: Twist Conditioning, Inc. University of Maryland Medical Center.com

Workout Australia

Thank You to:

My Husband
Model
For his support through my battle with cancer and while writing this and previous books.
Also, for the patience and hours he put in modeling for this book.

My Daughter
For giving me artistic inspiration and providing artwork for my previous books.

My Grandchildren
Just Because

God
For giving me the strength to overcome cancer and the wisdom to write these books.

Certifications, Continuing Education and License

Physical Therapist Assistant – L/PTA – 30 years in both Home Therapy and Short-Term Rehab facilities

ACE Certified Personal Trainer – CPT
- o **Functional Training Specialist**
- o **Therapeutic Exercise Specialist**
- o **Senior Fitness Specialist**
- o **Nutrition and Fitness Specialist**

©Klose Education
- o **Certified Lymphedema Therapist – CLT**
- o **Strength After Breast Cancer – Strength ABC**
- o **Breast Cancer Rehabilitation**

©Cancer Exercise Specialist Institute – CETI
- o **Cancer Exercise Specialist – CES**
- o **Breast Cancer Recovery BOSU(R) Specialist Advanced Qualification**
- o **Pilates Mat Certificate**

©MedFit
- o **Medical Fitness Specialist**
- o **Parkinson's Disease Fitness Specialist**
- o **Arthritis Fitness Specialist**

©Pink Ribbon Program

©The BioMechanics Method - Corrective Exercise Specialist

©ISSA - DNA-Based Fitness Coach

Lost Temple Fitness

www.ingramcontent.com/pod-product-compliance
Lightning Source LLC
Chambersburg PA
CBHW052107020426

42335CB00021B/2673